Intelligent Control and Learning Systems

Volume 10

The Springer book series Intelligent Control and Learning Systems addresses the emerging advances in intelligent control and learning systems from both mathematical theory and engineering application perspectives. It is a series of monographs and contributed volumes focusing on the in-depth exploration of learning theory in control such as iterative learning, machine learning, deep learning, and others sharing the learning concept, and their corresponding intelligent system frameworks in engineering applications. This series is featured by the comprehensive understanding and practical application of learning mechanisms. This book series involves applications in industrial engineering, control engineering, and material engineering, etc.

The Intelligent Control and Learning System book series promotes the exchange of emerging theory and technology of intelligent control and learning systems between academia and industry. It aims to provide a timely reflection of the advances in intelligent control and learning systems. This book series is distinguished by the combination of the system theory and emerging topics such as machine learning, artificial intelligence, and big data. As a collection, this book series provides valuable resources to a wide audience in academia, the engineering research community, industry and anyone else looking to expand their knowledge in intelligent control and learning systems.

Hao Jiang · Wai-Ki Ching

Kernel Methods for Omics Data Mining

Theory and Applications

Springer

Hao Jiang
School of Mathematics
Renmin University of China
Beijing, China

Wai-Ki Ching
Department of Mathematics
The University of Hong Kong
Pokfulam, Hong Kong

ISSN 2662-5458 ISSN 2662-5466 (electronic)
Intelligent Control and Learning Systems
ISBN 978-981-95-3128-8 ISBN 978-981-95-3129-5 (eBook)
https://doi.org/10.1007/978-981-95-3129-5

This Springer imprint is published by the registered company Springer Nature Singapore Pte Ltd.
The registered company address is: 152 Beach Road, #21-01/04 Gateway East, Singapore 189721, Singapore

Preface

The field of genomics has experienced an unprecedented surge in data generation, driven by advances in genome sequencing technologies and methodological developments. A wide variety of omics data, including genomic, proteomic, transcriptomic, and metabolomic information, is now readily accessible.

Genomics data are extensively utilized in biological research for diverse applications, such as elucidating complex molecular mechanisms, analyzing genetic variation, profiling gene expression, performing functional annotation, and conducting phylogenetic and evolutionary studies. Furthermore, they play an increasingly important role in identifying potential drug targets and biomarkers for disease diagnosis and prognosis, particularly in the realm of personalized medicine.

Key characteristics of genomics data include high variability, inherent complexity, and high dimensionality. A thorough understanding of these traits is essential for effectively processing, analyzing, and interpreting such data in both research and clinical settings. To address these challenges, a range of computational techniques, including machine learning, statistical methods, and metaheuristic algorithms, have been developed to facilitate the processing, normalization, integration, and interpretation of omics data.

In this monograph, we focus on the critical properties of nonlinearity and sparsity inherent in diverse types of genomics data. Kernel methods serve as elegant and powerful tools for capturing complex nonlinear relationships, making them particularly well-suited for characterizing and analyzing multi-omics data. The capability of kernel-based approaches to model intricate and higher-order interactions is consistently demonstrated across the various applications presented in this work.

In Chap. 1, we provide a comprehensive introduction to genomics data and elucidate its intrinsic characteristics, including high dimensionality, noise, heterogeneity, and sparsity, that pose both challenges and opportunities for computational analysis. The remainder of the monograph is dedicated to a detailed exposition of the fundamental theory underlying kernel methods, along with practical techniques for leveraging these tools to model, represent, and interpret relationships within genomics datasets. Subsequent chapters demonstrate the versatility and power of kernel methods through diverse applications in omics data mining. These case studies exemplify the unique advantages and contextual specificity of kernel-based approaches in tackling key biological challenges, such as improving disease diagnosis, uncovering cellular heterogeneity, identifying novel biomarkers, enabling network-driven data integration, and facilitating predictive modeling, highlighting their pivotal role in advancing genomic research.

The authors would like to express their sincere gratitude to Prof. Luonan Chen, Prof. Shihua Zhang, and Prof. Haiyan Huang for their insightful vision, fruitful discussions, and valuable suggestions, which greatly enhanced the quality of this research.

We wish to extend our sincere gratitude to a number of collaborators from around the world for their invaluable contributions. We are especially grateful to Prof. Wai-Shun Cheung for providing theoretical justification for our proposed kernel matrix, and to Prof. Ming Yi for his continued collaboration. We also thank Dr. Wenpin Hou, Dr. Hong Yin, Dr. Yushan Qiu, Dr. Xiaoqing Cheng, and Dr. ManYi Yim for fruitful discussions and collaborative efforts in omics data mining. We appreciate Dr. Chi Wing Wong for his significant help in polishing the whole draft.

We would like to extend our heartfelt gratitude to the excellent students who have made significant contributions to this monograph. In particular, we wish to acknowledge Senwen Zhan and Mengjie Wang, among others, for their dedicated efforts and unwavering commitment throughout the research process. Their hard work on data modelling, algorithm development, and theoretical analysis is evidently invaluable to the completion of this work.

Beijing, China Hao Jiang
Pokfulam, Hong Kong Wai-Ki Ching

Acknowledgements We are pleased to thank the support of the National Natural Science Foundation of China under grants 12271522 and 11901575.We sincerely appreciate the publishers Elsevier, IEEE, Springer Nature,Wiley, and Oxford University Press for granting us the permission to reuse materials in the copyrighted papers.

Competing Interests The authors have no competing interests to declare that are relevant to the content of this manuscript.

Contents

Chapter 1
Omics Data: Acquisition and Mining

1.1 Introduction

In the past few years, the field of genomics has experienced an unprecedented surge in data generation, driven by extraordinary advancements in genome sequencing technologies and computational methodologies (Goodwin et al. 2016). The astonishing growth in genomic data has not only revolutionized our understanding of biological systems but has also transformed various domains (Satam et al. 2023). By elucidating the genetic blueprint of organisms, genomic data unravels the intricate molecular mechanisms underlying cellular processes (Jagadeesh 2022) and pathways (Ramanan et al. 2012). Additionally, it empowers clinicians to tailor treatments based on individual genetic profiles (Wang and Wheeler 2014), guides more effective diagnostic and treatment strategies, drives innovation in biopharmaceuticals (Walsh and Walsh 2022), and fuels groundbreaking discoveries and applications across various sectors, thereby catalyzing advancements in medicine, biotechnology, and beyond.

The emergence of next-generation sequencing (NGS) (Hawkins et al. 2010) technologies has significantly expedited the pace and scope of genomic data generation. Unlike conventional Sanger sequencing methods, NGS platforms allow for swift and cost-effective sequencing of entire genomes. This capability facilitates large-scale genomic projects (Carrasco et al. 2017) and population-level studies, empowering researchers to delve deeper into the intricacies of genomics on an unprecedented scale.

Continuous advancements in sequencing technologies, alongside enhanced automation and parallelization, have led to a substantial reduction in per-base sequencing expenses (Gibbs 2020). This significant cost reduction has democratized access to genomic sequencing, empowering researchers globally to embark on genomic investigations spanning various species and populations. The significance of genomic data generation transcends basic research, extending into various applied domains. In medicine, genomic data plays a pivotal role in personalized healthcare and precision medicine. Furthermore, large-scale genomic initiatives, such as

H. Jiang and W.-K. Ching, *Kernel Methods for Omics Data Mining*, Intelligent Control and Learning Systems 10, https://doi.org/10.1007/978-981-95-3129-5_1

the Human Genome Project (Marshall 2012) and the Precision Medicine Initiative (Sankar and Parker 2016), have catalyzed collaborative efforts to decipher the genetic basis of complex diseases and accelerate the development of targeted therapies. Beyond healthcare, genomic data also underpins advancements in biotechnology. Biotechnological applications of genomic data encompass synthetic biology, bioinformatics, and gene editing, paving the way for innovations in biomanufacturing, drug discovery, and environmental remediation.

The proliferation of genomic data generation represents a transformative force in modern biology and beyond. By unraveling the intricacies of genetic information, genomic studies offer profound insights into the complexities of life, from the molecular mechanisms governing cellular processes to the evolutionary dynamics shaping biodiversity. Harnessing the power of genomic data holds the potential to revolutionize healthcare and various other fields, driving innovation, and addressing pressing global challenges.

1.2 Omics Data

The emergence of omics data (Schneider and Orchard 2011) provides us with a novel perspective, aiding us in a deeper understanding of the mysteries of life. Omics data involves the comprehensive analysis of biological systems at different levels, encompassing genomics, transcriptomics, proteomics, metabolomics, and others.

- Genomics Data
  Genomics is the study of genetic information within organisms. Genomics data provides rich information about the genetic composition of organisms (Oleksyk et al. 2015), including gene sequences, positions, functions, and more. By utilizing genomics data, we can identify and understand the roles and regulatory mechanisms of genes within organisms, thereby revealing the relationship between genes and phenotypes, exploring the mechanisms of disease onset, and even developing novel gene therapy approaches.
- Transcriptomics Data
  The regulated transcription of genes plays important role in determining cell identity and function. This involves an intricate regulation of gene expression, which primarily occurs during the transcription of genes into RNA (Cramer 2019). Transcriptomics investigates the transcriptional activities of genes within organisms, i.e., the production and expression of RNA. Transcriptomics data provides information on gene expression levels, aiding in the understanding of gene expression patterns and regulatory networks under different conditions. Through the analysis of transcriptomics data, we can discover new genes, understand the regulatory mechanisms of cellular signaling pathways, identify biomarkers associated with diseases, and more.

- Proteomics Data
  The proteome (Lualdi and Fasano 2019), including all "proteoforms", exhibits high level of complexity of biomolecules compared to genome and transcriptome. Proteomics is the study of the protein composition and functions within organisms. Proteomics data provides information about protein types, structures, expression levels, and more. By analyzing proteomics data, we can understand protein functions and interactions within organisms, uncover regulatory mechanisms of cellular signaling pathways and metabolic pathways, provide crucial insights for drug development and clinical diagnosis.
- Metabolomics Data
  Metabolomics (Lamichhane et al. 2018) is a comprehensive analysis of metabolites produced by biological systems or derived from other external sources. Metabolomics focuses on the study of metabolites and their dynamic changes. Metabolomics data provides information about the types, concentrations, metabolic pathways, and more of metabolites. Through the analysis of metabolomics data, we can understand the regulatory mechanisms of metabolic pathways within organisms, discover new biomarkers, explore diagnostic and therapeutic methods for diseases, and evaluate the toxicity and efficacy of drugs.
- Other Omics Fields
  In addition to genomics, transcriptomics, proteomics, and metabolomics, there exist several other omics disciplines. These include epigenomics (Stricker et al. 2016), glycomics (Raman et al. 2005), lipidomics (Dennis 2009), and interactomics (Davey et al. 2023), each with its specific focus: epigenomics delves into epigenetic modifications, glycomics investigates carbohydrate structures, lipidomics explores lipid molecules, and interactomics examines molecular interactions. Each of these omics fields offers distinct insights into unraveling the intricacies of biological systems.

1.3 Single Cell Omics Data

Single-cell genomics data (Lee et al. 2020) represents a paradigm shift in our understanding of cellular heterogeneity and function within complex biological systems. By dissecting individual cells and profiling their genomic, transcriptomic, epigenomic, and proteomic landscapes, single-cell technologies offer unprecedented insights into cellular diversity, dynamics, and interactions. This high-resolution characterization of cellular states and trajectories holds immense potential for deciphering developmental processes, unraveling disease mechanisms, and advancing personalized medicine. At the heart of single-cell genomics lies the ability to capture the molecular signatures of individual cells, transcending the limitations of bulk analyses that mask cellular heterogeneity. Through techniques such as single-cell RNA sequencing (scRNA-seq), researchers can unravel the transcriptional diversity within tissues, identify rare cell types, and delineate cell lineage trajectories during cellular development and disease progression. With the first release of scRNA-seq technology in 2009 (Lao et al. 2009), the development of scRNA-seq technology has undergone several key milestones. Initial scRNA-seq methods were limited by low throughput and high cost. However, with continuous technological improvements and cost reductions, modern scRNA-seq approaches have become increasingly high-throughput, sensitive, and cost-effective. Currently, there are many commercial scRNA-seq platforms and reagent kits available, making this technology more user-friendly and widely applicable across various research fields. The highly parallel scRNA-seq methods such as Drop-seq (Bageritz and Raddi 2019) and Microwell-seq (Han et al. 2018; Ye et al. 2024) have made the analysis of human cell atlas (HCA) feasible. Single-cell amplification and sequencing of full-length RNAs by Nanopore platform (SCAN-seq) could detect the full-length transcripts in single cells with high precision (Fan et al. 2020). With the maturation and widespread adoption of scRNA-seq technology, researchers have made numerous significant scientific discoveries. For example, scRNA-seq has been utilized to identify and characterize rare cell subpopulations within various tissues and organs, revealing transcriptional differences and gene regulatory networks among different cell types. Additionally, scRNA-seq has been widely applied to study processes such as cellular differentiation during development (Teschendorff and Enver 2017), tumor heterogeneity (Jiang et al. 2018), and immune responses (Zhang et al. 2020), addressing critical biological questions.

Moreover, single-cell epigenomic profiling enables the mapping of chromatin accessibility, DNA methylation patterns, and histone modifications at single-cell resolution, shedding light on the regulatory mechanisms underlying cellular identity and plasticity. Single-cell epigenomic profiling has emerged as a powerful technique for dissecting the complex landscape of epigenetic modifications at single-cell resolution. Traditionally, bulk epigenomic assays provided valuable insights into chromatin states and regulatory elements averaged across a population of cells. However, these approaches mask the considerable heterogeneity that exists among individual cells within a population. Single-cell epigenomic profiling techniques, such as single-cell ATAC-seq (Trevino et al. 2020), and single-cell DNA methylation sequencing (Smallwood et al. 2014), have overcome this limitation by enabling the interrogation of chromatin accessibility and DNA methylation patterns in individual cells. The development of single-cell epigenomic profiling methods has faced unique challenges due to the inherently low amounts of starting material and the stochastic nature of epigenetic processes. Nonetheless, innovative experimental protocols and computational algorithms have been developed to overcome these hurdles. For example, single-cell combinatorial indexing methods have been devised to barcode individual chromatin fragments or DNA molecules from single cells, allowing for high-throughput and cost-effective profiling of epigenomic features across thousands of cells (Cao et al. 2018; Rotem et al. 2015). Single-cell epigenomic profiling has unveiled novel insights into cellular heterogeneity and dynamics across various biological contexts. These techniques have been instrumental in identifying rare cell populations, characterizing cell type-specific regulatory elements, and elucidating the epigenetic basis of cellular differentiation and disease pathogenesis. Moreover, single-cell epigenomic studies have provided critical insights into the role of epigenetic plasticity in cellular

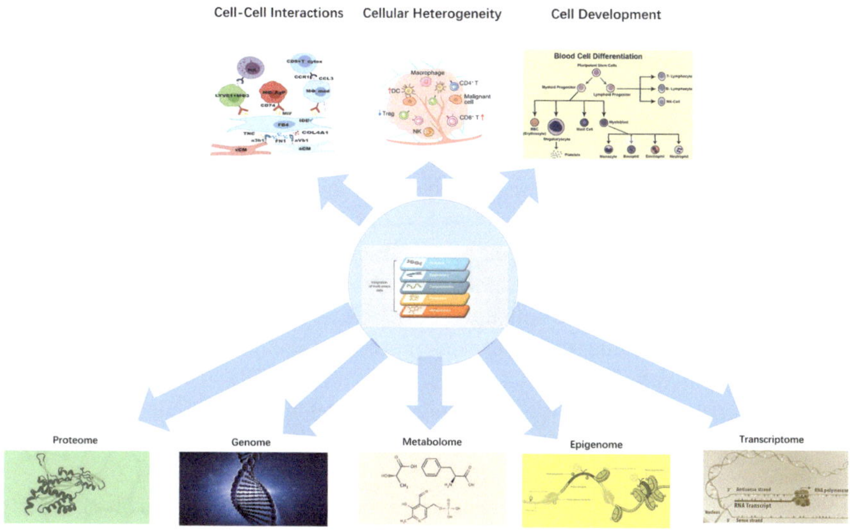

Fig. 1.1 Single cell omics layers and applications

reprogramming and lineage commitment during development (Angermueller et al. 2015). Moving forward, continued advancements in single-cell epigenomic profiling technologies are expected to further our understanding of epigenetic regulation in health and disease. Integrating single-cell epigenomic data with other omics modalities (Danese et al. 2019), such as single-cell transcriptomics and single-cell proteomics, promises to provide a comprehensive view of cellular identity and function, ultimately paving the way for the development of targeted therapies and precision medicine approaches.

1.4 Single Omics Data Mining

Building on scRNA-seq technologies, multi-omics technologies (Baysoy et al. 2023) maintain the progress made in profiling transcriptomic information while simultaneously capturing other modalities. Representative multi-omics technology G&T-seq (Macaulay et al. 2015) captures both the genome and the transcriptomic information in single cells. Cellular indexing of transcriptomes and epitopes by sequencing (CITE-seq) (Stoeckius et al. 2017; Rivello et al. 2021) labels single cells with antibody conjugates bound to biotinylated DNA barcodes. scNMT (Clark et al. 2018) realizes parallel quantification of chromatin accessibility, DNA methylation and transcriptome. These single-cell multi-omics technologies can uncover cellular heterogeneity across multiple molecular layers within a population of cells (see Fig. 1.1). They can also elucidate how the variation is interconnected or independent across different omics layers. The datasets produced by these techniques have the potential to facilitate deeper understanding of the fundamental biological processes and mechanisms underlying cellular heterogeneity. Furthermore, they can shed light on their association with normal development, aging, and the onset of diseases.

A central task in omics data mining is to extract meaningful biological patterns and associations from high-dimensional and heterogeneous data. In omics data analysis, traditional machine learning methods such as Principal Component Analysis (PCA), t-Stochastic Neighborhood Embedding (tSNE) have been widely used for dimensionality reduction, Linear Discriminant Analysis (LDA), Support Vector Machines (SVM), and Logistic Regression have been widely used for classification problems. For multi-omics integration, typical approaches include multi-view clustering, matrix factorization-based models, which can, harmonize data from different sources and reveal cross-omics regulatory relationships. Omics data particularly single-cell data often exhibit highly nonlinear, sparse structures, such as continuous nonlinear changes along developmental trajectories. Conventional linear methods often struggle to fully capture these intricate relationships. Therefore, machine learning approaches better suited for nonlinear problems such as graph-based models, deep autoencoders, and kernel methods adapted to single-cell contexts will more effectively uncover cellular heterogeneity, infer differentiation trajectories, and thereby advancing deeper applications of single-cell omics in precision medicine and systems biology.

In the following chapters, we will focus on the development and application of kernel methods in omics data mining. We will systematically explore how kernel-based techniques known for their flexibility in capturing complex, nonlinear relationships have been adapted and extended to address the unique challenges posed by modern biological data. This discussion will cover fundamental kernel design principles tailored to various types of omics data, introduce representative kernel-based models for tasks such as classification, clustering, and integration analysis, and examine their use in both single-omics and multi-omics settings.

References

Angermueller C, Clark SJ, Lee HJ, Macaulay IC, Teng MJ, Hu TX, Krueger F, Smallwood SA, Ponting CP, Voet T, Kelsey G, Stegle O, Reik W (2015) Parallel single-cell sequencing links transcriptional and epigenetic heterogeneity. Nat Methods 13:229–232

Bageritz J, Raddi G (2019) Single-cell RNA sequencing with drop-seq. In: Single cell methods: sequencing and proteomics, pp 73–85

Baysoy A, Bai Z, Satija R, Fan R (2023) The technological landscape and applications of single-cell multi-omics. Nat Rev Mol Cell Biol, 1–19 (2023)

Cao J, Cusanovich DA, Ramani V, Aghamirzaie D, Pliner HA, Hill AJ, Daza RM, McFaline-Figueroa JL, Packer JS, Christiansen L, Steemers FJ, Adey AC, Trapnell C, Shendure J (2018) Joint profiling of chromatin accessibility and gene expression in thousands of single cells. Science 361(6409):1380–1385

Carrasco-Ramiro F, Peiró-Pastor R, Aguado B (2017) Human genomics projects and precision medicine. Gene Ther 24:551–561

Clark SJ, Argelaguet R, Kapourani CA, Stubbs TM, Lee HJ, Alda-Catalinas C, Krueger F, Sanguinetti G, Kelsey G, Marioni JC, Stegle O, Reik W (2018) scNMT-seq enables joint profiling of chromatin accessibility DNA methylation and transcription in single cells. Nat Commun 9
Cramer P (2019) Organization and regulation of gene transcription. Nature 573:45–54
Danese A, Richter ML, Fischer DS, Theis FJ, Colomé-Tatché M (2019) Episcanpy: integrated single-cell epigenomic analysis. Nat Commun 12:5228
Davey NE, Simonetti L, Ivarsson Y (2023) The next wave of interactomics: mapping the slim-based interactions of the intrinsically disordered proteome. Curr Opin Struct Biol 80(102):593. DOIurl10.1016/j.sbi.2023.102593, https://www.sciencedirect.com/science/article/pii/S0959440X23000672
Dennis EA (2009) Lipidomics joins the omics evolution. Proc Natl Acad Sci 106:2089–2090
Fan X, Tang D, Liao Y, Li P, Zhang Y, Wang M, Liang F, Wang X, Gao Y, Wen L, Wang D, Wang Y, Tang F (2020) Single-cell RNA-SEQ analysis of mouse preimplantation embryos by third-generation sequencing. PLoS Biol 18 (2020)
Gibbs RA (2020) The human genome project changed everything. Nat Rev Genet 21:575–576
Goodwin S, McPherson JD, McCombie WR (2016) Coming of age: ten years of next-generation sequencing technologies. Nat Rev Genet 17:333–351
Han X, Wang R, Zhou Y, Fei L, Sun H, Lai S, Saadatpour A, Zhou Z, Chen H, Ye F, Huang D, Xu Y, Huang W, Jiang M, Jiang X, Mao J, Chen Y, Lu C, Xie J, Fang Q, Wang Y, Yue R, Li T, Huang H, Orkin SH, Yuan G, Chen M, Guo G (2018) Mapping the mouse cell atlas by microwell-seq. Cell 172:1091-1107.e17
Hawkins R, Hon GC, Ren B (2010) Next-generation genomics: an integrative approach. Nat Rev Genet 11:476–486
Jagadeesh KA, Dey KK, Montoro DT, Mohan R, Gazal S, Engreitz JM, Xavier RJ, Price AL, Regev A (2022) Identifying disease-critical cell types and cellular processes by integrating single-cell RNA-sequencing and human genetics. Nat Genet 54:1479–1492
Jiang H, Sohn LL, Huang H, Chen L (2018) Single cell clustering based on cell-pair differentiability correlation and variance analysis. Bioinformatics 34(21):3684–3694
Lamichhane S, Sen P, Dickens AM, Hyötyläinen T, Orešič M (2018) Chapter Fourteen—An overview of metabolomics data analysis: current tools and future perspectives. In: Jaumot J, Bedia C, Tauler R (eds) Data analysis for Omic sciences: methods and applications. Comprehensive analytical chemistry, vol 82, pp 387–413. Elsevier
Lao K, Tang F, Barbacioru CC, Wang Y, Nordman E, Lee CC, Xu N, Wang D, Tuch B, Bodeau JP, Siddiqui AS, Surani A (2009) mRNA-SEQ whole-transcriptome analysis of a single cell. Nat Methods 6:377–382
Lee J, Hyeon DY, Hwang D (2020) Single-cell multiomics: technologies and data analysis methods. Exp Mol Med 52:1428–1442
Lualdi M, Fasano M (2019) Statistical analysis of proteomics data: a review on feature selection. J Proteomics 198:18–26
Macaulay IC, Haerty W, Kumar P, Li YI, Hu TX, Teng MJ, Goolam M, Saurat N, Coupland P, Shirley LM, Smith M, der Aa NV, Banerjee R, Ellis PD, Quail MA, Swerdlow HP, Zernicka-Goetz M, Livesey FJ, Ponting CP, Voet T (2015) G&t-seq: parallel sequencing of single-cell genomes and transcriptomes. Nat Methods 12:519–522
Marshall J (2012) Human genome project. In: Chadwick R (ed) Encyclopedia of applied ethics, 2nd ed. Academic Press, San Diego, pp 636–643 (2012). https://doi.org/10.1016/B978-0-12-373932-2.00391-4, https://www.sciencedirect.com/science/article/pii/B9780123739322003914
Oleksyk T, AG C, Auton A, Abecasis GR, Altshuler DM, Durbin R, Bentley DR, Chakravarti A, Clark AG, Donnelly P, Eichler EE, Flicek P, Gabriel S, Gibbs RA, Green ED, Hurles ME, Knoppers BM, Korbel JO, Lander ES, Lee C, Lehrach H, Mardis ER, Marth GT, McVean G, Nickerson DA, Schmidt J, Sherry ST, Wang J, Wilson RK, Barnes KC, Beiswanger CM, Burchard EG, Bustamante CD, Cai H, Cao H, Gerry NP, Gharani N, Gignoux CR, Gravel S, Henn BM, Jones DA, Jorde LB, Kaye J, Keinan A, Kent A, Kerasidou A, Li Y, Mathias RA, Moreno-Estrada A, Ossorio PN, Parker M, Resch AM, Rotimi CN, Royal CD, Sandoval K, Su Y, Sudbrak R, Tian

Z, Tishkoff SA, Toji LH, Tyler-Smith C, Via M, Wang Y, Yang H, Yang L, Zhu J, Brooks LD, Felsenfeld AL, Mcewen JE, Vaydylevich Y, Duncanson A, Dunn M, Schloss JA, Garrison EP, Kang HM, Marchini J, McCarthy SA, (2015) A global reference for human genetic variation. Nature 526:68–74

Raman R, Raguram S, Venkataraman G, Paulson JC, Sasisekharan R (2005) Glycomics: an integrated systems approach to structure-function relationships of glycans. Nat Methods 2:817–824

Ramanan VK, Shen L, Moore JH, Saykin AJ (2012) Pathway analysis of genomic data: concepts, methods, and prospects for future development. Trends Genet, TIG 28(7):323–332

Rivello F, van Buijtenen E, Matuła K, van Buggenum JA, Vink PM, van Eenennaam H, Mulder KW, Huck WTS (2021) Single-cell intracellular epitope and transcript detection reveals signal transduction dynamics. Cell Rep Methods 1

Rotem A, Ram O, Shoresh N, Sperling RA, Schnall-Levin M, Zhang H, Basu A, Bernstein BE, Weitz DA (2015) High-throughput single-cell labeling (HI-SCL) for RNA-SEQ using drop-based microfluidics. PLoS One 10 (2015)

Sankar PL, Parker LS (2016) The precision medicine initiative s all of us research program: an agenda for research on its ethical, legal, and social issues. Genet Med 19:743–750 (2016). https://api.semanticscholar.org/CorpusID:4818256

Satam H, Joshi K, Mangrolia U, Waghoo S, Zaidi G, Rawool S, Thakare RP, Banday S, Mishra AK, Das G, Malonia SK (2023) Next-generation sequencing technology: current trends and advancements. Biology 12(7). https://www.mdpi.com/2079-7737/12/7/997

Schneider MV, Orchard S (2011) Omics technologies, data and bioinformatics principles. Humana Press, Totowa, NJ, pp 3–30

Smallwood SA, Lee HJ, Angermueller C, Krueger F, Saadeh H, Peat JR, Andrews SR, Stegle O, Reik W, Kelsey G (2014) Single-cell genome-wide bisulfite sequencing for assessing epigenetic heterogeneity. Nat Methods 11:817–820

Stoeckius M, Chattopadhyay Pratip K, Houck-Loomis B, Stephenson W, Swerdlow H (2017) Simultaneous epitope and transcriptome measurement in single cells. Nat Methods 14:865–868

Stricker SH, Köferle A, Beck S (2016) From profiles to function in epigenomics. Nat Rev Genet 18:51–66

Teschendorff AE, Enver T (2017) Single-cell entropy for accurate estimation of differentiation potency from a cell's transcriptome. Nat Commun 8

Trevino AE, Sinnott-Armstrong N, Andersen J, Yoon SJ, Huber N, Pritchard JK, Chang HY, Greenleaf WJ, PasÌ§ca SP (2020) Chromatin accessibility dynamics in a model of human forebrain development. Science 367(6476):eaay1645

Walsh G, Walsh E (2022) Biopharmaceutical benchmarks 2022. Nat Biotechnol 40:1722–1760

Wang L, Wheeler DA (2014) Genomic sequencing for cancer diagnosis and therapy. Ann Rev Med 65:33–48

Ye F, Zhang S, Fu Y, Yang L, Zhang G, Wu Y, Pan J, Chen H, Wang X, Ma L, Niu H, Jiang M, Zhang T, Jia D, Wang J, Wang Y, Han X, Guo G (2024) Fast and flexible profiling of chromatin accessibility and total RNA expression in single nuclei using microwell-seq3. Cell Discov **10** (2024)

Zhang J, Wang XM, Xing X, Xu Z, Zhang C, Song J, Fan X, Xia P, Fu J, Yu Wang S, Xu R, Dai XP, Shi L, Huang L, Jun Jiang T, Shi M, Zhang Y, Zumla A, Maeurer M, Bai F, Wang FS (2020) Single-cell landscape of immunological responses in patients with Covid-19. Nat Immunol 21:1107–1118

Chapter 2
Kernels and Indefinite Kernel Optimizations

2.1 Introduction

Support vector machines (SVMs), a set of powerful supervised machine learning algorithms was introduced by Vapnik (1995, 1998). By using structural risk minimization strategy, SVMs (Carrizosa and Morales 2013) are traditionally regarded as one of the best algorithms in machine learning area. Kernel SVM works by embedding data in high dimensional or infinite feature space and an optimal separating hyperplane is constructed in the space (Scholkopf et al. 2004). Kernel methods for their strong capability in dealing with nonlinear data modelling, have been widely applied in the field of bioinformatics. In Pan et al. (2016), an incremental kernel ridge regression model was proposed to predict soft-tissue deformations after craniomaxillofacial surgery. In Liu et al. (2009), a new kernel was developed for kernel-based Linear Discriminant Analysis (LDA) method to address the problem of face recognition under illumination variations. In order to address the problem of complex and nonlinear data distribution, authors in Pan et al. (2011) presented a nonlinear non-negative matrix factorization (NMF) based on a self-constructed Mercer kernel which preserves the non-negative constraints on both bases and coefficients in kernel feature space. Being positive semi-definite (PSD) is crucial (Scholkopf and Smola 2001) for a kernel matrix induced by kernel functions in SVMs. It is required to ensure the existence of a Reproducing Kernel Hilbert Space (RKHS). A convex optimization problem can be formulated to obtain an optimal solution in RKHS. In real-world applications however, similarity matrices generated for practical use cannot ensure such a PSD property. For instance, in pair-wise similarity evaluation between DNA or protein sequences, general tools include BLAST and Dynamic Time Warping often generate indefinite matrices (Altschul et al. 1990; Saigo et al. 2004; Shimodaira et al. 2002). The popular generalized histogram intersection(GHI) kernel that is conditionally positive definite is not usually PSD (Boughorbel et al. 2005). Hyperbolic tangent kernels/Sigmoid kernels (Lin and Lin 2003; Smola et al. 2001) that perform well in practice sometimes are indefinite as well. There is still no

H. Jiang and W.-K. Ching, *Kernel Methods for Omics Data Mining*, Intelligent Control and Learning Systems 10, https://doi.org/10.1007/978-981-95-3129-5_2

fixed rule on how to effectively deal with indefinite kernels in the SVM framework. Training indefinite SVMs therefore forms challenging problems since global optimal solutions are no longer valid in this learning scenario for standard SVMs (Hassdonk 2005).

To deal with indefinite kernel, a number of Euclideanization methods including multidimensional scaling and pseudo-euclidean space have been proposed in Munoz and Diego (2006). Representative methods tackle such problem by altering the spectrum of an indefinite kernel matrix so as to generate a PSD one. Denoising method in Pekalska et al. (2002) considered negative eigenvalues as noise and substitutes them with zero. The flipping method by flipping the sign of negative eigenvalues (Graepel et al. 1998) constituted another effective method for transforming indefinite kernel into PSD one. In Wu et al. (2005), data distribution was taking into consideration in the diffusion method and the eigenvalues were replaced with exponential form. In the shifting method (Roth et al. 2000), eigenvalues were shifted by introducing new parameters to guarantee the non-negativity of all the eigenvalues. Authors in Lin and Lin (2003) investigated non-PSD kernels in the perspective of separability, and developed a method in order to find stationary points under non-convex dual formulation of SVMs with sigmoid kernels. In Ong et al. (2004), indefinite kernel learning was considered as a minimization problem in a pseudo-Euclidean space. In Luss and D'Aspremont (2009), a max-min optimization problem was further proposed so as to find a proxy kernel for the indefinite kernel. Based on confidence function, a simple generalization of SVMs was suggested in Guo and Schuurmans (2009). Kernel principal component analysis was developed as a kernel transformation method to deal with indefinite kernels (Gu and Guo 2012).

In this chapter, we develop a superior and effective method, i.e., projection method, to transform an indefinite kernel into a PSD one. The proposed method demonstrates flexibility and effectiveness. Popular flipping methods and denoising methods are special cases by varying its parameter λ in the proposed method. Furthermore, our suggested λ under LogDet Divergence and perturbed von-Neumann Divergence can always yield near optimal performance, which can be regarded as a good choice for dealing with indefinite kernels. Besides, our suggested optimal projection matrix also has certain special mathematical properties. The connection between our projection method and spectrum method can be investigated through eigenvalue analysis.

The rest of this chapter is organized as follows. Firstly, we present the projection method and the associated theoretical analysis. The optimal λ determination in the projection matrix is modeled under unconstrained optimization framework. Indefinite kernels on real world data sets are introduced for method evaluation. The theoretical validity of the suggested optimal λ is demonstrated with the experimental data. Discussions of the experimental validation on the suggested optimal λ under LogDet Divergence and perturbed von-Neumann Divergence are provided as well.

2.2 Methodology

Assume $(\mathbf{X}_i, y_i)_{i=1}^n$, where $\mathbf{X}_i \in \mathbf{R}^p$, and $y_i \in \{1, -1\}$ is a given list of labeled patterns. Function k is defined as follows:

$$k : \chi \times \chi \to \mathbf{R}$$

which can be regarded as a kernel function where $\chi \subset \mathbf{R}^p$ represents the input space. The kernel induced by the kernel function is defined element-wise by

$$K(i, j) = k(\mathbf{X}_i, \mathbf{X}_j), \qquad i, j \in \{1, 2, \ldots, n\}. \tag{2.1}$$

However, in view of Mercer's theorem (Mercer 1909), only PSD kernels are deemed valid because they can be written as eigenfunction series. Thus, to deal with invalid kernels, kernel transformation strategy is increasingly popular. In the case of a non-PSD kernel K, one may decompose it into this form:

$$K = P \cdot D \cdot P'.$$

Here D is a diagonal matrix and not all the diagonal entries are non-negative, P is orthonormal matrix with the jth column corresponding to the eigenvector for jth eigenvalue in D and P' is the transpose of matrix P. Eigenvalue transform is the representative method in kernel transformation (Pekalska et al. 2002; Graepel et al. 1998; Wu et al. 2005; Roth et al. 2000).

In the following, we present our projection method for transforming an indefinite kernel to a PSD one.

Lemma 2.1 *Let K be a real symmetric matrix and let m be the negative inertial index of K. Suppose that $m \geq 1$. Then for any real λ, there exists an $n \times m$ matrix B satisfying $B'B = I_m$ such that $(I_n - \lambda BB')$ has $1 - \lambda$ and 1 as its eigenvalues, the multiplicities for whom are m and $n - m$, respectively. Besides, it shares the same set of eigenvectors with K.*

Proof Consider that K is a real and symmetric matrix, we decompose it as $K = P \cdot D \cdot P'$ where $P = [\mathbf{p}_1, \mathbf{p}_2, \ldots, \mathbf{p}_n]$ is orthogonal and $D = \text{diag}[d_1, d_2, \ldots, d_n]$ is a diagonal matrix with the diagonal elements $d_i, i = 1, 2, \ldots, n$. W.L.O.G, we may assume all the eigenvalues are sorted in ascending order. We further assume the negative inertia index is m.

Denote $B = [\mathbf{p}_1, \mathbf{p}_2, \ldots, \mathbf{p}_m]$, we have $B'B = I_m$ because $\mathbf{p}_1, \ldots, \mathbf{p}_n$ are orthonormal. Then, we have

$$(I_n - \lambda BB')\mathbf{p}_i = \begin{cases} (1 - \lambda)\mathbf{p}_i, & i \in \{1, 2, \ldots, m\} \\ \mathbf{p}_i, & i \in \{m + 1, m + 2, \ldots, n\} \end{cases} \tag{2.2}$$

Thus, it has 1 and $(1-\lambda)$ as its eigenvalues. The multiplicity of $(1-\lambda)$ is m and for 1 the multiplicity is $n-m$. Furthermore, the eigenvectors of $(I_n-\lambda BB')$ are exactly the same as the kernel K. □

Theorem 2.1 *Let K be an $n \times n$ real symmetric matrix which is indefinite and let λ be the regularization parameter. Then there exists an $n \times m$ $(1 \le m < n)$ matrix B satisfying $B'B = I_m$ such that $(I_n - \lambda BB')K$ is a PSD kernel provided that $\lambda \ge 1$.*

Proof Denote $B = [\mathbf{p}_1, \mathbf{p}_2, \ldots, \mathbf{p}_m]$, where the definitions of $\mathbf{p}_i, i = 1, 2, \ldots, m$ are the same as denoted in Lemma 2.1. Note that $1 \le m < n$ as K is indefinite. By Eq. (2.2), we have

$$\begin{aligned} &(I_n - \lambda BB')K \\ &= P\text{diag}\{1-\lambda, \ldots, 1-\lambda, 1, \ldots, 1\}P' \cdot P\text{diag}\{d_1, d_2, \ldots, d_n\}P' \\ &= P\text{diag}\{(1-\lambda)d_1, \ldots, (1-\lambda)d_m, \underbrace{0, \ldots, 0}_{n-m-l}, d_{n-l+1}, \ldots, d_n\}P'. \end{aligned} \tag{2.3}$$

Since $\lambda \ge 1$, we have $(1-\lambda)d_i \ge 0$ for $1 \le i \le m$. This will guarantee the kernel matrix $(I_n - \lambda BB')K$ is positive semi-definite. □

The denoising method and the flipping method are particular cases of the projection method, and they are recovered by setting $\lambda = 1$ and $\lambda = 2$ respectively in Eq. (2.3).

Determination of Optimal λ. Considering that λ is an embedded parameter in the projection method, it is necessary to study optimal λ determination which can demonstrate excellent prediction power for $\lambda > 0$. To this end, we begin with the definition of Bregman matrix divergence (Brian et al. 2006).

Definition 2.1 (Bregman Matrix Divergences) Let ϕ be a strictly convex differentiable function over the set of all real symmetric $n \times n$ matrices. The Bregman Matrix Divergence with respect to ϕ is defined as follows:

$$D_\phi(K, K_0) = \phi(K) - \phi(K_0) - \text{tr}\left[(\nabla\phi(K_0))'(K - K_0)\right].$$

Here $\text{tr}(K)$ means the trace of matrix K and $\nabla\phi = \begin{pmatrix} \frac{\partial\phi}{\partial k_{11}} & \cdots & \frac{\partial\phi}{\partial k_{1n}} \\ \vdots & & \vdots \\ \frac{\partial\phi}{\partial k_{n1}} & \cdots & \frac{\partial\phi}{\partial k_{nn}} \end{pmatrix}$ is the gradient of ϕ in matrix form.

A number of matrix divergences can be found in Brian et al. (2006); Nock et al. (2013).

1. Mahalanobis Divergence ($p = 2$):

$$D_\phi(K, K_0) = \text{tr}(K^2 - 2KK_0 + K_0^2). \tag{2.4}$$

2. Frobenius Divergence ($\phi(K) = \|K\|_F^2$):

$$D_\phi(K, K_0) = \|K - K_0\|_F^2. \tag{2.5}$$

3. von-Neumann Divergence ($\phi(K) = \mathrm{tr}(K \log(K) - K)$):

$$D_\phi(K, K_0) = \mathrm{tr}(K \log K - K \log K_0 - K + K_0). \tag{2.6}$$

4. LogDet Divergence ($\phi(K) = -\log\det(K)$ for positive-definite matrix K):

$$D_\phi(K, K_0) = \mathrm{tr}(K K_0^{-1}) - \log\det(K K_0^{-1}) - n. \tag{2.7}$$

Inspired by the work in Li et al. (2009) where authors proposed a framework of kernel learning (Conforti and Guido 2010) by using unconstrained optimization, we re-formulate the optimal λ determination problem as a kernel learning one in a similar manner. The optimal λ can be obtained by the minimization of $D_\phi(\tilde{K}, K)$ where $\tilde{K}$ is the optimal PSD kernel which is close to original kernel K in terms of divergence.

To be precise, if $K = \sum_{i=1}^{n} d_i \mathbf{p}_i \mathbf{p}_i'$ is an arbitrary fixed real symmetric and indefinite matrix, we let B be defined as in Lemma 2.1 (or the theorem following it) and let

$$\tilde{K}_\lambda = (I - \lambda B B')K = \sum_{i=1}^{m} (1 - \lambda) d_i \mathbf{p}_i \mathbf{p}_i' + \sum_{i=m+1}^{n} d_i \mathbf{p}_i \mathbf{p}_i', \qquad \lambda \geq 1.$$

Then the optimal λ is determined by solving the following minimization problem

$$\min_{\lambda \geq 1} D_\phi(\tilde{K}_\lambda, K).$$

For Mahalanobis Divergence, by Definition 2.1, we know that $K\tilde{K}_\lambda = \tilde{K}_\lambda K$ as they share the same set of eigenvectors. Therefore, the minimization problem can be expressed as

$$\min_\lambda \lambda^2 \mathrm{tr}(B B' K)^2. \tag{2.8}$$

The optimal λ can be quickly obtained as 0.

For Frobenius Divergence, the minimization problem in finding optimal λ as derived from Eq. (2.5) is

$$\min_\lambda \lambda \|B B' K\|_F^2. \tag{2.9}$$

It is easy to see that the optimal λ is 0.

For von Neumann Divergence, we can deduce the minimization problem to be

$$\min_{\lambda} \sum_{i=1}^{m} d_i((1-\lambda)\log(1-\lambda)+\lambda). \tag{2.10}$$

Applying differentiation to Eq. (2.10), we obtain the optimal value of $\lambda = 0$.

The optimal $\lambda = 0$ does not make any perturbation to the original kernel matrix which is not reasonable. Hence we focus on LogDet Divergence (Li et al. 2009), the optimal λ can be determined through the following formula

$$-\frac{m}{1-\lambda} - \sum_{i=1}^{m} d_i \mathrm{tr}(K^{-1}\mathbf{p}_i\mathbf{p}_i') = 0. \tag{2.11}$$

Considering that the calculation involves inverse of matrix K, where K is not necessarily positive definite, we use Moore-Penroses inverse K^+ instead. Thus, the final theoretical optimal λ becomes:

$$\lambda_{\text{opt}} = 1 + \frac{m}{\sum_{i=1}^{m} d_i \mathrm{tr}(K^+\mathbf{p}_i\mathbf{p}_i')}. \tag{2.12}$$

2.3 Results

2.3.1 *Materials*

To empirically assess our approach, we selected various life science datasets that meet the criterion of producing indefinite kernels, with a predominant focus on cancer-related datasets. Among these, three datasets were sourced from lib-svm datasets (NCBI 2017). One of these datasets comprises sonar data, featuring 208 instances, with 97 labeled as positive and 111 as negative. The Liver disorder dataset consists of 345 instances, with 145 classified as positive and 200 as negative. The Breast Cancer dataset encompasses 683 instances, with 444 classified as negative and 239 as positive, and comprises 10 attributes. Additionally, two other datasets are relevant to cystic fibrosis and leukemia. The cystic fibrosis dataset comprises 177 glycan structures, including 89 associated with cystic fibrosis, 107 with respiratory mucin, and 101 with bronchial mucin. The leukemia-related dataset includes 355 structures originating from four human blood components: leukemic cells, erythrocytes, serum, and plasma, with respective examples numbering 162, 111, 85, and 73. All the glycan structures are retrieved from the KEGG/GLYCAN database (Hashimoto et al. 2006), where annotations are retrieved from CarbBank/CCSD database (Doubet and Albersheim 1992). If the glycan data set contains N glycans $\{g_1, g_2, \ldots, g_N\}$, we denote the set of all q-grams existing in these N glycans to be a q-gram set: $\Phi_q = \{\phi_q^1, \phi_q^2, \ldots, \phi_q^{n_q}\}$. For a specific glycan g_i in the data set, $q-$gram representation is a column vector $x_i^q = [x_{1i}^q, x_{2i}^q, \ldots, x_{n_q i}^q]^T$ where x_{li}^q means the number of lth q-gram in the glycan g_i. The number of attributes within the dataset depends on the

Table 2.1 Data set information

Data set	Number of instances	Number of attributes
Sonar	208	60
Liver disorder	345	6
Breast cancer	683	10
Cystic fibrosis	177	Depends on q
Leukemia	355	Depends on q
Lung cancer	91	54675

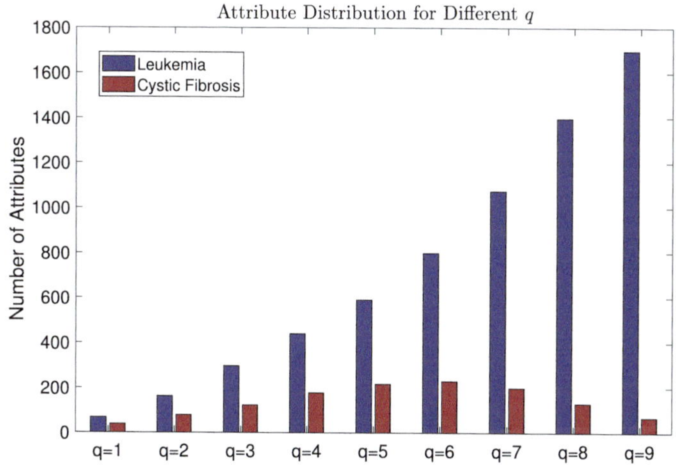

Fig. 2.1 Attribute distribution for different values of q in leukemia data and cystic fibrosis data

value of q ($q = 1$ to 9), where we have 9 datasets derived from cystic fibrosis data and leukemia data respectively. The last data set is about lung cancer and we obtained it from NCBI (National Center of Biotechnology Information) GEO (Gene Expression Omnibus) (NCBI 2017). Affymetrix Human Genome U133 Plus 2.0 Array experiments were carried out in a set of 91 non-small cell lung cancer (NSCLC) samples, containing 46 tumors and 45 controls. Detailed information on the data sets can be found in Table 2.1.

Attribute Distribution Information for different q is provided in Fig. 2.1 for Leukemia Data and Cystic Fibrosis Data. We can see that the number of attributes in Leukemia Data is increasing with the increment of q while it is not the case in Cystic Fibrosis Data. In Cystic Fibrosis Data set, the number of the attributes firstly increases then decreases with the increment of q. The possible reason is that the glycan structures in Leukemia Data set is more complicated than that in Cystic Fibrosis Data set.

2.3.2 Experiments

The LogDet divergence is used in these experiments, with the optimal λ determined by Eq. (2.12). We perform the experiments in fivefold cross-validation setting and evaluate model performance using the Area Under Curve (AUC), a widely adopted metric calculated as the area under the Receiver Operating Characteristic (ROC) curve. To robustly assess model performance, we compute the average AUC values across 10 iterations of fivefold cross-validation. In this study, we introduce two kernels: the Generalized Histogram Intersection (GHI) kernel (Boughorbel et al. 2005) and the cosine kernel, chosen for illustrative purposes. Notably, these kernels are predominantly indefinite, shown in Table 2.2. It is worth mentioning that these kernels have not been previously utilized in biological applications such as glycan classification or cancer prediction.

GHI kernel is frequently used in image classification and the definition is as follows:

$$k(\mathbf{X}_j, \mathbf{X}_k) = \sum_{i=1}^{p} \min(|\mathbf{X}_{ji}|^{\alpha}, |\mathbf{X}_{ki}|^{\beta})$$

where $\mathbf{X}_j$ represents data vector and $\mathbf{X}_{ji}$ represents the ith element of $\mathbf{X}_j$, $j = 1, 2, \ldots, n$. In addition, α and β are usually positive parameters.

When $\alpha = \beta$, the kernel can be proved to be a positive semi-definite matrix. Experimental results in Table 2.2 also show consistence with the statement the minimal eigenvalue in GHI kernel is 0 when $\alpha = \beta$. We in experimental settings use different values of $\alpha, \beta \in \{1, 2, 3\}$, $\alpha \neq \beta$ to evaluate the performance of our proposed projection method.

The cosine kernel function is defined by:

$$k(\mathbf{X}_j, \mathbf{X}_k) = \cos(||\mathbf{X}_j - \mathbf{X}_k||),$$

which is different from the usual definition of cosine similarity: $\frac{\mathbf{X}_j'\mathbf{X}_k}{||\mathbf{X}_j||\cdot||\mathbf{X}_k||}$. The reason we did not consider the usual definition is that the corresponding kernel matrix induced by it is PSD, which fails to satisfy our requirements.

2.3.2.1 Experiments on GHI Kernel

The performance of projection method and the original GHI Kernel SVM was summarized in Tables 2.3, 2.4 and 2.5. Values marked in bold face represent best performance and no marks are made when both methods showing comparable performance. When α differs from β, GHI kernel is indefinite (see Table 2.2), one can see that projection method outperforms GHI Kernel method.

The performance for sonar data set is reported in Table 2.3. For example, when $(\alpha, \beta) = (1, 2)$, projection method shows the averaged AUC value 81.47% with standard deviation 0.99% while in GHI kernel method the averaged AUC value is

Table 2.2 Maximum and minimum eigenvalues with considered kernels in the considered datasets

Data methods	GHI kernel						Cosine kernel
	$\alpha = 1, \beta = 1$	$\alpha = 1, \beta = 2$	$\alpha = 1, \beta = 3$	$\alpha = 2, \beta = 2$	$\alpha = 2, \beta = 3$	$\alpha = 3, \beta = 3$	
Liver disorder	$1 \times 10^5(0)$	$1 \times 10^5(-2.3)$	$1 \times 10^5(-4.1)$	$1 \times 10^9(0)$	$1 \times 10^9(-1.2)$	$1 \times 10^{13}(0)$	$243.8(-28)$
Sonar	$1 \times 10^4(0)$	$1 \times 10^4(-2.3)$	$1 \times 10^4(-5.1)$	$1 \times 10^8(0)$	$1 \times 10^8(-0.8)$	$1 \times 10^{12}(0)$	$39.5(-110)$
Breast	$4.6 \times 10^3(0)$	$4.2 \times 10^3(-5.3)$	$3.9 \times 10^3(-6.4)$	$3.9 \times 10^3(0)$	$3.7 \times 10^3(-1)$	$3.5 \times 10^3(0)$	$432.8(-253.5)$
Cystic ($q = 1$)	498.4(0)	498.4(−0.08)	498.4(−0.08)	561.9(0)	561.9(0)	759.6(0)	35.6(−111)
Cystic ($q = 2$)	303.8(0)	303.8(0)	303.8(0)	315.1(0)	315.1(0)	347.5(0)	30.2(−125.2)
Cystic ($q = 3$)	196.1(0)	196.1(0)	196.1(0)	196.8(0)	196.8(0)	198.7(0)	32.2(−131.5)
Cystic ($q = 4$)	102.3(0)	102.3(0)	102.3(0)	102.4(0)	102.4(0)	102.6(0)	52.7(−119.4)
Cystic ($q = 5$)	47.3(0)	47.3(0)	47.3(0)	47.3(0)	47.3(0)	47.3(0)	77.2(−94)
Cystic ($q = 6$)	32.5(0)	32.5(0)	32.5(0)	32.5(0)	32.5(0)	32.5(0)	104.4(−65.4)
Cystic ($q = 7$)	30.3(0)	30.3(0)	30.3(0)	30.3(0)	30.3(0)	30.3(0)	129.4(−38.5)
Cystic ($q = 8$)	25.0(0)	25.0(0)	25.0(0)	25.0(0)	25.0(0)	25.0(0)	149.6(−38.5)
Cystic ($q = 9$)	18.0(0)	18.0(0)	18.0(0)	18.0(0)	18.0(0)	18.0(0)	165.8(−5.8)
Leukemia ($q = 1$)	$2.3 \times 10^3(0)$	$2.4 \times 10^3(-14.0)$	$2.4 \times 10^3(-14.0)$	$5.6 \times 10^3(0)$	$6.3 \times 10^3(-151.4)$	$1.7 \times 10^4(0)$	114.9(−178.8)
Leukemia ($q = 2$)	$2.0 \times 10^3(0)$	$2.0 \times 10^3(-4.1)$	$2.0 \times 10^3(-4.1)$	$3.5 \times 10^3(0)$	$3.9 \times 10^3(-55.7)$	$8.3 \times 10^3(0)$	80.8(−222.4)
Leukemia ($q = 3$)	$2.0 \times 10^3(0)$	$2.0 \times 10^3(-4.0)$	$2.0 \times 10^3(-4.0)$	$2.5 \times 10^3(0)$	$2.6 \times 10^3(-16.7)$	$3.5 \times 10^3(0)$	57.6(−188.8)
Leukemia ($q = 4$)	$2.3 \times 10^3(0)$	$2.3 \times 10^3(0)$	$2.3 \times 10^3(0)$	$2.4 \times 10^3(0)$	$2.4 \times 10^3(0)$	$2.4 \times 10^3(0)$	67.9(−178.9)
Leukemia ($q = 5$)	$2.8 \times 10^3(0)$	$2.8 \times 10^3(0)$	$2.8 \times 10^3(0)$	$2.8 \times 10^3(0)$	$2.8 \times 10^3(0)$	$2.8 \times 10^3(0)$	120.7(−188.4)
Leukemia ($q = 6$)	$3.2 \times 10^3(0)$	$3.2 \times 10^3(0)$	$3.2 \times 10^3(0)$	$3.2 \times 10^3(0)$	$3.2 \times 10^3(0)$	$3.2 \times 10^3(0)$	120.6(−157.0)
Leukemia ($q = 7$)	$3.4 \times 10^3(0)$	$3.4 \times 10^3(0)$	$3.4 \times 10^3(0)$	$3.4 \times 10^3(0)$	$3.4 \times 10^3(0)$	$3.4 \times 10^3(0)$	180.2(−170.0)
Leukemia ($q = 8$)	$3.4 \times 10^3(0)$	$3.4 \times 10^3(0)$	$3.4 \times 10^3(0)$	$3.4 \times 10^3(0)$	$3.4 \times 10^3(0)$	$3.4 \times 10^3(0)$)	169.2(−146.2)
Leukemia ($q - 9$)	$3.1 \times 10^3(0)$	$3.1 \times 10^3(0)$	$3.1 \times 10^3(0)$	$3.1 \times 10^3(0)$	$3.1 \times 10^3(0)$	$3.1 \times 10^3(0)$	198.6(−131.7)
NSCLC	$2.5 \times 10^7(0)$	$2.7 \times 10^7(-883.8)$	$2.7 \times 10^7(-877.3)$	$1.5 \times 10^8(0)$	$1.6 \times 10^8(-1.4 \times 10^4)$	$1.0 \times 10^9(0)$	13.9(−11.8)

Table 2.3 Averaged AUC values (%) of projection method and GHI kernel using sonar data, liver disorder data, breast cancer data and NSCLC data

Data sets	Parameters	Projection method	GHI kernel
Sonar	$\alpha = 1, \beta = 1$	82.87 ± 0.99	82.87 ± 0.99
	$\alpha = 1, \beta = 2$	**81.47 ± 0.99**	53.42 ± 4.94
	$\alpha = 1, \beta = 3$	**84.02 ± 1.19**	54.10 ± 4.92
	$\alpha = 2, \beta = 2$	84.29 ± 1.54	84.29 ± 1.54
	$\alpha = 2, \beta = 3$	**84.31 ± 1.56**	83.06 ± 2.04
	$\alpha = 3, \beta = 3$	83.62 ± 1.17	83.62 ± 1.17
Live	$\alpha = 1, \beta = 1$	82.87 ± 0.99	82.87 ± 0.99
	$\alpha = 1, \beta = 2$	**81.47 ± 0.99**	53.42 ± 4.94
	$\alpha = 1, \beta = 3$	**84.02 ± 1.19**	54.10 ± 4.92
	$\alpha = 2, \beta = 2$	84.29 ± 1.54	84.29 ± 1.54
	$\alpha = 2, \beta = 3$	**84.31 ± 1.56**	83.06 ± 2.04
	$\alpha = 3, \beta = 3$	83.62 ± 1.17	83.62 ± 1.17
Breast	$\alpha = 1, \beta = 1$	96.73 ± 0.11	96.73 ± 0.11
	$\alpha = 1, \beta = 2$	**97.06 ± 0.01**	90.12 ± 4.78
	$\alpha = 1, \beta = 3$	**97.01 ± 0.01**	75.61 ± 7.44
	$\alpha = 2, \beta = 2$	96.71 ± 0.11	96.71 ± 0.11
	$\alpha = 2, \beta = 3$	96.92 ± 0.01	96.96 ± 0.01
	$\alpha = 3, \beta = 3$	96.63 ± 0.10	96.63 ± 0.10
NSCLC	$\alpha = 1, \beta = 1$	100 ± 0	100 ± 0
	$\alpha = 1, \beta = 2$	**99.72 ± 0.01**	64.07 ± 7.42
	$\alpha = 1, \beta = 3$	**61.46 ± 1.57**	51.47 ± 5.53
	$\alpha = 2, \beta = 2$	100 ± 0	100 ± 0
	$\alpha = 2, \beta = 3$	**99.99 ± 0**	73.07 ± 8.17
	$\alpha = 3, \beta = 3$	100 ± 0	100 ± 0

53.42% with standard deviation 4.94%. When $(\alpha, \beta) = (1, 3)$, projection method shows 84.02% in the averaged AUC value, with standard deviation 1.19%. However, the averaged AUC value for GHI kernel method is only 54.10% with standard deviation 4.92%. When $(\alpha, \beta) = (2, 3)$, the averaged AUC value for projection method is 84.31%, larger than the averaged AUC value for GHI Method 83.06%. The standard deviation in projection method is 1.56%, while in GHI kernel method the standard deviation is 2.04%. This implies that projection method is more powerful and stable compared to the original GHI kernel method.

For Liver Disorder data set, we can see from Table 2.3 that projection method performs significantly better than the GHI kernel method when $\alpha \neq \beta$. The best performance of indefinite GHI kernel achieves around 60% in AUC value which is not satisfying. When $\alpha = \beta$, both methods show comparable performance.

For breast cancer data set, results in Table 2.3 indicate that when $(\alpha, \beta) = (1, 2)$ and $(\alpha, \beta) = (1, 3)$, projection method is clearly superior to the GHI kernel method while comparable performance is detected in both methods when $(\alpha, \beta) = (2, 3)$. This illustrates the fact that indefinite kernels sometimes can also perform well. However, the superiority of projection method over the original GHI kernel method is clearly shown in this data set.

In cystic fibrosis data set, we obtain 9 different comparison results when values of q vary from 1 to 9 as shown in Table 2.4. There is no clear difference between projection method and GHI kernel method, as GHI kernel is PSD for almost all considered pairs of α and β (see Table 2.2). The only 2 cases when the GHI kernel is indefinite are $(\alpha, \beta) = (1, 2)$ and $(\alpha, \beta) = (1, 3)$ for q = 1, and the minimal eigenvalue in these 2 cases is only -0.08, which is quite close to 0, demonstrating that the generated kernel is almost PSD.

Results for Leukemia Data are summarized in Table 2.5. Similar to the results in cystic fibrosis data, projection method and GHI kernel method show similar performance in most of the cases for q from 1 to 9. From Table 2.2 we can see that, GHI kernel is indefinite when $\alpha \neq \beta$ for $q = 1, 2, 3$. When $q = 1, 2$, projection method is better than GHI kernel method for $(\alpha, \beta) = (1, 2)$ and $(\alpha, \beta) = (1, 3)$; However, GHI kernel method is comparable to projection method for $(\alpha, \beta) = (2, 3)$.

Some interesting results can be found for NSCLC data as shown in Table 2.3. Projection method and GHI kernel method show exact performance when $\alpha = \beta$, yielding 100% in AUC values. We note that projection method does not make any perturbation to the original kernel when the GHI kernel is PSD ($\alpha = \beta$), we can conclude that GHI kernel is a preferred kernel for tumor differentiation with NSCLC data. When α differs from β, different results are shown. When $(\alpha, \beta) = (1, 2)$, projection method shows 99.72% in averaged AUC values with 0.01% standard deviation, while GHI kernel method only can obtain 64.07% in averaged AUC values with a large standard deviation 7.42%. When $(\alpha, \beta) = (2, 3)$, projection method shows 99.99% in averaged AUC values with 0 standard deviation, while GHI kernel method can obtain 73.07% in averaged AUC values with a large standard deviation 8.17%. When $(\alpha, \beta) = (1, 3)$, the projection method can only obtain 61.46% in averaged AUC values and GHI kernel method is even worse, achieving only 51.47% in averaged AUC values.

We can conclude that the performance of projection method is not always similar for different pairs (α, β). There exists a best pair of (α, β) for inducing best projection method for a given data set, but different data sets may be suitable to different pairs. Sometimes GHI kernel method also performs well even though the kernel is indefinite. But in general, projection method is clearly better than the GHI kernel for the above considered data sets.

2.3.2.2 Experiments on Cosine Kernel

Table 2.6 compares the performance of projection method with Cosine Kernel method for the considered datasets. Our projection method demonstrates visible better performance compared to Cosine Kernel method in terms of averaged AUC values. From the bold text on the left column of table, we can see that projection method is

Table 2.4 Averaged AUC values (%) of projection method and GHI kernel using cystic fibrosis data

Parameters	Projection method ($q = 1$)	GHI ($q = 1$)	Projection method ($q = 2$)	GHI ($q = 2$)
$\alpha = 1, \beta = 1$	78.57 ± 1.75	78.57 ± 1.75	81.32 ± 1.25	81.32 ± 1.25
$\alpha = 1, \beta = 2$	78.94 ± 1.86	78.94 ± 1.86	81.74 ± 1.60	81.74 ± 1.60
$\alpha = 1, \beta = 3$	78.64 ± 1.01	78.63 ± 1.01	80.82 ± 1.30	80.82 ± 1.29
$\alpha = 2, \beta = 2$	79.33 ± 1.42	79.33 ± 1.41	80.53 ± 1.72	80.53 ± 1.72
$\alpha = 2, \beta = 3$	79.32 ± 1.19	79.32 ± 1.19	81.06 ± 1.37	81.06 ± 1.36
$\alpha = 3, \beta = 3$	78.14 ± 1.11	78.13 ± 1.11	80.79 ± 1.12	80.78 ± 1.12
Parameters	Projection method ($q = 3$)	GHI ($q = 3$)	Projection method ($q = 4$)	GHI ($q = 4$)
$\alpha = 1, \beta = 1$	80.77 ± 1.44	80.76 ± 1.44	83.10 ± 2.10	83.09 ± 2.10
$\alpha = 1, \beta = 2$	80.98 ± 1.81	80.97 ± 1.81	82.11 ± 1.77	82.13 ± 1.77
$\alpha = 1, \beta = 3$	81.20 ± 1.95	81.19 ± 1.94	83.54 ± 1.46	83.51 ± 1.48
$\alpha = 2, \beta = 2$	81.32 ± 1.26	81.30 ± 1.27	82.75 ± 2.14	82.79 ± 2.15
$\alpha = 2, \beta = 3$	81.10 ± 1.10	81.09 ± 1.11	83.62 ± 1.61	83.65 ± 1.65
$\alpha = 3, \beta = 3$	81.06 ± 1.39	81.04 ± 1.39	83.49 ± 0.77	83.56 ± 0.82
Parameters	Projection method ($q = 5$)	GHI ($q = 5$)	Projection method ($q = 6$)	GHI ($q = 6$)
$\alpha = 1, \beta = 1$	74.03 ± 2.18	74.00 ± 2.18	72.30 ± 1.93	72.50 ± 1.87
$\alpha = 1, \beta = 2$	71.67 ± 2.52	71.62 ± 2.58	73.62 ± 2.69	73.80 ± 2.70
$\alpha = 1, \beta = 3$	74.77 ± 2.27	74.73 ± 2.28	71.94 ± 1.77	72.11 ± 1.65
$\alpha = 2, \beta = 2$	73.73 ± 1.36	73.73 ± 1.38	71.49 ± 2.78	71.60 ± 2.84
$\alpha = 2, \beta = 3$	72.62 ± 2.97	72.61 ± 2.92	72.81 ± 1.91	73.01 ± 1.92
$\alpha = 3, \beta = 3$	75.23 ± 2.64	75.20 ± 2.55	73.53 ± 2.62	73.80 ± 2.67
Parameters	Projection method ($q = 7$)	GHI ($q = 7$)	Projection method ($q = 8$)	GHI ($q = 8$)
$\alpha = 1, \beta = 1$	67.99 ± 2.78	67.60 ± 2.87	60.65 ± 4.20	60.90 ± 4.36
$\alpha = 1, \beta = 2$	68.28 ± 3.51	67.89 ± 3.60	58.19 ± 3.72	58.33 ± 3.77
$\alpha = 1, \beta = 3$	67.75 ± 2.20	67.25 ± 2.19	58.98 ± 3.67	59.28 ± 3.69
$\alpha = 2, \beta = 2$	67.90 ± 3.11	67.23 ± 3.04	58.28 ± 4.20	58.34 ± 4.13
$\alpha = 2, \beta = 3$	67.58 ± 2.91	66.96 ± 2.88	58.66 ± 2.40	58.86 ± 2.37
$\alpha = 3, \beta = 3$	68.85 ± 2.28	68.44 ± 2.13	59.62 ± 3.34	59.77 ± 3.37
Parameters	Projection method ($q = 9$)	GHI ($q = 9$)		
$\alpha = 1, \beta = 1$	53.25 ± 3.99	53.25 ± 3.99		
$\alpha = 1, \beta = 2$	52.12 ± 4.28	52.12 ± 4.28		
$\alpha = 1, \beta = 3$	52.54 ± 3.22	52.54 ± 3.22		
$\alpha = 2, \beta = 2$	51.16 ± 2.37	51.16 ± 2.37		
$\alpha = 2, \beta = 3$	51.62 ± 4.18	51.62 ± 4.18		
$\alpha = 3, \beta = 3$	51.96 ± 5.01	51.96 ± 5.01		

Table 2.5 Averaged AUC values (%) of projection method and GHI kernel using leukemia data

Parameters	Projection method ($q = 1$)	GHI ($q = 1$)	Projection method ($q = 2$)	GHI ($q = 2$)
$\alpha = 1, \beta = 1$	93.68 ± 0.62	93.68 ± 0.62	95.90 ± 0.84	95.90 ± 0.84
$\alpha = 1, \beta = 2$	$\mathbf{93.75 \pm 0.59}$	87.00 ± 4.10	$\mathbf{95.85 \pm 0.41}$	94.93 ± 0.81
$\alpha = 1, \beta = 3$	$\mathbf{93.34 \pm 0.91}$	86.94 ± 3.37	$\mathbf{95.41 \pm 0.64}$	94.53 ± 0.89
$\alpha = 2, \beta = 2$	93.33 ± 0.74	93.32 ± 0.74	95.61 ± 0.46	95.61 ± 0.46
$\alpha = 2, \beta = 3$	93.31 ± 0.47	93.51 ± 0.46	95.17 ± 0.69	95.66 ± 0.85
$\alpha = 3, \beta = 3$	93.54 ± 0.66	93.54 ± 0.66	95.77 ± 0.40	95.77 ± 0.40
Parameters	Projection method ($q = 3$)	GHI ($q = 3$)	Projection method ($q = 4$)	GHI ($q = 4$)
$\alpha = 1, \beta = 1$	95.07 ± 0.64	95.08 ± 0.65	93.51 ± 0.54	93.54 ± 0.54
$\alpha = 1, \beta = 2$	95.13 ± 0.46	95.10 ± 0.471	93.86 ± 0.77	93.88 ± 0.77
$\alpha = 1, \beta = 3$	94.83 ± 0.41	94.77 ± 0.42	94.13 ± 0.52	94.15 ± 0.52
$\alpha = 2, \beta = 2$	95.13 ± 0.53	95.13 ± 0.53	94.05 ± 0.49	94.06 ± 0.49
$\alpha = 2, \beta = 3$	94.84 ± 0.67	94.85 ± 0.67	93.81 ± 0.69	93.82 ± 0.69
$\alpha = 3, \beta = 3$	94.77 ± 0.61	94.77 ± 0.61	93.98 ± 0.36	93.99 ± 0.36
Parameters	Projection method ($q = 5$)	GHI ($q = 5$)	Projection method ($q = 6$)	GHI ($q = 6$)
$\alpha = 1, \beta = 1$	93.40 ± 0.58	93.44 ± 0.58	93.23 ± 0.26	93.38 ± 0.26
$\alpha = 1, \beta = 2$	93.12 ± 0.70	93.16 ± 0.70	93.07 ± 0.75	93.21 ± 0.74
$\alpha = 1, \beta = 3$	93.20 ± 0.27	93.25 ± 0.28	93.05 ± 0.63	93.18 ± 0.63
$\alpha = 2, \beta = 2$	93.61 ± 0.73	93.64 ± 0.74	93.21 ± 0.48	93.35 ± 0.48
$\alpha = 2, \beta = 3$	93.78 ± 0.56	93.83 ± 0.56	93.26 ± 0.70	93.41 ± 0.72
$\alpha = 3, \beta = 3$	93.71 ± 0.72	93.75 ± 0.73	93.38 ± 0.65	93.51 ± 0.67
Parameters	Projection method ($q = 7$)	GHI ($q = 7$)	Projection method ($q = 8$)	GHI ($q = 8$)
$\alpha = 1, \beta = 1$	92.15 ± 0.68	92.37 ± 0.67	90.10 ± 0.71	90.36 ± 0.70
$\alpha = 1, \beta = 2$	92.33 ± 0.57	92.53 ± 0.59	90.68 ± 1.14	90.92 ± 1.13
$\alpha = 1, \beta = 3$	92.11 ± 0.86	92.31 ± 0.86	90.72 ± 0.73	90.96 ± 0.73
$\alpha = 2, \beta = 2$	92.01 ± 0.50	92.23 ± 0.50	90.67 ± 1.06	90.93 ± 1.04
$\alpha = 2, \beta = 3$	92.06 ± 0.45	92.27 ± 0.43	90.31 ± 0.90	90.53 ± 0.89
$\alpha = 3, \beta = 3$	92.28 ± 0.71	92.48 ± 0.73	90.66 ± 0.65	90.92 ± 0.67
Parameters	Projection method ($q = 9$)	GHI ($q = 9$)		
$\alpha = 1, \beta = 1$	88.92 ± 0.59	89.20 ± 0.62		
$\alpha = 1, \beta = 2$	89.61 ± 0.62	89.86 ± 0.63		
$\alpha = 1, \beta = 3$	89.33 ± 0.68	89.60 ± 0.67		
$\alpha = 2, \beta = 2$	89.54 ± 0.96	89.80 ± 0.96		
$\alpha = 2, \beta = 3$	88.57 ± 0.67	88.82 ± 0.68		
$\alpha = 3, \beta = 3$	88.56 ± 0.63	88.84 ± 0.63		

Table 2.6 Averaged AUC values (%) of projection method and cosine kernel for the considered datasets

Dataset	Projection method	Cosine kernel
Live disorder data	**73.71 ± 1.21**	65.63 ± 2.75
Sonar data	**89.57 ± 1.37**	67.46 ± 4.32
Breast data	**99.37 ± 0.06**	97.99 ± 3.09
Cystic ($q = 1$)	**79.25 ± 1.80**	76.89 ± 3.24
Cystic ($q = 2$)	**80.55 ± 1.38**	79.80 ± 1.84
Cystic ($q = 3$)	**78.27 ± 1.59**	70.10 ± 4.01
Cystic ($q = 4$)	**73.24 ± 2.15**	58.52 ± 4.95
Cystic ($q = 5$)	**64.38 ± 3.85**	52.13 ± 4.30
Cystic ($q = 6$)	**69.26 ± 2.11**	60.72 ± 5.36
Cystic ($q = 7$)	**64.6 ± 2.38**	58.54 ± 3.80
Cystic ($q = 8$)	63.17 ± 2.89	63.66 ± 3.21
Cystic ($q = 9$)	**54.21 ± 2.30**	43.05 ± 2.38
Leukemia ($q = 1$)	**94.36 ± 0.43**	90.73 ± 1.94
Leukemia ($q = 2$)	**94.38 ± 0.79**	69.45 ± 4.81
Leukemia ($q = 3$)	**95.20 ± 0.49**	69.97 ± 6.58
Leukemia ($q = 4$)	**94.73 ± 0.45**	73.33 ± 5.99
Leukemia ($q = 5$)	**91.23 ± 0.44**	71.81 ± 9.62
Leukemia ($q = 6$)	**93.19 ± 0.66**	79.08 ± 6.96
Leukemia ($q = 7$)	**90.56 ± 1.25**	65.26 ± 6.90
Leukemia ($q = 8$)	**87.81 ± 0.98**	58.31 ± 2.87
Leukemia ($q = 9$)	**87.52 ± 1.20**	55.88 ± 3.82
NSCLC	**52.91 ± 4.45**	48.64 ± 5.30

superior for almost all the cases (except $q = 8$ where the two methods show comparable performance with each other). Apart from that, projection method is more stable than Cosine Kernel method because the standard deviation of AUC values for each data set is smaller in Projection method. In Liver Disorder Data set, the averaged AUC values of Cosine Kernel method is 65.63% with standard deviation 2.75%, and projection method is much better than Cosine Kernel method, achieving 73.71% AUC values in average. The superiority of projection method over Cosine Kernel method is clearly demonstrated in Sonar Data as well. The averaged AUC value for Cosine Kernel method is 67.46% but 89.57% for projection method. For Cystic Fibrosis Data and Leukemia Data, projection method shows a general decrement in performance with the increment of q. However, in Cosine Kernel method there is no obvious correlation between the performance and the value of q within the data sets. In NSCLC Data set, both projection method and Cosine Kernel method show unsatisfying performance though projection method is clearly better than the original Cosine Kernel method.

2.4 Discussions on the Optimality of λ

Experimental results show that projection method is better or comparable with the compared kernel methods: GHI kernel and Cosine kernel. Despite the fact that GHI kernel and Cosine kernel can sometimes yield good performance when the kernel is indefinite, projection method still demonstrates comparable performance. The necessity of projection as a transformation for the considered indefinite kernels is clearly demonstrated. Projection method (when $\lambda \geq 1$) can transform an indefinite kernel into a PSD one. The optimal λ determination in projection method focusing on four different divergences is also considered. We focus on the optimality of the λ given by Eq. (2.11) for the LogDet Divergence as it is more realistic.

In the following, we will conduct experiments on the considered data sets, to confirm if the suggested optimal λ of projection method can show optimal performance in various values of $\lambda > 0$.

2.4.1 Optimal λ in the Projection Method

2.4.1.1 Optimal λ in the Projection Method for Sonar Data

We set parameters $\alpha \neq \beta \in \{1, 2, 3\}$ for GHI kernel and consider $\lambda \in [0.1, 200]$ with step size 0.1. Figure 2.2 plots the performance of projection method with different $\lambda \in [0.1, 200]$. The '$\star$' shape in black marks the performance of the projection method with the suggested optimal λ obtained under LogDet Divergence. The red line represents projected GHI kernel with $(\alpha, \beta) = (1, 2)$. The green line represents projected GHI kernel with $(\alpha, \beta) = (1, 3)$. The blue line represents projected GHI kernel with $(\alpha, \beta) = (2, 3)$. The cyan line plots the performance of projected Cosine Kernel.

The suggested optimal λ is 2.0 in Projected GHI kernel for all pairs of (α, β), $\alpha \neq \beta$, and it is marked by '$\star$' in Fig. 2.2. The performance of projection method shows a steady decrement when $\lambda > 2$, implying that $\lambda = 2$ is a good choice for projection method. When λ is small, the performance of projection method is quite unstable because the PSD property cannot be guaranteed.

It is very interesting to see that the suggested optimal λ is uniformly the same in the two considered kernels. Take projected GHI kernel with different (α, β) for comparison, we can see that projected method with $\alpha = 1, \beta = 3$ shows best performance with suggest optimal λ is 0.8733 while the experimental best performance is shown to be 0.8735 achieving at $\lambda = 1.9$. When $(\alpha, \beta) = (1, 2)$, the projection method with suggested optimal λ achieves 0.8246 in averaged AUC value, and the experimental best result is 0.8276. When $(\alpha, \beta) = (2, 3)$, the projection method with suggested optimal λ achieves 0.8540 in averaged AUC value, and the experimental best result is 0.8557. Considering the projected Cosine Kernel, the experimental best AUC value for Projected Cosine Kernel 0.9126 is achieved at $\lambda = 3.8$, while our suggested optimal $\lambda = 2$ yielding AUC value 0.9051, the difference between the two

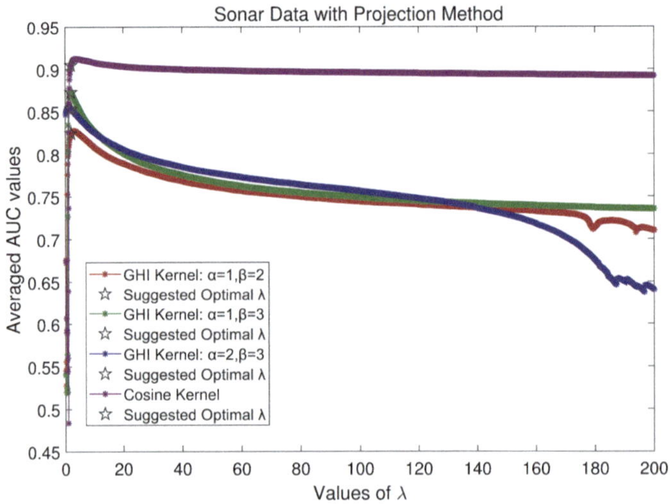

Fig. 2.2 Averaged AUC values for different values of λ in projection method with two considered kernels using sonar data set

values is little: 0.0075. We can conclude that the suggested optimal λ can guarantee at least an near optimal performance.

2.4.1.2 Optimal λ in the Projection Method for Liver Disorder Data

Figure 2.3 shows the performance of Projection Method in different kernels for Liver Disorder Data. The experimental optimal λ for GHI kernel with $(\alpha, \beta) = (1, 2)$ is 1.8, achieving averaged AUC value 0.7570. Our suggested λ under LogDet Divergence is 2.38, achieving averaged AUC value 0.7566. The performance difference in projection method with theoretical optimal $\lambda = 2.38$ and experimental optimal $\lambda = 1.8$ is very small: 0.0004. When $(\alpha, \beta) = (1, 3)$, the experimental optimal λ for GHI kernel is 1.6, with the average AUC value equaling 0.7381. Our suggested optimal λ is 2.37, with averaged AUC value 0.7333. The performance difference of the projection method with suggested optimal $\lambda = 2.37$ and experimental optimal $\lambda = 1.6$ is also very small: 0.0048. The experimental best AUC value 0.7417 in Cosine kernel is achieved at $\lambda = 0.4$, while our suggested optimal $\lambda = 2.17$ yielding an AUC value 0.7292. It can be seen that when $\lambda > 120$, the performance of projected method with the two considered kernels fluctuates. When $\lambda < 120$, the performance of projected method increases firstly and then decreases. The suggested optimal λ can guarantee at least an near optimal performance.

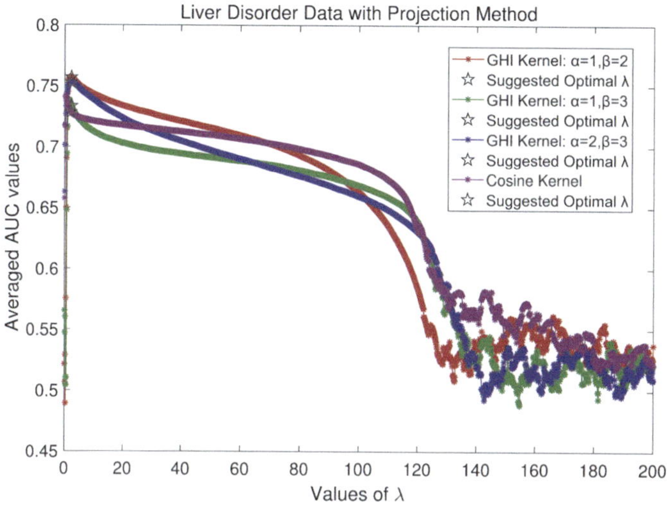

Fig. 2.3 Averaged AUC values for different values of λ in projection method with two considered kernels using liver disorder data set

2.4.1.3 Optimal λ in Projection Method for Breast Cancer Data

Figure 2.4 records the performance of projection method for Breast Cancer Data. The experimental optimal λ is 1.1 for GHI kernel with $(\alpha, \beta) = (1, 2)$, achieving averaged AUC value 0.9713. Our suggested optimal λ is 4.5957, with the averaged AUC value 0.9693. The performance becomes slightly worse with increment of λ. The performance difference of projection method with suggested optimal $\lambda = 4.5957$ and experimental optimal $\lambda = 1.1$ is subtle: 0.0018. Similar results are shown for GHI kernel with other (α, β) pairs. The experimental best AUC value 0.9941 is achieved at $\lambda = 0.8$ for Cosine Kernel, while our suggested optimal $\lambda = 4.29$ yielding AUC value 0.9939. Comparing projected GHI kernel and Cosine Kernel, we can see that projected cosine kernel shows visible better performance than projected GHI kernel, suggesting that we should choose projected Cosine kernel for breast cancer prediction. When all the kernels are considered, the suggested optimal λ is preferable in obtaining optimal performance for different values of λ.

2.4.1.4 Optimal λ in Projection Method for Cystic Fibrosis Data

Figures 2.5, 2.6, 2.7 and 2.8 record the performance of Projection method with the 2 considered kernels. We can see that in almost all cases, projection method shows identical performance for $\lambda \in (0, 200]$ except for $q = 1$ when $(\alpha, \beta) = (1, 2)$ and $(\alpha, \beta) = (1, 3)$. One possible explanation might be that GHI kernel is PSD already before projection. When $q = 1$ and $(\alpha, \beta) = (1, 2)$, the best AUC value when $\lambda \in$

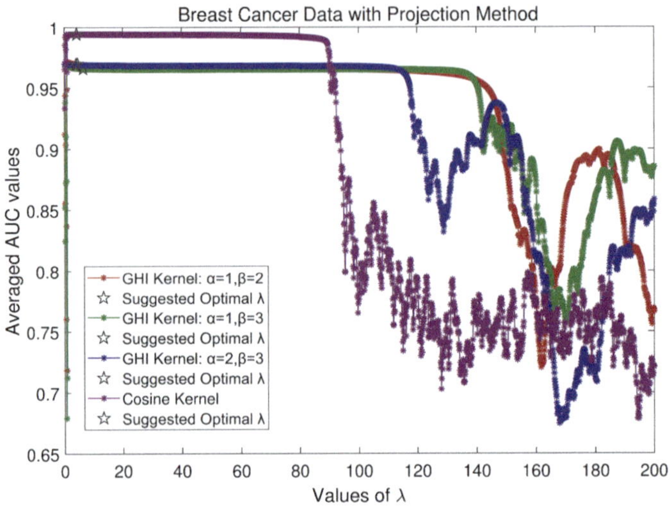

Fig. 2.4 Averaged AUC values for different values of λ in projection method with two considered kernels using breast cancer data set

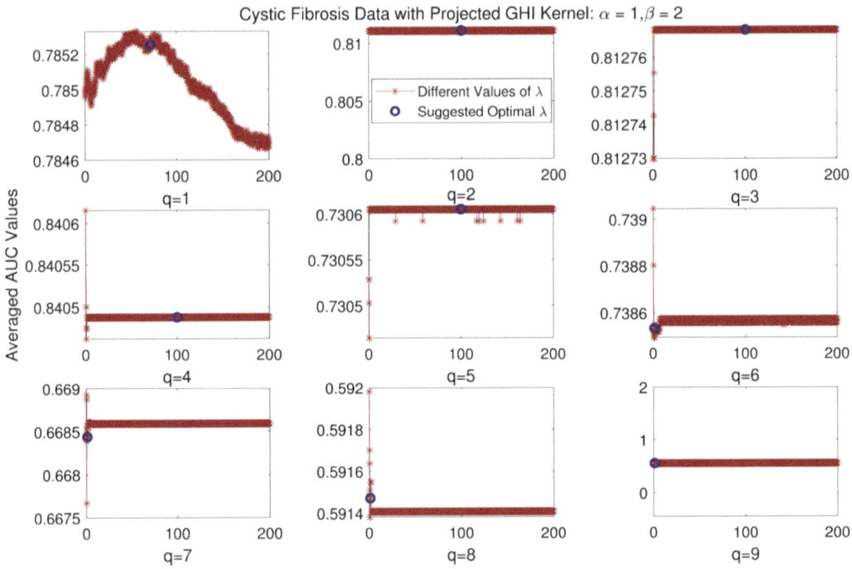

Fig. 2.5 Averaged AUC values for different values of λ in projection method with two considered kernels using cystic fibrosis data set: GHI kernel with $\alpha = 1$ and $\beta = 2$

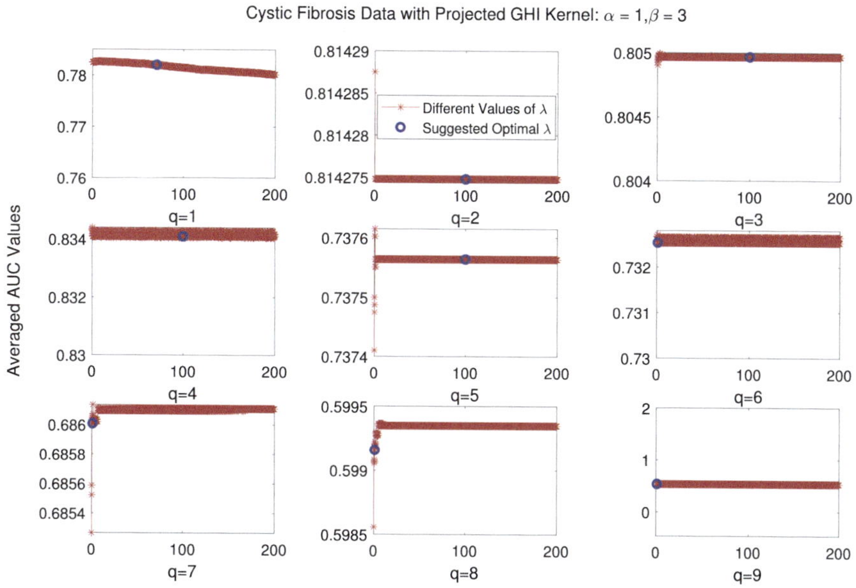

Fig. 2.6 Averaged AUC values for different values of λ in projection method with two considered kernels using cystic fibrosis data set: GHI kernel with $\alpha = 1$ and $\beta = 3$

(0, 200] is 0.7908, and the smallest AUC value is 0.7890, while theoretical optimal λ yields 0.7905 in AUC value which is near optimal. When $(\alpha, \beta) = (1, 3)$, the smallest AUC value is 0.7831 as λ approach 200, the best AUC value is 0.7841 when $\lambda = 22.5$, and the suggested optimal λ through LogDet Divergence yields 0.7840, which is also near optimal.

Considering Cosine kernel, the performance of projection method firstly improves and then descends gradually for $q = 1, 2$ and 3. For example, the best performance in experiment for $q = 1$ is achieved at $\lambda = 77$, with the AUC value 0.7987, while our suggested optimal $\lambda = 5.8$ obtains 0.7955 in AUC value, which is near optimal.

When q increases, the performance of projection method improves firstly and stays relatively stable afterwards. For example, when $q = 4$, with the suggested optimal $\lambda = 3.67$ one can obtain 0.7846 in AUC value and the experimental best performance 0.8012 is obtained when $\lambda = 26.7$. It can be seen that denoising method when $\lambda = 1$ achieves 0.6574 and flipping method when $\lambda = 2$ achieves 0.7441, implying that projection method with suggested λ is better than these two methods. Although it is not optimal, the performance of projection method is satisfactory, which is slightly inferior to the experimental optimal.

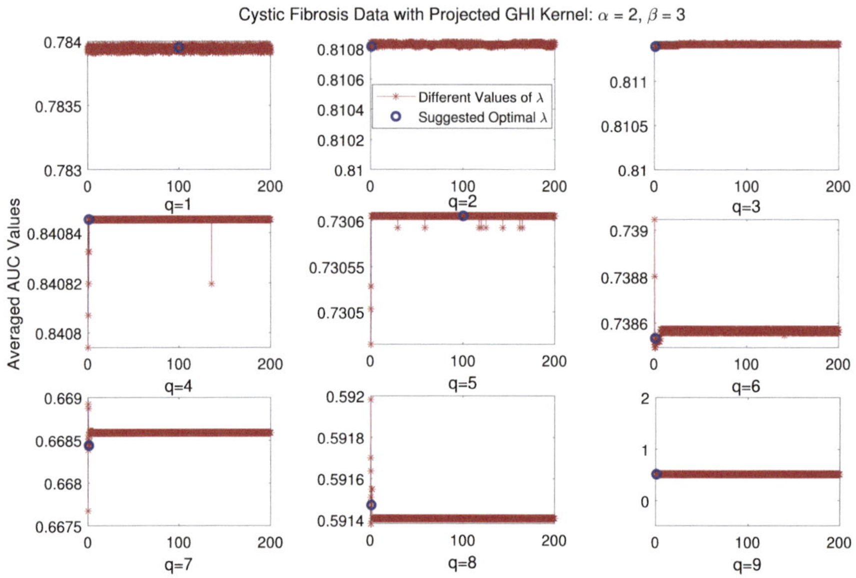

Fig. 2.7 Averaged AUC values for different values of λ in projection method with two considered kernels using cystic fibrosis data set: GHI kernel with $\alpha = 2$ and $\beta = 3$

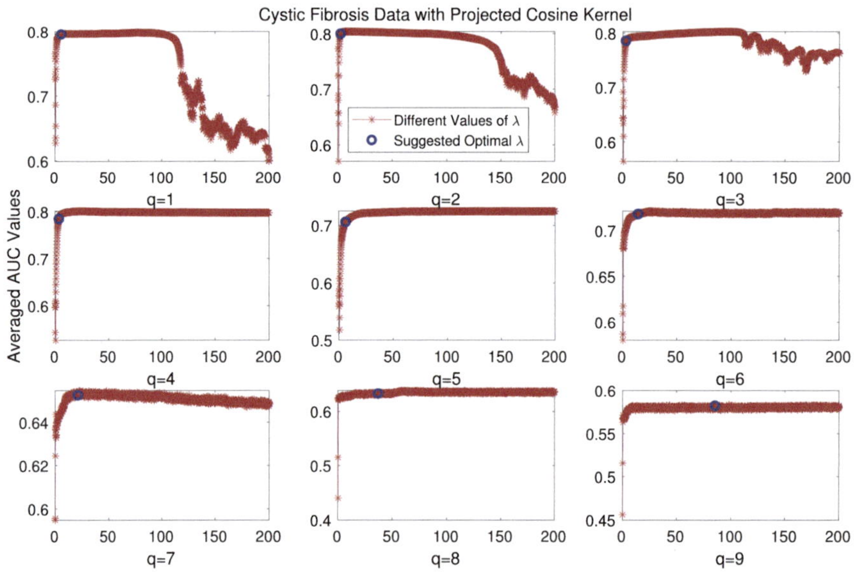

Fig. 2.8 Averaged AUC values for different values of λ in projection method with two considered kernels using cystic fibrosis data set: cosine kernel

2.4.1.5 Optimal λ in Projection Method for Leukemia Data

Experimental Results for projection method with GHI kernel and Cosine kernel in leukemia data for $q \in \{1, 2, \ldots, 9\}$ are demonstrated in Figs. 2.9, 2.10, 2.11 and 2.12. Similar to Cystic Fibrosis Data, projection method in GHI kernel shows almost identical performance for $\lambda \in (0, 200]$ for $q \in \{4, 5, 6, 7, 8, 9\}$. This is consistent with the results in Table 2.2 where original GHI kernel is positive semi-definite when $q \geq 4$, as the minimal eigenvalues of the kernel matrix is 0. When $q = 1$, the experimental best AUC value is 0.9364 for $(\alpha, \beta) = (1, 2)$, and our suggested optimal λ yields 0.9342. When $q = 2$, the experimental best AUC value is 0.9545 for $(\alpha, \beta) = (1, 2)$, and our suggested optimal λ yields 0.9542. When $q = 3$, the experimental best AUC value is 0.9539 for $(\alpha, \beta) = (1, 2)$, and our suggested optimal λ yields 0.9539. Experimental results are similar for other pairs of (α, β). Results for projected GHI kernel show that our suggested optimal λ can induce a near optimal projection method. In the case of Cosine kernel, we can obtain some information from Fig. 2.12. For all the considered q, there is no overall tendency when $\lambda \leq 2$, but the averaged AUC values will slowly increase in a steady manner when the optimal performance is achieved. Some interesting phenomenon can be detected where projection method always shows poor performance when $\lambda = 1$ (Denoising Method). For example, when $q = 2$ the averaged AUC value of projection method is 0.6134 for $\lambda = 1$, but 0.7450 for $\lambda = 0.9$ and 0.9318 for $\lambda = 1.1$. When $q = 3$ the averaged AUC value of projection method is 0.4221 for $\lambda = 1$, but 0.7784 for

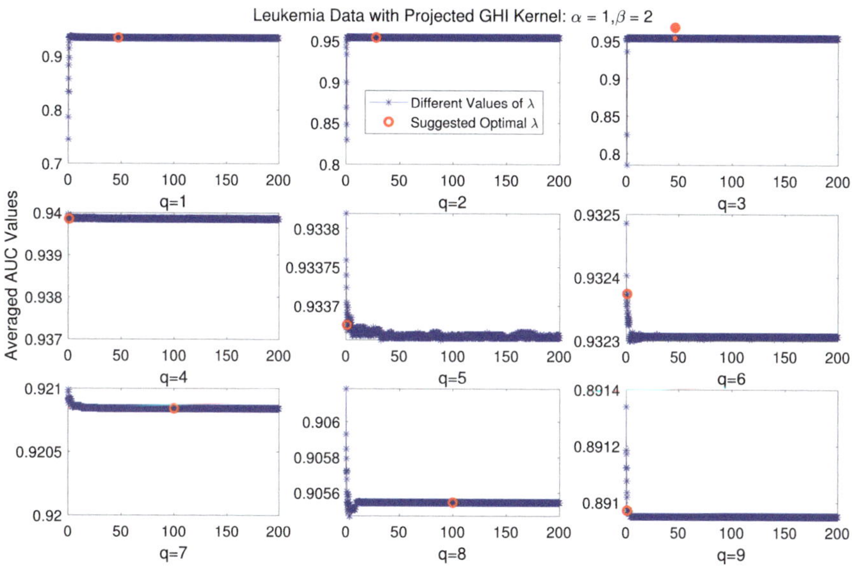

Fig. 2.9 Averaged AUC values for different values of λ in projection method with two considered kernels using leukemia data set: GHI kernel with $\alpha = 1$ and $\beta = 2$

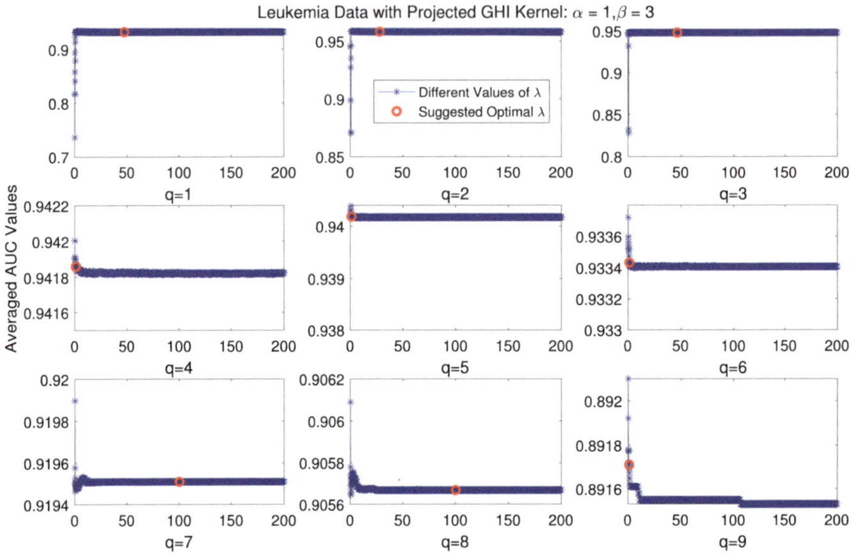

Fig. 2.10 Averaged AUC values for different values of λ in projection method with two considered kernels using leukemia data set: GHI kernel with $\alpha = 1$ and $\beta = 3$

$\lambda = 0.9$ and 0.9151 for $\lambda = 1.1$. This probably can be explained that denoising strategy neglects some hidden information embedded in the negative eigenvalues and eigenvectors which is critical for describing the Leukemia Data. Regarding to the suggested optimal λ in projected Cosine Kernel, we can see that projection method with the suggested optimal λ can always obtain at least near optimal performance for all $q \in \{1, 2, \ldots, 9\}$.

2.4.1.6 Optimal λ in Projection Method with NSCLC Data

The performance of Projection Method with GHI kernel and Cosine Kernel in NSCLC Data is shown in Fig. 2.13. When $(\alpha, \beta) = (1, 2)$, the optimal averaged AUC value in experiment is 0.9979 and projection method with our suggested optimal $\lambda = 2$ can produce the same value. When $(\alpha, \beta) = (1, 3)$, the experimental optimal averaged AUC value 0.6145 and projection method with $\lambda = 2$ can also ensure best performance 0.6145. When $(\alpha, \beta) = (2, 3)$, the optimal averaged AUC value 1 in experiment and projection method with our suggested optimal $\lambda = 2$ can also ensure equivalent best performance. Another conclusion can be made is that projection method with GHI kernel in different pairs of (α, β) may perform significantly different. In this experiment, we can see that $(\alpha, \beta) = (1, 3)$ is not fit for the task. Taking into consideration of the projected Cosine Kernel method, we can also conclude that cosine kernel is not suitable for dealing with tumor differentiation in NSCLC data.

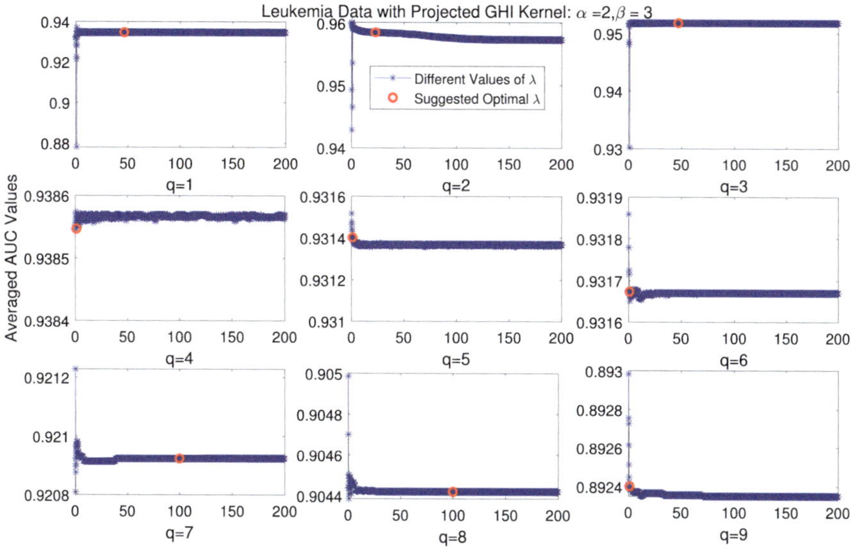

Fig. 2.11 Averaged AUC values for different values of λ in projection method with two considered kernels using leukemia data set: GHI kernel with $\alpha = 2$ and $\beta = 3$

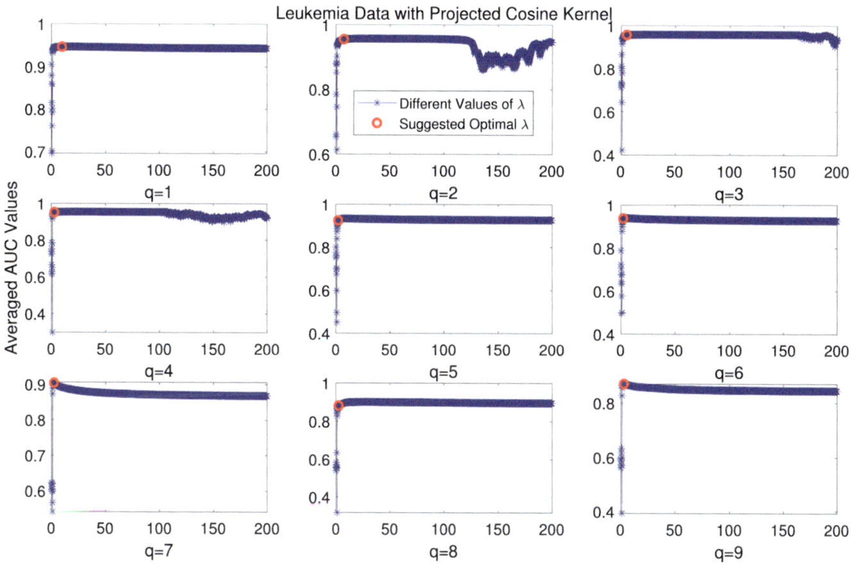

Fig. 2.12 Averaged AUC values for different values of λ in projection method with two considered kernels using leukemia data set: cosine kernel

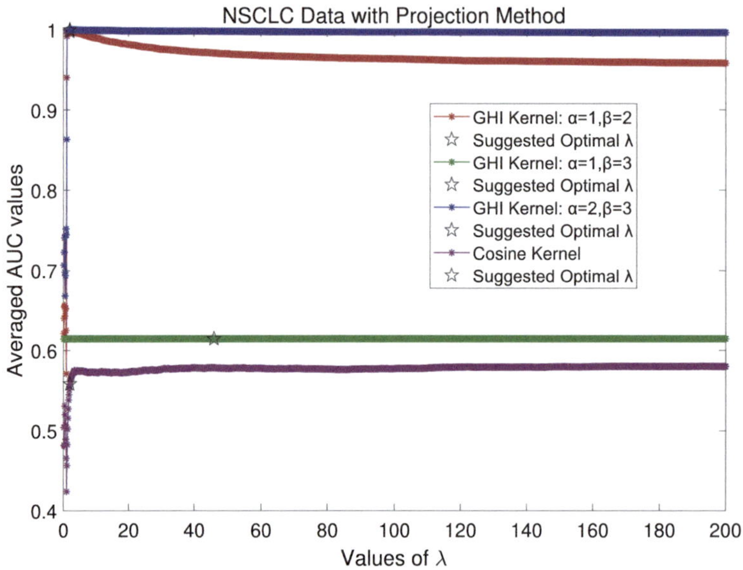

Fig. 2.13 Averaged AUC values for different values of λ in projection method with two considered kernels using NSCLC data set

2.4.1.7 Theoretical Optimal λ Under LogDet Divergence

Table 2.7 lists the optimal λ under LogDet Divergence with considered kernels for all the considered data sets. The first 3 columns refer to suggested optimal λ in Projected GHI kernel method. It is interesting to see that for cystic fibrosis data set, the suggested optimal λ is either 1 or 100 in most cases (except for $q = 1$ when $(\alpha, \beta) = (1, 2)$ and $(\alpha, \beta) = (1, 3)$). The situation is similar for leukemia data set, where the suggested optimal λ in most cases is either 1 or 100 ($q \geq 4$). Note that our suggested optimal λ has the formula $1 + \frac{m}{\sum_{i=1}^{m} d_i \operatorname{tr}(K^{+}\mathbf{p}_i\mathbf{p}_i')}$ (Please refer to Eq. (2.12)). Computational error may occur when calculating the optimal λ as $\lambda \to \pm\infty$ which is not realistic. We therefore make the amendments accordingly where optimal λ is defined to be 1 when approaching $-\infty$ and 100 when approaching $+\infty$. The last column lists the theoretical optimal λ for the considered data sets with Cosine kernel. Computational error does not have influence on projection method with Cosine Kernel in cystic fibrosis data as $\frac{m}{\sum_{i=1}^{m} d_i \operatorname{tr}(K^{-1}\mathbf{p}_i\mathbf{p}_i')}$ is not close to 0. We can draw some conclusions from the table. Firstly, when kernels are different, the suggested optimal λ in most of the cases are different within the same data set. Secondly, when data sets are different, the suggested optimal λ in most of the cases are different even under the same kernel type. Focusing on the GHI kernel, we can see that the suggested optimal λ for different (α, β) differ from each other in most of the cases. Comparing GHI kernel and Cosine kernel, we can see that even for the

Table 2.7 Optimal λ suggested in projection method with considered kernels

Dataset methods	GHI kernel			Cosine Kernel
	$\alpha = 1, \beta = 2$	$\alpha = 1, \beta = 3$	$\alpha = 2, \beta = 3$	
Liver disorder data	2.38	2.37	2.45	2.17
Sonar data	2	2	2	2
Breast data	4.6	6.57	4.06	4.29
Cystic ($q = 1$)	71	71	100	5.8
Cystic ($q = 2$)	100	100	1	2.5
Cystic ($q = 3$)	100	100	1	2.8
Cystic ($q = 4$)	100	100	1	3.67
Cystic ($q = 5$)	100	100	100	6.2
Cystic ($q = 6$)	1	1	1	14
Cystic ($q = 7$)	1	1	1	21
Cystic ($q = 8$)	1	1	1	37
Cystic ($q = 9$)	1	1	1	85
Leukemia ($q = 1$)	47.33	47.33	46.67	10
Leukemia ($q = 2$)	28.25	28.25	22.80	7.4
Leukemia ($q = 3$)	46.5	46.5	47	5.42
Leukemia ($q = 4$)	1	1	1	3.06
Leukemia ($q = 5$)	1	1	1	2.33
Leukemia ($q = 6$)	1	1	1	2.39
Leukemia ($q = 7$)	100	100	100	2.56
Leukemia ($q = 8$)	100	100	100	2.67
Leukemia ($q = 9$)	1	1	1	2.98
NSCLC	2.0	46	2	2

same data set, it may happen that one type of kernel is positive semi-definite while the other type is indefinite, this can also partly explain why the suggested optimal λ is different.

2.4.2 Improvement of the Optimal λ for Projection Method

As stated above, we can see that under LogDet divergence, we can determine a near optimal λ for projection method. In this subsection, we are considering if there is any way to improve the projection method, in terms of improving the optimal λ. Recall that Von Neumann divergence has the formula $D_\phi(K, K_0) = \mathrm{tr}(K \log K - K \log K_0 - K + K_0)$, we here make an adjustment to the formula $D_\phi(K, K_0) = \mathrm{tr}K\,\mathrm{tr}(\log K - \log K_0) + \mathrm{tr}(-K + K_0)$. Then we can determine optimal λ through minimizing the following function

$$
\begin{aligned}
V(\lambda) = &\left(\sum_{i=1}^{m}(1-\lambda)d_i + \sum_{i=m+1}^{n} d_i\right)\\
&\times\left(\sum_{i=1}^{m}(1-\lambda)d_i \mathrm{tr}\left(K_0^{-1}\mathbf{p}_i\mathbf{p}_i' + \sum_{i=m+1}^{n} d_i \mathrm{tr}(K_0^{-1}\mathbf{p}_i\mathbf{p}_i')\right)\right)\\
&+\sum_{i=1}^{m} d_i
\end{aligned}
$$

where $\{\mathbf{p}_1, \ldots, \mathbf{p}_n\}$ is an orthonormal eigenbasis of K and m is the negative inertial index of K. We can easily obtain

$$
V'(\lambda) = -2(1-\lambda)\sum_{i=1}^{m} d_i \sum_{i=1}^{m} \mathrm{tr}(K_0^{-1}\mathbf{p}_i\mathbf{p}_i') - 2\sum_{i=1}^{m} d_i \cdot \sum_{i=m+1}^{n} d_i \mathrm{tr}(K_0^{-1}\mathbf{p}_i\mathbf{p}_i') + \sum_{i=1}^{m} d_i.
$$

Therefore, the new optimal λ_{opt1} is of the following formula:

$$
\lambda_{\mathrm{opt1}} = \frac{\sum_{i=1}^{n} d_i \mathrm{tr}(K_0^{-1}\mathbf{p}_i\mathbf{p}_i') - 0.5}{\sum_{i=1}^{m} d_i \mathrm{tr}(K_0^{-1}\mathbf{p}_i\mathbf{p}_i')}.
$$

We next conducted experiments on all the considered data sets to compare the performance of the optimal λ from LogDet divergence λ_{opt} and the newly proposed λ_{opt1} in conjunction with projection method.

- Comparison with Projection Method in Sonar Data, Liver Disorder Data, Breast Cancer Data and NSCLC Data
  As shown in the table (Table 2.8), we can see that the newly determined optimal λ through perturbed Von Neumann Divergence shows similar performance with the optimal λ generated by LogDet divergence. The only clear difference can be detected for Sonar data in GHI kernel when $(\alpha, \beta) = (2, 3)$ and Cosine Kernel. For GHI kernel with $(\alpha, \beta) = (2, 3)$ we can see that λ_{opt} is superior to λ_{opt1} in the sense of greater AUC value, while for Cosine kernel, λ_{opt1} is superior to λ_{opt}. Regarding the determined optimal λ under different divergences, we can see that λ_{opt} differs from λ_{opt1}. For GHI kernel case, the determined optimal λ under LogDet

Table 2.8 Optimal λ comparison in projection method with considered kernels in sonar data, liver disorder data, breast cancer data and NSCLC data

		$\alpha = 1, \beta = 2$	$\alpha = 1, \beta = 3$	$\alpha = 2, \beta = 3$	Cosine
Sonar	(λ_{opt},AUC$_{opt}$)	(2.00, 0.8266)	(2.00, 0.8787)	**(2.00, 0.8585)**	(2.00, 0.9034)
	(λ_{opt1},AUC$_{opt1}$)	(2.59, 0.8284)	(2.16, 0.8784)	(4.32, 0.8486)	**(8.30, 0.9118)**
Live	(λ_{opt},AUC$_{opt}$)	(2.38, 0.7559)	(2.37, 0.7397)	(2.45, 0.7543)	(2.17, 0.7292)
	(λ_{opt1},AUC$_{opt1}$)	(2.08, 0.7571)	(2.04, 0.7415)	(2.09, 0.7542)	(6.70, 0.7249)
Breast	(λ_{opt},AUC$_{opt}$)	(4.60, 0.9689)	(6.57, 0.9659)	(4.06, 0.9684)	(4.29, 0.9937)
	(λ_{opt1},AUC$_{opt1}$)	(2.03, 0.9702)	(2.02, 0.9675)	(2.20, 0.9686)	(13.04, 0.9936)
NSCLC	(λ_{opt},AUC$_{opt}$)	(2.00, 0.9996)	(2.00, 0.9959)	(2.00, 0.9903)	(2.00, 0.4059)
	(λ_{opt1},AUC$_{opt1}$)	(4.96, 0.9990)	(3.58, 0.9978)	(2.69, 0.9910)	(2.30, 0.4010)

Divergence and perturbed von-Neumann Divergence is similar to each other in Live data set but quite different in other data sets. For cosine kernel case, λ_{opt} and λ_{opt1} are quite different from each other. We can see that though the determined optimal λ under LogDet Divergence and perturbed von-Neumann Divergence is different, the performance is comparable. Therefore, by comparing both kernels, we can see that Cosine kernel with λ_{opt1} is a preferred option.

- Comparison with Projection Method in Cystic Fibrosis Data
  From Table 2.9, we can obtain some conclusions. For GHI kernel, it is obvious that projection method shows almost identical performance with λ_{opt} and λ_{opt1}. It is interesting to see that in GHI kernel case, λ_{opt} and λ_{opt1} are equal to each other expect when $q = 1$ for $(\alpha, \beta) = (1, 2)$ and $(\alpha, \beta) = (1, 3)$. From Table 2.2, we know that GHI kernel in these 2 cases is indefinite. Although the values of λ_{opt} and λ_{opt1} are quite different from each other when $q = 1$ for $(\alpha, \beta) = (1, 2)$ and $(\alpha, \beta) = (1, 3)$, the performances are similar to each other. When it comes to Cosine kernel, we can see that projection method with λ_{opt1} tends to perform better for $q \in \{1, 2, 3, 4, 5, 6, 9\}$. Clear differences can be detected when $q = 3, 4, 5$ that are marked in bold face. Besides, λ_{opt1} in Cosine kernel is larger than λ_{opt} for most cases ($q \in \{1, 2, \ldots, 7\}$), meaning that projection method with Cosine kernel tends to show better performance for relatively large λ. When we compare GHI kernel and Cosine kernel, we find that GHI kernel in general tends to show better performance for small q, and Cosine kernel shows better performance when q is large.
- Comparison with Projection Method in Leukemia Data
  We can obtain similar conclusions for Leukemia data. As shown in the table (Table 2.10), projection method shows almost identical performance with λ_{opt} and λ_{opt1} though different optimal λ values are obtained (Please check $q = 1, 2, 3$ respectively). When $q = 1$, λ_{opt1} is smaller than λ_{opt}. When $q = 2, 3$ respectively, λ_{opt1} is larger than λ_{opt}. Though values of optimal λ differ from each other, the performances are quite similar, meaning that projection method with GHI kernel for Leukemia data is less sensitive in the optimal λ. When $q \in \{4, 5, 6, 7, 8, 9\}$, λ_{opt} and λ_{opt1} are identical, we can see from Table 2.2 that GHI kernel in these cases

Table 2.9 Optimal λ comparison in projection method with considered kernels in cystic fibrosis data

		$\alpha = 1, \beta = 2$	$\alpha = 1, \beta = 3$	$\alpha = 2, \beta = 3$	Cosine
$q = 1$	(λ_{opt},AUC$_{opt}$)	$(71, 0.7771)$	$(71, 0.7711)$	$(100, 0.7829)$	(5.8, 0.7889)
	(λ_{opt1},AUC$_{opt1}$)	(36.5, 0.7775)	(36.5, 0.7713)	$(100, 0.7829)$	(28.3, 0.7912)
$q = 2$	(λ_{opt},AUC$_{opt}$)	$(100, 0.8031)$	$(100, 0.8114)$	$(1, 0.8209)$	(2.5, 0.7951)
	(λ_{opt1},AUC$_{opt1}$)	$(100, 0.8031)$	$(100, 0.8114)$	$(1, 0.8209)$	(43.38, 0.7959)
$q = 3$	(λ_{opt},AUC$_{opt}$)	$(100, 0.8103)$	$(100, 0.8140))$	$(1, 0.8033)$	(2.8, 0.7978)
	(λ_{opt1},AUC$_{opt1}$)	$(100, 0.8103)$	$(100, 0.8140)$	$(1, 0.8033)$	(**34.3**, **0.8111**)
$q = 4$	(λ_{opt},AUC$_{opt}$)	$(100, 0.8296)$	$(100, 0.8356)$	$(1, 0.8286)$	(3.67, 0.7825)
	(λ_{opt1},AUC$_{opt1}$)	$(100, 0.8296)$	$(100, 0.8356)$	$(1, 0.8286)$	(**26.58**, **0.7979**)
$q = 5$	(λ_{opt},AUC$_{opt}$)	$(100, 0.7400)$	$(100, 0.7272)$	$(100, 0.7405)$	(6.2, 0.6973)
	(λ_{opt1},AUC$_{opt1}$)	$(100, 0.7400)$	$(100, 0.7272)$	$(100, 0.7405)$	(**27**, **0.7137**)
$q = 6$	(λ_{opt},AUC$_{opt}$)	$(1, 0.7173)$	$(1, 0.7164)$	$(1, 0.7224)$	(14, 0.7144)
	(λ_{opt1},AUC$_{opt1}$)	$(1, 0.7173)$	$(1, 0.7164)$	$(1, 0.7224)$	(34.16, 0.7156)
$q = 7$	(λ_{opt},AUC$_{opt}$)	$(1, 0.6702)$	$(1, 0.6721)$	$(1, 0.6713)$	(21, 0.6620)
	(λ_{opt1},AUC$_{opt1}$)	$(1, 0.6702)$	$(1, 0.6721)$	$(1, 0.6713)$	(22.17, 0.6616)
$q = 8$	(λ_{opt},AUC$_{opt}$)	$(1, 0.5928)$	$(1, 0.5791)$	$(1, 0.5935)$	(37, 0.6388)
	(λ_{opt1},AUC$_{opt1}$)	$(1, 0.5928)$	$(1, 0.5791)$	$(1, 0.5935)$	(19.25, 0.6387)
$q = 9$	(λ_{opt},AUC$_{opt}$)	$(1, 0.5146)$	$(1, 0.5107)$	$(1, 0.5254)$	(85, 0.5637)
	(λ_{opt1},AUC$_{opt1}$)	$(1, 0.5146)$	$(1, 0.5107)$	$(1, 0.5254)$	(17.5, 0.5688)

are PSD already. For Cosine Kernel, optimal λ determined by LogDet Divergence and perturbed Von-Neumann Divergence differs. Projection method with λ_{opt1} performs slightly better than projection method with λ_{opt}. Besides, λ_{opt1} in Cosine kernel is larger than λ_{opt}, implying that projection method tends to show better performance for large λ. When we focus on the performance of projection method with λ_{opt1}, we can find that different from Cystic Fibrosis data set, the performance of projected cosine kernel with λ_{opt1} tends to show better performance for small q while projected GHI kernel with λ_{opt} tends to show better performance for large q.

In summary, when $\lambda \in (0, 1)$, the positive semi-definiteness of the projected kernel matrix cannot be assured, and the performance tends to be extremely unstable. The suggested optimal λ in Projection method is related to the eigenvalues in original kernel matrix, and thus varies in different data sets. Besides, the suggested optimal λ under LogDet Divergence and perturbed Von-Neumann Divergence differs from each other in the same data sets in most cases. Even in that case, projection method under the two different cases can still guarantee near optimal performance. It can be seen that when optimal λ under LogDet Divergence and optimal λ under perturbed Von-Neumann Divergence is very different, the performance of projection method in both cases is still similar, showing that in this case projection method is relatively insensitive to the values of suggested optimal λ (projection method with a large

Table 2.10 Optimal λ comparison in projection method with considered kernels in leukemia data

		$\alpha = 1, \beta = 2$	$\alpha = 1, \beta = 3$	$\alpha = 2, \beta = 3$	Cosine
$q = 1$	$(\lambda_{\text{opt}}, \text{AUC}_{\text{opt}})$	(47.3, 0.9418)	(47.3, 0.9377)	(46.7, 0.9365)	(10, 0.9469)
	$(\lambda_{\text{opt1}}, \text{AUC}_{\text{opt1}})$	(26.8, 0.9419)	(26.8, 0.9377)	(27.8, 0.9367)	(16.6, 0.9472)
$q = 2$	$(\lambda_{\text{opt}}, \text{AUC}_{\text{opt}})$	(28.3, 0.9551)	((28.3, 0.9551)	(22.8, 0.9582)	(7.4, 0.9541)
	$(\lambda_{\text{opt1}}, \text{AUC}_{\text{opt1}})$	(35.9, 0.9550)	(35.9, 0.9551)	(29.3, 0.9582)	(24.7, 0.9555)
$q = 3$	$(\lambda_{\text{opt}}, \text{AUC}_{\text{opt}})$	(46.5, 0.9512)	(46.5, 0.9540)	(47, 0.9500)	(5.42, 0.9573)
	$(\lambda_{\text{opt1}}, \text{AUC}_{\text{opt1}})$	(87.8, 0.9512)	(87.8, 0.9551)	(88.8, 0.9500)	(23.1, 0.9593)
$q = 4$	$(\lambda_{\text{opt}}, \text{AUC}_{\text{opt}})$	(1, 0.9427)	(1, 0.9416)	(1, 0.9405)	(3.06, 0.9485)
	$(\lambda_{\text{opt1}}, \text{AUC}_{\text{opt1}})$	(1, 0.9427)	(1, 0.9416)	(1, 0.9405)	(18.6, 0.9522)
$q = 5$	$(\lambda_{\text{opt}}, \text{AUC}_{\text{opt}})$	(1, 0.9352)	(1, 0.9362)	(1, 0.9363)	(2.33, 0.9175)
	$(\lambda_{\text{opt1}}, \text{AUC}_{\text{opt1}})$	(1, 0.9352)	(1, 0.9362)	(1, 0.9363)	**(11.08, 0.9259)**
$q = 6$	$(\lambda_{\text{opt}}, \text{AUC}_{\text{opt}})$	(1, 0.9310)	(1, 0.9319)	(1, 0.9311)	(2.39, 0.9333)
	$(\lambda_{\text{opt1}}, \text{AUC}_{\text{opt1}})$	(1, 0.9310)	(1, 0.9319)	(1, 0.9311)	(7.74, 0.9337)
$q = 7$	$(\lambda_{\text{opt}}, \text{AUC}_{\text{opt}})$	(100, 0.9201)	(100, 0.9236)	(1, 0.9212)	(2.56, 0.8993)
	$(\lambda_{\text{opt1}}, \text{AUC}_{\text{opt1}})$	(100, 0.9201)	(100, 0.9236)	(1, 0.9212)	(5.03, 0.8921)
$q = 8$	$(\lambda_{\text{opt}}, \text{AUC}_{\text{opt}})$	(100, 0.9035)	(100, 0.9096)	(100, 0.9059)	(2.67, 0.8795)
	$(\lambda_{\text{opt1}}, \text{AUC}_{\text{opt1}})$	(100, 0.9035)	(100, 0.9096)	(100, 0.9059)	(3.56, 0.8845)
$q = 9$	$(\lambda_{\text{opt}}, \text{AUC}_{\text{opt}})$	(1, 0.8936)	(1, 0.8915)	(1, 0.8899)	(2.98, 0.8734)
	$(\lambda_{\text{opt1}}, \text{AUC}_{\text{opt1}})$	(1,0.8936)	(1, 0.8915)	(1, 0.8899)	(3.72, 0.8735)

range of λ values can suggest near optimal performance). Our suggested theoretical λ under LogDet Divergence and perturbed Von-Neumann Divergence sometimes cannot guarantee the best performance. There are two possible reasons. One possible reason is that the optimal λ determination by unconstrained optimization in framework of kernel learning hypothesized the positive definiteness of the kernels, but we use indefinite kernels in this case. Another possible reason is that the inverse of kernel was substituted by pseudo inverse.

2.5 Conclusions

In this chapter, we propose projection method for addressing indefinite kernel learning problems. The projection method is constructed from an eigen-space perspective. It is very flexible by varying the parameter λ, to change from the denoising method to the flipping method. These two spectrum based methods are well-known techniques in dealing with indefinite kernels. Two kernels that are not generally PSD are introduced for comparison: GHI kernel method and the Cosine kernel method. We show better performance for projection method in terms of AUC values under fivefold cross-validations. The optimal λ embedded in projection method can be determined by solving an unconstrained optimization problem. Experimental studies show consistence with theoretical analysis as projection method with our suggested λ can always guarantee at least near optimal performance for $\lambda > 0$. In the pursuit of precise optimal λ determination method, we also compared optimal λ determination with LogDet Divergence and perturbed von-Neumann Divergence, aiming at finding better λ in the projection method. The determined optimal λ differs from each other for different kernels and data sets involved, and the results obtained are in general similar. Our proposed projection method may be regarded as a good choice for dealing with indefinite kernels. Future work may contribute to the development of more precise optimal λ determination method and the development of more variants of projection method for indefinite kernels, hoping to be applied in other areas.

References

Altschul S et al (1990) A basic local alignment search tool. J Mol Biol 215:403–410

Boughorbel S, Tarel J, Bougemaa N (2005) Generalized histogram intersection kernel for image recognition. In: Proceeding of the IEEE the 2005 international conference on image processing. Genoa, pp III–161–164

Brian K, Sustik MA, Dhillon I (2006) Learning low-rank kernel matrices. In: Proceedings of the 23rd international conference on machine learning. Pittsburgh, pp 505–512

Carrizosa E, Morales DR (2013) Supervised classification and mathematical optimization. Comput Oper Res 40:150–165

Conforti D, Guido R (2010) Kernel based support vector machine via semidefinite programming: application to medical diagnosis. Comput Oper Res 37(8):1389–1394

Doubet S, Albersheim P (1992) Carbbank. Glycobiology 2(6):505–507

Graepel T, Herbrich R, Bollmann-Sdorra P, Obermayer K (1998) Classification on pairwise proximity data. Adv Neural Inf Process Syst 11:438–444

Gu S, Guo Y (2012) Learning SVM classifiers with indefinite kernels. In: Proceedings of the twenty-sixth conference on artificial intelligence. Toronto

Guo Y, Schuurmans D (2009) A reformulation of support vector machines for general confidence functions. In: Proceedings of Asian conference on machine learning: advances in machine learning. Nanjing, China, pp 109–119

Hashimoto K, Goto S, Kawano S, Aokikinoshita KF, Ueda N, Hamajima M, Kawasaki T, Kanehisa M (2006) KEGG as a glycome informatics resource. Glycobiology 16(5):63R-70R

Hassdonk B (2005) Feature space interpretation of SVMs with indefinite kernels. IEEE Trans Pattern Anal Mach Intell 27:298–482

Li F, Fu Y, Dai Y, Cristian S, Wang J (2009) Kernel learning by unconstrained optimization. In: In Proceedings of international conference on artificial intelligence and statistics, pp 328–335

Lin H, Lin C (2003) A study on sigmoid kernel for SVM and the training of non-PSD kernels by SMO-type methods. National Taiwan University, Taipei, Taiwan, Technical report

Liu X, Yuen P, Feng G, Chen W (2009) Learning kernel in kernel-based LDA for face recognition under illumination variations. IEEE Signal Process Lett 16:1019–1022

Luss R, D'Aspremont A (2009) Support vector machine classification with indefinite kernels. Math Program Comput 1(2):97–118

Mercer J (1909) Functions of positive and negative type and their connection with the theory of integral equations. Phil Trans R Soc A 209(441–458):415–446

Muñoz A, Diego IM (2006) From indefinite to positive semi-definite matrices. Springer, Berlin Heidelberg

NCBI(National Center of Biotechnology Information) GEO(Gene Expression Omnibus) Repository. https://www.ncbi.nlm.nih.gov/gds/. Accessed 2 Mar 2017

Nock R, Magdalou B, Briys E, Nielsen F (2013) Mining matrix data with Bregman matrix divergences for portfolio selection. Matrix Inf Geom 373–402
Ong C, Mary X, Canu S, Smola A (2004) Learning with non-positive kernels. In: International conference on machine learning. Banff, pp 639–646
Pan B, Lai J, Chen W (2011) Nonlinear nonnegative matrix factorization based on mercer kernel construction. Pattern Recogn 44:2800–2810
Pan B, Zhang G, Xia J, Yuan P, Ip H, He Q, Lee P, Chow B, Zhou X (2016) Prediction of soft tissue deformations after CMF surgery with incremental kernel ridge regression. Comput Biol Med 75:1–9
Pekalska E, Paclik P, DuinA R (2002) A generalized kernel approach to dissimilarity-based classification. J Mach Learn Res 2(2):175–211
Roth V, Laub J, Kawanabe M (2000) Optimal cluster preserving embedding of non-metric proximity data. IEEE Trans Pattern Anal Mach Intell 25:1540–1551
Saigo H, Vert J, Ueda N, Akutsu T (2004) Protein homology detection using string alignment kernels. Bioinformatics 11:1682–1689
Scholkopf B, Smola A (2001) Learning with kernels. MIT Press, London
Scholkopf B, Koji T, Jean P (2004) Kernel methods in computational biology. MIT Press, London
Shimodaira H, Noma KI, Nakai M, Sagayama S (2002) Dynamic time-alignment kernel in support vector machine. In: Advances in neural information processing systems, vol 14. MIT Press, London, pp 921–928
Smola AJ, Óvári ZL, Williamson RC (2001) Regularization with dot-product kernels. In: Advances in neural information processing systems, vol 13. MIT Press, London, pp 308–314
Vapnik V (1995) The nature of statistical learning theory, 2nd edn. Springer, New York
Vapnik V (1998) Statistical learning theory. Wiley, New York
Wu G, Chang E, Zhang Z (2005) An analysis of transformation on non-positive semidefinite similarity matrix for kernel machines. In: International conference on machine learning. Bonn, pp 1682–1689

Chapter 3
Kernels and Spectrum Perturbations

3.1 Introduction

Kernel Methods are part of a category of algorithms used for pattern analysis. The most well-known member within this class is the Support Vector Machine (SVM). Kernels operate by transforming the data into a high-dimensional feature space, where each axis corresponds to a specific feature of the data points. Kernel method can effectively convert the gathered data into a collection of points within the Euclidean space. Kernels facilitate operations within the feature space by simply calculating the inner products between all pairs of data points instead of directly computing the coordinates of the data within that space. Very often, this approach is proved to be more computationally efficient than explicitly computing the coordinates. The Positive Semi-Definite (PSD) property of a kernel matrix is necessary to ensure the existence of a Reproducing Kernel Hilbert Space (RKHS), as noted in Schalkopf and Smola (2002), where a convex optimization formulation can be derived to obtain an optimal solution.

The spectrum perturbation in the context of kernel methods often involves computing the eigenvalues and eigenvectors of the kernel matrix. The eigenvalues and eigenvectors of kernel provide insights into the spectral properties of the data set. Specifically, the eigenvalues indicate the variance or importance of different directions in the feature space, while the eigenvectors represent the corresponding directions or principal components. Traditional methods for generating appropriate kernels from the perspective of spectrum include the following types.

- Shifting Method. It involves adding a small positive shift to the kernel matrix. This shift is often represented as a diagonal matrix λI, where λ is a small positive constant and I is the identity matrix. Adding this shift ensures that all eigenvalues of the kernel matrix are positive, which can lead to more stable spectral decomposition and better separation of clusters.

H. Jiang and W.-K. Ching, *Kernel Methods for Omics Data Mining*, Intelligent Control and Learning Systems 10, https://doi.org/10.1007/978-981-95-3129-5_3

- Denoising Method. It is applied to the kernel matrix to mitigate the effects of noise. It works by setting negative eigenvalues to zero and this can effectively remove noise components from the spectrum.
- Diffusion Method. The diffusion strategy shifts the eigenvalues of the kernel matrix to the exponential of them
- Flipping Method. The flipping strategy typically involves identifying negative eigenvalues and regarded these elements as noise, outliers, or inconsistencies in the data. It selectively flips the signs of these elements to alter their contribution to the spectral decomposition.

The emergence of innovative computational techniques enriches the advancement and evolution of research in computational biology area. Spectrum perturbations in kernels for their concise expressions and clear theoretical framework have been applied extensively in bioinformatics areas, in particular for applications in high-dimensional data analysis (Jiang and Ching 2012; Jiang et al. 2011). When confronted with datasets featuring an extensive array (tens of thousands) of attributes, an increase in predictors may compromise the efficacy of the classifier. According to the "ugly duckling" theorem, the inclusion of irrelevant predictors may unintentionally obscure the distinctions between different classes, thereby reducing classification accuracy. Thus, a reduction in predictors becomes imperative to attain heightened precision in prediction.

Protein function prediction as a typical scenario for high-dimensional data analysis has been considered from a classification point of view (Borgwardt and Kriegel 2005). With the increasing popularity of kernel-based methods for pattern classification (Shawe and Cristianini 2003; Jaakkola et al. 2000), a variety of string kernels have been proposed in protein function prediction area, namely spectrum kernel (Leslie et al. 2001), mismatch spectrum kernel (Leslie et al. 2004) and kernel based on latent semantic analysis (Yuan et al. 2005). The weighted degree kernel (Ratsch et al. 2005) has been applied in the recognition of alternatively spliced exons. However, the above string kernels assume independence among different features which may lead to a biased result from the physico-chemical perspective. AAindex Based Kernel therefore has been developed (Webb et al. 2010) for pairwise protein homology detection. A novel kernel based on the K-Spectrum Kernel, which incorporates both physico-chemical and biological information in the protein sequences for the captured protein classification problem has been proposed (Jiang and Ching 2012). The main innovation of the proposed method lies in the Eigen-matrix translation technique. The main idea and effect of this technique is to add a rank one PSD matrix to the original kernel matrix. In general, the effect of the technique is to increase the number of positive eigenvalues in the kernel matrix while bringing little perturbation to the original positive eigenvalues that are critical to fulfill the classification problem (Horn and Johnson 1985). We let

$$X = [\mathbf{x}_1, \mathbf{x}_2, \ldots, \mathbf{x}_N] \quad \text{and} \quad P = \mathrm{Diag}\,(0, \ldots, 0, \lambda_1, \ldots, \lambda_m)$$

respectively to be the original eigen-matrix and the corresponding eigenvalues of the kernel matrix where

$$Ker = X \cdot P \cdot X^T \text{is the kernel matrix.}$$

Then the new kernel after making an Eigen-matrix translation will be

$$Ker_{new} = N\lambda \mathbf{v} \cdot \mathbf{v}^T + X \cdot P \cdot X^T$$

where λ is the translation parameter and the vector

$$\mathbf{v} = \frac{1}{\sqrt{N}} \left[\sum_{i=1}^{N} x_{1i}, \ldots, \sum_{i=1}^{N} x_{Ni} \right]^T$$

exhibits a nice property: the inner products of the vector $\mathbf{v}$ with all the eigenvectors in the old kernel Ker are the same.

We shall investigate the major role of the Eigen-matrix translation. Focusing on the characteristics of the data sets, the number of data instances is 40–50 while the number of features can be up to 7000–8000. This gives us a clue on the potential power of the Eigen-matrix translation in dimension reduction. High-dimensional data sets give us many mathematical challenges as well as opportunities for new theoretical developments (Donoho et al. 2000). Traditional algorithms in machine learning and pattern recognition are often susceptible to the well-known problem of the curse of dimensionality (Hammer 1962), while certain computationally expensive novel methods (Breiman 2001) can construct predictive models with high accuracy from high-dimensional data. Therefore it is still of interest in many applications to reduce the dimension of the original data set before the analysis of the data and this serves as a data pre-processing step. In a machine learning method (Dy and Brodley 2000), feature selection, is a useful technique for selecting a subset of relevant features in building robust learning models. When applied to a biology domain, the technique is also known as discriminative gene selection. Subset selection algorithms can be categorized into three types: Wrappers, Filters and Embedded. Wrapper induction uses supervised learning to learn rules from manually labeled training examples. The disadvantages of wrapper induction are that the labeling process is time-consuming and the maintenance of wrapper is difficult. Filters select subsets of variables as a pre-processing step, independently of the chosen predictor. Embedded methods perform variable selection in the process of training and are usually specific to the given learning machine.

In this chapter, we put forward a novel perspective of feature selection technique. We suggest that the major role of Eigen-matrix translation lies in the feature selection within the huge size of feature dimensions. The remainder of this chapter is organized as follows. In Sect. 3.2, we give the formulation of the captured problem. The relationship between the Eigen-matrix translation and feature selection is then illustrated. Computational experiments on real biological data sets are then given to demonstrate the effectiveness of our proposed methods and models in Sects. 3.3 and 3.4. Finally, concluding remarks are given in Sect. 3.5.

3.2 Methodology

In this section, we present a relationship between the Eigen-matrix translation technique and feature selection in binary classification. Since the Eigen-matrix translation technique was first established on the spectrum kernel, it is more coherent to give a brief introduction on spectrum kernel. Details will be left for the illustration of internal connections of eigen-matrix translation and feature selection.

3.2.1 Spectrum Kernel

In protein classification, spectrum kernel is one of the outstanding representatives in string kernels. In K-spectrum kernel, where K is a positive integer, the input space χ consists of all finite K-length sequences from the alphabet $\Re$ with $|\Re| = n_K$. We assume the input data set contains N sequences $\{p_1, p_2, \ldots, p_N\}$. The K-spectrum of an input sequence p_i is the set of all the K-length (contiguous) subsequences that it contains. The K-mer representation of the sequence is denoted through a feature map from χ to R^{n^K}. Here, the ith protein p_i is expressed as

$$x_i^K = [x_{1i}^K, x_{2i}^K, \ldots, x_{n_K i}^K]^T,$$

where x_{li}^K is the occurrence of lth K-mer in the input data p_i and n_K is the dimensionality of features. If V_K is the K-mer representation matrix for the whole input data set of dimensionality $n_K \times N$, denoting the representations for the N protein sequences, then its K-spectrum kernel can be expressed as follows: $Ker_K = V_K^T \cdot V_K$.

3.2.2 Eigen-Matrix Translation

The PSD property is guaranteed by $Ker_K = V_K^T \cdot V_K$. The Eigen-matrix translation technique is an effective procedure to improve classification accuracy. It involves two steps:

Step 1: The Eigenvalue Decomposition:

$$Ker_K = X \cdot P \cdot X^T,$$

where X is the orthogonal matrix containing all the column eigenvectors of the matrix Ker_K and P is a diagonal matrix containing all the corresponding eigenvalues of Ker_K, see for instance (Horn and Johnson 1985).

Step 2: The Eigen-matrix translation technique:

$$Ker_{new} := X \cdot [P + \lambda \mathbf{w} \cdot \mathbf{w}^T] \cdot X^T.$$

The effect of this translation is to add a rank one PSD matrix to the kernel matrix where $\mathbf{w} = [1, 1, \ldots, 1]^T$. Following the Weyl's theorem (Horn and Johnson 1985) for two Hermitian matrices, it can be shown that if a given Hermitian matrix is modified by adding a rank one Hermitian matrix, the new and the original eigenvalues must be interlacing. We refer interested readers to Jiang et al. (2011) for details. More precisely, it turns a zero eigenvalue to positive but does not make much perturbation to the original positive eigenvalues while preserving their positivity. This means that if we assume $d_1 \leq d_2 \leq \cdots \leq d_n$ are the eigenvalues of the original Ker_K which are arranged in an increasing order, and $\tilde{d}_1 \leq \tilde{d}_2 \leq \cdots \leq \tilde{d}_n$ are the eigenvalues of the new kernel matrix Ker_{new} after performing the eigen-matrix translation. Then we have

$$d_1 \leq \tilde{d}_1 \leq d_2 \leq \tilde{d}_2 \leq \ldots \leq d_n \leq \tilde{d}_n.$$

This property is important in the classification problem. At the same time, we note that the PSD property is preserved automatically. Furthermore, from the interlacing theorem, if the number of the zero eigenvalue is m then it is straightforward to see that for the new kernel matrix,

$$\tilde{d}_1 = d_1 = \tilde{d}_2 = d_2 = \ldots = \tilde{d}_{m-1} = d_{m-1} = 0$$

it has $(m - 1)$ zero eigenvalues and $\tilde{d}_m \geq 0$. This means that $\tilde{d}_m$ can be zero or nonzero. Here it has been shown that the kernel matrix after adding a rank one matrix would change the mth eigenvalue into a nonzero one by a suitable rank one perturbation. Thus we aim to characterize those rank one symmetric matrices such that one zero eigenvalue would be changed into a nonzero one. In order to numerically verify our claim about the effect of the rank one symmetric matrix, we generate a kernel matrix which is rank deficient. Without loss of generality, we formulate a data set with 40 data instances and 2000 features. In particular, we generate the above data set in the following way. We first create a random matrix A of size 40×20 by ensuring that A is of full rank. We then construct a matrix B of size 40×1980 from A as follows: setting each column of B linearly dependent of the columns in A. Therefore, we have a desirable matrix C combining A and B, the rank of which is 20. This available data set provides us a platform to apply the Eigen-matrix translation technique to the constructed kernel matrix, i.e., $C \cdot C^T$. Furthermore, we try to add the following rank one matrices: $\mathbf{w}_1 \cdot \mathbf{w}_1^T, \mathbf{w}_2 \cdot \mathbf{w}_2^T, \cdots, \mathbf{w}_{19} \cdot \mathbf{w}_{19}^T$ where $\mathbf{w}_1 = [1, 0, \ldots, 0]^T, \mathbf{w}_2 = [1, 1, 0, \ldots, 0]^T, \cdots, \mathbf{w}_{19} = [\underbrace{1, 1, \ldots 1}_{19}, 0, \ldots, 0]^T$ to the kernel matrix and we find that the number of zero eigenvalues of the resulting matrix still remains the same. There are 20 zero eigenvalues for all the above cases which is exactly the same with the original kernel matrix. Therefore, the effect of the Eigen-matrix translation technique is closely related to the selection of the rank one matrix. One should determine the characteristic of those matrices of rank one such that they convert the original mth zero eigenvalue to a nonzero one. The following proposition addresses the above issue. In order to prove the proposition, we shall present a lemma about the eigenvalues under the perturbation of a rank one symmetric matrix.

Lemma 3.1 *He (2006) Let A be a $n \times n$ real symmetric matrix and $\mathbf{x}$ be a n-dimensional column vector. Let $M = \mathbf{x}\mathbf{x}^{\mathbf{T}}$. Suppose that $A = PDP^T$, where P is the eigen-matrix and D is a diagonal matrix with its diagonal elements being the eigenvalues. We have*

$$A + tM = PDP^T + tM = P(D + tP^T\mathbf{x}\mathbf{x}^{\mathbf{T}}P)P^T.$$

If we let $\mathbf{q} = P^T\mathbf{x}$, then $q_i = (P_i)^T\mathbf{x}$ for each $i = 1, 2, \ldots, n$ where P_i is the ith column of P and

$$A + tM = P(D + t\mathbf{q}\mathbf{q}^T)P^T.$$

Let $D(t) = D + t\mathbf{q}\mathbf{q}^T$, we have

$$\det(D + t\mathbf{q}\mathbf{q}^T - \tilde{\alpha}I) = \det(A - \tilde{\alpha}I)\left(1 + \sum_i \frac{tq_i^2}{\alpha_i - \tilde{\alpha}}\right),$$

where α_i is the diagonal elements of D and $\tilde{\alpha}$ is a perturbation parameter.

Then, we have the following proposition concerning about the selection of the rank one matrix.

Proposition 3.1 *If the mth eigenvalue of the original kernel matrix is 0 and mth entry of $\mathbf{w}$ is nonzero, then for the new kernel matrix after performing Eigen-matrix translation technique, the mth eigenvalue would be changed to nonzero.*

Proof Let $\tilde{X}$ be the orthogonal matrix containing all the column eigenvectors of the matrix $\tilde{K}er_K$ and $\tilde{P} = \text{Diag}\,(\mu_1, \ldots, \mu_n)$ is a diagonal matrix containing all the corresponding eigenvalues of $\tilde{K}er_K$. We then define $\mathbf{b} = \tilde{X}\mathbf{z}$, and we can obtain

$$\tilde{K}er_{new} = \tilde{X}[\tilde{P} + \lambda\mathbf{z}\mathbf{z}^T]\tilde{X}^T = \tilde{K}er_K + \lambda\mathbf{b}\mathbf{b}^T.$$

In general, we denote $\mathbf{z}$ as a n-dimensional column vector and $\mathbf{z} = [\xi_1, \xi_2, \ldots, \xi_n]^T$. We let

$$P(\lambda) = \tilde{P} + \lambda\mathbf{z}\mathbf{z}^T, \quad \lambda > 0.$$

Then by Lemma 3.1, which concerns about the determinant of $P(\lambda)$, we have

$$\det(\tilde{P} + \lambda\mathbf{z}\mathbf{z}^T - \tilde{\mu}I) = \det(\tilde{K}er_K - \tilde{\mu}I)\left(1 + \sum_i \frac{\lambda\xi_i^2}{\mu_i - \tilde{\mu}}\right).$$

Furthermore, if we denote

$$F_\lambda(\tilde{\mu}) = 1 + \sum_i \frac{\lambda \xi_i^2}{\mu_i - \tilde{\mu}},$$

then the roots of $F_\lambda(\tilde{\mu})$ are exactly the eigenvalues of $\tilde{Ker}_{new}$. If $\xi_i \neq 0$, it is straightforward to see that

$$\tilde{\mu}_i = \mu_i + \lambda \xi_i^2 > \mu_i \quad (\lambda > 0).$$

Here, we assume that the mth eigenvalue for the kernel matrix is zero and $\xi_m \neq 0$, the mth eigenvalue for the new kernel matrix must be nonzero. □

From the above proposition, we know that to ensure the mth zero eigenvalue to perturb to positive one, we should choose the rank one vector $\mathbf{z}$ with the mth entry which is positive. Here we choose $\mathbf{w} = [1, 1, \ldots, 1]^T$ which implies the mth entry is positive, we can thus guarantee the Eigen-matrix translation technique is effective in turning one zero eigenvalue to a nonzero one. Actually, this perturbation always preserves the positive definiteness when the real symmetric kernel matrix is positive definite or it increases the positive inertial index by one otherwise.

3.2.3 Problem Formulation

The Eigen-matrix translation technique is experimentally proved to be successful in improving classification accuracy for protein classification problem with few data instances but huge size of features. If we let the number of data instances is n and let the number of features for each data instance is p, then $n \ll p$.

Let S be a $p \times p$ matrix, then the original kernel matrix before making the Eigen-matrix translation can be re-written in the following form (from the perspective of similarities among different features):

$$Ker_K = V_K^T \cdot S \cdot V_K.$$

Here S is the identity matrix of dimension $p \times p$. In other words, the spectrum kernel assumes no similarity between two different features. Each feature is assumed to have equal importance and all of the features are used for classification.

We note that

$$Ker_{new} - Ker_K = X \cdot \lambda [1, 1, \ldots, 1]^T \cdot [1, 1, \ldots, 1] \cdot X^T$$

and we write $Ker_{new} - Ker_K$ in the following form:

$$Ker_{new} - Ker_K = V_K^T \cdot \Delta S \cdot V_K$$

where ΔS is also a diagonal matrix of size $p \times p$. The nonzero entries among the p diagonal entries are important in classification. As for those zero diagonal entries, it means that the corresponding features are invariable to the Eigen-matrix translation technique. On the other hand, for those nonzero ones, they indicate either strengthening or impairing the effect of features in classification. In this context, we have

$$Ker_{new} = V_K^T \cdot [S + \Delta S] \cdot V_K.$$

As a matter of fact, the above assumptions can be realized with the following construction procedures. Since $Ker_{new} - Ker_K$ is a rank one matrix, it can be represented as follows:

$$Ker_{new} - Ker_K = Y \cdot Y^T$$

where

$$Y = [y_1, y_2, \ldots, y_n]^T \quad \text{and} \quad y_i = \sqrt{\lambda} \sum_{j=1}^{N} x_{ij}, \quad i = 1, 2, \ldots, n.$$

If we denote $\Delta S = \text{diag}(S_{11}, \ldots, S_{pp})$, i.e.

$$\Delta S = \begin{bmatrix} S_{11} & & & \\ & S_{22} & & \\ & & \ddots & \\ & & & S_{pp} \end{bmatrix}$$

then we have

$$\begin{bmatrix} y_1^2 & y_1 y_2 & \cdots & y_1 y_n \\ y_2 y_1 & y_2^2 & \cdots & y_2 y_n \\ \vdots & \vdots & \ddots & \vdots \\ y_n y_1 & y_n y_2 & \cdots & y_n^2 \end{bmatrix} = \begin{bmatrix} v_{11} & v_{12} & \cdots & v_{1p} \\ v_{21} & v_{22} & \cdots & v_{2p} \\ \vdots & \vdots & & \vdots \\ v_{n1} & v_{n2} & \cdots & v_{np} \end{bmatrix} \begin{bmatrix} S_{11} & & & \\ & S_{22} & & \\ & & \ddots & \\ & & & S_{pp} \end{bmatrix} \cdot \begin{bmatrix} v_{11} & v_{21} & \cdots & v_{n1} \\ v_{12} & v_{22} & \cdots & v_{n2} \\ \vdots & \vdots & & \vdots \\ v_{1p} & v_{2p} & \cdots & v_{np} \end{bmatrix}.$$

The symmetric property of the matrix on both sides ultimately turns the problem of n^2 linear equations of p unknowns to a problem of $n(n+1)/2$ linear equations of p unknowns. Since $n \ll p$, $n(n+1)/2 < p$ still holds, there exist infinitely many least-square solutions with the sparse structure of the solution being guaranteed. The problem is then transformed into the problem of solving a linear system of $n(n+1)/2$ equations and p unknowns:

Table 3.1 The glycan structure

NeuAca2-8NeuAca2-8NeuAca2-8NeuAca2-3(GalNAcb1-4)Galb1-4Glcb-Sp0

$$\begin{bmatrix} v_{11}^2 & \cdots & v_{1p}^2 \\ \vdots & \vdots & \vdots \\ v_{n1}^2 & \cdots & v_{np}^2 \\ v_{21}v_{11} & \cdots & v_{2p}v_{1p} \\ \vdots & \vdots & \vdots \\ v_{n1}v_{11} & \cdots & v_{np}v_{1p} \\ \vdots & \vdots & \vdots \\ v_{n1}v_{n-11} & \cdots & v_{np}v_{n-1p} \end{bmatrix} \begin{bmatrix} S_{11} \\ S_{22} \\ \vdots \\ \vdots \\ \vdots \\ \vdots \\ S_{pp} \end{bmatrix} = \begin{bmatrix} y_1^2 \\ \vdots \\ y_n^2 \\ y_2 y_1 \\ \vdots \\ y_n y_1 \\ \vdots \\ y_n y_{n-1} \end{bmatrix}.$$

We utilize the linear system solver under the condition of least square errors. Suppose that

$$I_{irrelevant} = \{i : S_{ii} = 0, i \in \{1, 2, \ldots, p\}\} \text{ and } I_{relevant} = \{i : S_{ii} \neq 0, i \in \{1, 2, \ldots, p\}\}.$$

We have

$$I_{irrelevant} \cap I_{relevant} = \emptyset \quad \text{and} \quad I_{relevant} \cup I_{relevant} = \{1, 2, \ldots, p\}.$$

The indices in $I_{relevant}$ represent the features essential for classification. Hence we choose those features for classification. We note that the new kernel in this context becomes

$$Ker_1 = [V_K(I_{relevant}, :)]^T \cdot V_K(I_{relevant}, :).$$

3.3 Experimental Results

3.3.1 Data Source

We employ glycan-binding related protein data to demonstrate the effectiveness of our proposed method. Glycan structures, lectin-glycan binding affinity, lectin sequences are retrieved from the the glycan database of Functional Glycomics Gateway (CFG) (FGG 2025). We assume a lectin binds to a glycan if the binding affinity exceeds 10000. Here we focus on the glycan structures with a relatively large number ($\geq$20) of binding lectins. The glycan structure is illustrated in Table 3.1.

In the captured three glycan structures, glycan-binding protein prediction can be regarded as a classification problem to assess the binding property of a protein sequence. In the glycan, 20 positive data constitute the positive part, and the same number of the negative data from the data set is then chosen to ensure the balance of positive and negative data. The dimension of the features of the data is 7815, a typical example of small $n = 40$ and large $p = 7815$.

3.3.2 Experiments

The focus of our study is the role of the Eigen-matrix translation technique in classification, we therefore concentrate on the data sets whose classification accuracies are improved after making an Eigen-matrix translation. In the following experiments, 4-spectrum kernel is adopted for making comparisons. The reason for employing 4-mer as a feature is following. It was suggested in a number of research works (Leslie et al. 2001, 2004; Yang et al. 2008) that 4-mers is superior for string kernel.

In performing the eigen-matrix translation, $\lambda = 0.1$ was chosen as suggested in Jiang and Ching (2012) which guaranteed that for λ in $[0.01, 1]$, a better classification result can be obtained. To some extent it renders λ a free tuning parameter. We therefore employ 0.1 as the value of λ.

However, different value of λ may have different effects on selection of predictor variables in the final model. Therefore, it is necessary to conduct a sensitivity analysis on λ for feature selections. Figure 3.1 describes the number of features selected for different values of λ. We use the same step size as in Jiang and Ching (2012), in addition, we use 0.001 as the step size for λ in $[0.001, 0.01]$. It can be shown through experiments that for λ in $[0.001, 1]$, the same number of features are selected. Furthermore, we find that the set of the selected features remain the same. Hence we observe the variation of λ would not change the final selected features. Thus we adopt $\lambda = 0.1$ in the following settings. Secondly, in order to demonstrate the effectiveness of our proposed method, numerical experiments are conducted on the selected data sets. The effectiveness of our method is then evaluated through comparison with the 4-spectrum kernel method in terms of AUC values. The experimental results indicate that the proposed method is an effective tool for dimension reduction in classification. In the data set, 110 out of 7815 features are selected for classification. The AUC values are also larger than the original 4-spectrum kernel, see Fig. 3.3 for instance. This further confirms the effectiveness of our developed method for classification.

We also concerned that if the Eigen-matrix translation technique, as a feature selector, can outperform other feature selectors. Therefore, we conduct a study on the comparison of our method with other feature selectors. We employ two famous feature selectors for making a comparison. The first one ranks the features in the data set using a two-sample t-test for the binary classification. The other criterion tries to maximize the area under the ROC curve to assess the significance of every feature for separating two labeled groups. Since these two feature ranking algorithms cannot determine the number of significant features automatically, we use the same number of features in our proposed model for the comparison study. Figure 3.2 clearly illustrates the superiority of our proposed model as a feature selector.

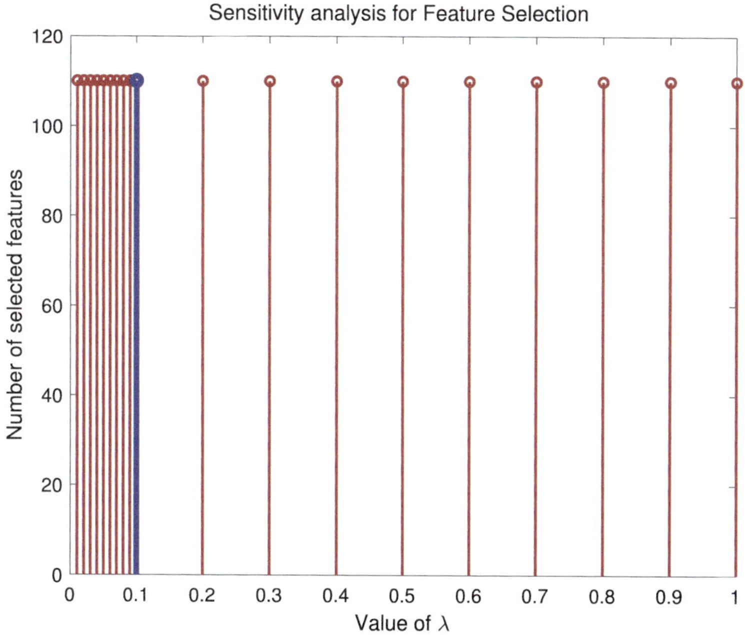

Fig. 3.1 A sensitivity analysis on Glycan data. A step size of 0.001 is used for λ in [0.001, 0.01] and 0.01 is used for λ in [0.01, 0.1], step size 0.1 is used for λ in [0.1, 1]. 110 features are selected for all the values of λ. This indicates the insensitivity of λ to the selection of features in the final model

To show the importance of the selected features in classification, we test the selected features based on the proposed method. After we get the solutions for the above linear system, we rank the nonzero entries of the solutions for each λ. As the nonzero entries involve both positive and negative ones, the top 10 features are selected for those rank top 5 and the last 5. A subset of the features is selected in a similar manner to test the importance of the features obtained in solving linear system. For instance, we use the top 10, 20, 30, ..., 110 features for classification, where the features are selected following the same rule of the top 10 features. Results are then given in Fig. 3.4 which confirm the importance of the selected features obtained from our proposed method. One can see that the general increment of classification accuracy with respect to the increase of number of features. When the number of subset of features is close to the total number of the selected features chosen by our proposed method, the classification accuracy tends to be the best.

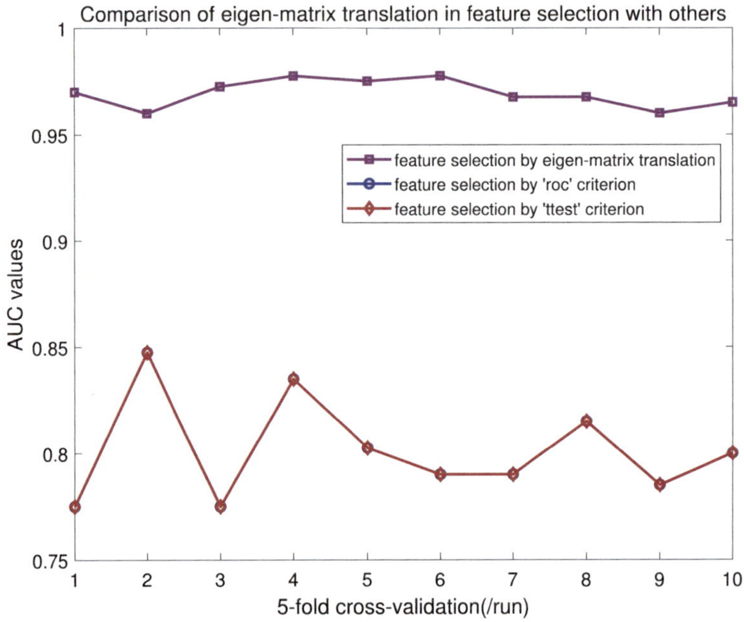

Fig. 3.2 A comparison of different feature selectors on Glycan 3 related data. The solid line with '□' is the performance of using selected features by Eigen-matrix translation based model, with solid line in '○' standing for the performance of feature selectors by 'roc' criterion. Solid line in '◇' stands for the performance of feature selectors by 'ttest' criterion. Our model performs the best in the 10 times fivefold cross-validations. Around 0.96 AUC values are achieved in average. For feature selectors by 'roc' and 'ttest' criterion, similar performance can be obtained, reaching on average 0.8 AUC values

3.3.3 A Simulation Study

In this subsection, we conduct a simulation study to demonstrate that the Eigen-matrix translation technique is an effective feature selector. We generate a data set with 40 data instances and 2000 features, 20 of the data instances are positive and 20 are negative. Among the 2000 features, 1970 features are the same for all the data instances. For simplicity, we use 0 for all feature values. Then we perturb the 30 features with randomly generated vectors of length 10. Actually this kind of data set has 30 important features for classification. All the other 1970 features can be regarded as noises as they bring no difference between positive and negative data. After generating the data set, we apply the Eigen-matrix translation technique to the original linear kernel constructed and select a subset of features for classification. The results indicate that Eigen-matrix translation can indeed select the exact 30 features for classification.

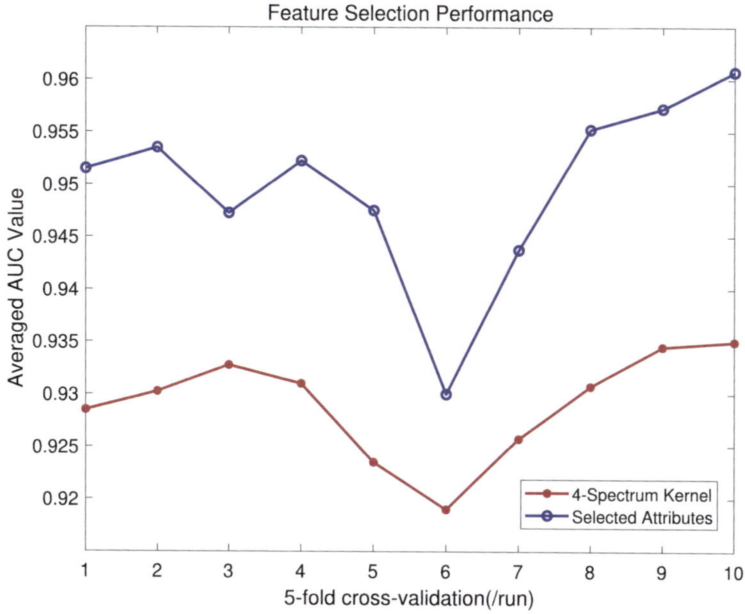

Fig. 3.3 A comparison of performance on Glycan 3 related data in mer4. This figure compares the performance of 4-spectrum kernel with the new kernel constructed on selected features where the features are selected through the framework of Eigen-matrix translation technique, with our proposed method. 10 times fivefold cross validation are performed as well, introducing Averaged AUC values as criterion. For Glycan Data set, with our proposed method, the new kernel on the selected 110 features out of 7815 features achieves better classification accuracy. The averaged AUC values for 4-spectrum kernel are about 0.93 while for the kernel on selected features, averaged AUC values improve to 0.95

3.4 Discussions

Experimental results have further validated the effective role of our proposed method in feature selection. The selected features used in classification show their superiority when compared to the whole set of features. In Glycan data set with 4-mer features, the number of features reduces from 7815 to 110. This is a drastic improvement particularly in data sets with massive number of features. The Eigen-matrix translation technique plays an important role in the feature selection, the newly constructed kernel after feature selection outperformed the original k-mer kernel in terms of classification accuracy.

For human breast cancer data set, the number of the features (24481) is extremely larger than that of the data instances (78). This motivates us to apply the Eigen-matrix translation technique associated with the feature selection to validate the performance of the classification. We utilize the Eigen-matrix translation technique, it has been shown that classification accuracy keeps in a steady manner. Focusing on breast cancer data set, we find that all the eigenvalues of the kernel matrix are positive, the

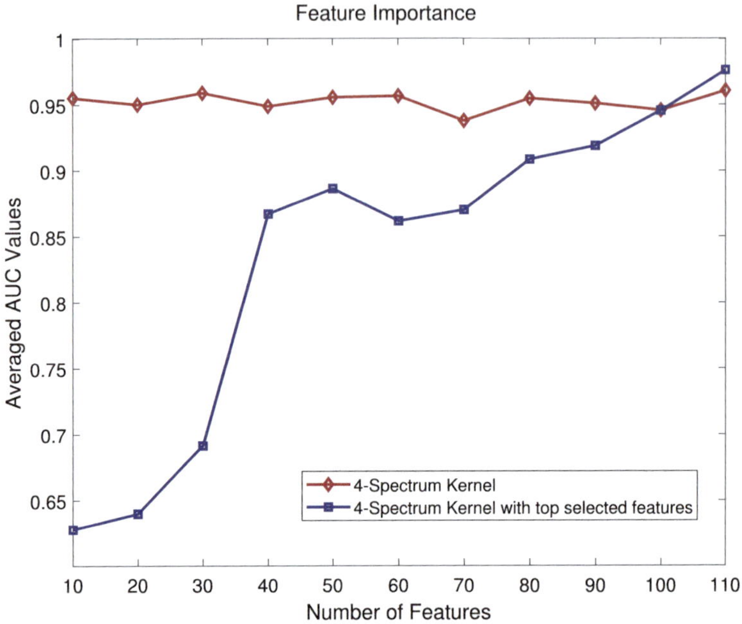

Fig. 3.4 A comparison of performance on Glycan data. A subset of features is selected to perform classification in order to test the importance of the selected features by our proposed method. The X-axis is the number of features selected for classification, the Y-axis represents the averaged AUC values for classification each time. Comparison is made with the whole set of features within the data set. The solid line with '□' is the selected features, with solid line in '◇' standing for the whole set of features. One can see general increment of accuracy with the increase of the number of features. In Glycan 3 related data set, top 10, 20, 30, ..., 110 features are selected. The averaged AUC values increase stably from 0.4 with 10 features to 0.95 with 110 features

perturbation of the rank one matrix does not have much effect on the classification. Even we conduct the proposed feature selection technique, the number of features is reduced from 24481 to 3004. When we use the 3004 features conduct classification, not much improvement is obtained, see Fig. 3.5. Compared with the Glycan data sets, we find that the breast cancer data set is highly dense and many features are linearly independent. This means most of them can be useful features and they may play a role in the classification. Thus, when it occurs to a data set that has massive number of features and many of them are linearly independent, then our proposed method is less effective than the case where the features are individually correlated. As a conclusion, through mathematical formulation, we developed a relationship between Eigen-matrix translation and feature selection. And the effectiveness of the model is assured by the experiment results.

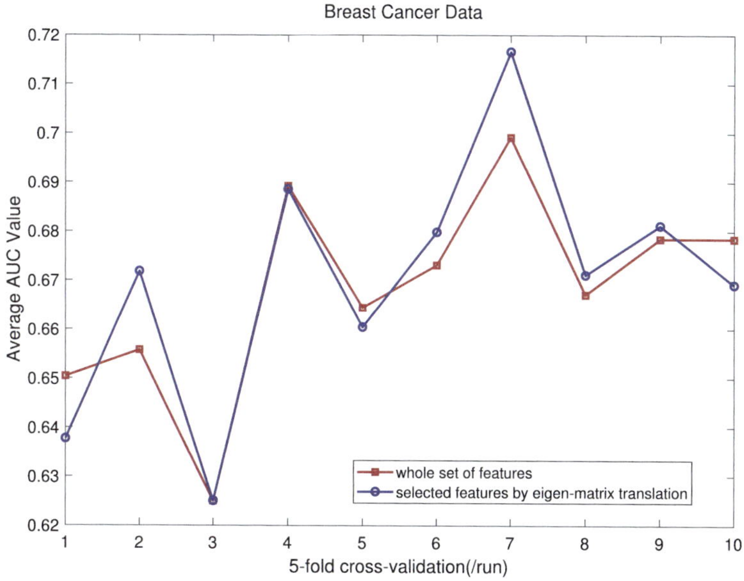

Fig. 3.5 This figure compares the performance of the original kernel matrix with the new kernel constructed on the selected features where the features are selected through the framework of Eigen-matrix translation technique, with our proposed method. 10 times fivefold cross validation are performed as well, introducing Averaged AUC values for criterion. For the breast cancer data set, with our proposed method, the new kernel on the selected 3004 features out of 24481 features can not effectively improve the classification accuracy

3.5 Concluding Remarks

In this chapter, we investigate the major role of the Eigen-matrix translation technique in SVM for classification. Through mathematical formulation of the problem, we suggest the effective role of the technique in feature selection. Different from the traditional algorithms in feature selection, our method realizes the task of dimension reduction in an automatic way. And the sparsity of the selected subset of features is guaranteed. Furthermore, the selected features used for classification tend to be optimal in the sense of classification performance of AUC values. Experimental results further validate the effectiveness of our proposed method. This also provides another perspective in dimension reduction for data sets of huge size of features.

References

Borgwardt KM, Kriegel PH (2005) Kernel methods for protein function prediction

Breiman L (2001) Random forests. Mach Learn 45:5–32

Donoho DL, Averbuch A, Hastie TJ, Johnstone I, Owen AL, Scott D, Stine B, Tibshirani R, University SFX, Willinger W, Gregory S, Xchange PS, Bosch E, Army US, Eng T, Ctr J, Elder, Inselberg A, Starck JL, 'Astronomie CED, Weinberger P, Flesia AG, Levi O, Jennings KS (2000) High-dimensional data analysis: the curses and blessings of dimensionality

Dy JG, Brodley CE (2000) Feature subset selection and order identification for unsupervised learning. In: International conference on machine learning

Functional glycomics gateway. http://www.functionalglycomics.org

Hammer PC (1962) Adaptive control processes: a guided tour (R. Bellman). SIAM Rev 4(2):163. https://doi.org/10.1137/1004050

He HL (2006) Eigenvectors and reconstruction. Electron J Comb 14

Horn RA, Johnson CR (1985) Matrix analysis

Jaakkola T, Diekhans ME, Haussler D (2000) A discriminative framework for detecting remote protein homologies. J Comput Biol J Comput Mol Cell Biol 7(1–2):95–114

Jiang H, Ching WK (2012) Physico-chemically weighted kernel for SVM protein classification. Appl Mech Mater 195–196:385–390

Jiang H, Ching WK, Zheng Z (2011) Kernel techniques in support vector machines for classification of biological data. Int J Inf Technol Comput Sci 3:1–8

Leslie CS, Eskin E, Cohen A, Weston J, Noble WS (2004) Mismatch string kernels for discriminative protein classification. Bioinformatics 20(4):467–476

Leslie CS, Eskin E, Noble WS (2001) The spectrum kernel: a string kernel for SVM protein classification. In: Pacific symposium on biocomputing: pacific symposium on biocomputing, pp 564–575

Rätsch G, Sonnenburg S, Schölkopf B (2005) RASE: recognition of alternatively spliced exons in C. Elegans. Bioinformatics 21(suppl1):i369–i377. https://doi.org/10.1093/bioinformatics/bti1053

Schälkopf B, Smola A (2002) A short introduction to learning with kernels. In: Machine learning summer school

Shawe-Taylor J, Cristianini N (2003) Kernel methods for pattern analysis. In: IEEE international conference on tools with artificial intelligence

Webb-Robertson BJM, Ratuiste KG, Oehmen CS (2010) Physicochemical property distributions for accurate and rapid pairwise protein homology detection. BMC Bioinform 11:145

Yang Y, Tantoso E, Li KB (2008) Remote protein homology detection using recurrence quantification analysis and amino acid physicochemical properties. J Theor Biol 252(1):145–154

Yuan Y, Lin L, Dong Q, Wang X, Li M (2005) A protein classification method based on latent semantic analysis*. In: 2005 IEEE engineering in medicine and biology 27th annual conference, pp 7738–7741

Chapter 4
Hadamard Kernel SVM with Applications

4.1 Introduction

It is a well-established fact that 13% of deaths worldwide were attributed to cancer (DeSantis et al. 2011). Among women, breast cancer stands out as a leading cause of death globally. Breast cancer claimed 670,000 lives globally in 2022. Approximately half of all breast cancer cases occur in women with no identifiable risk factors other than gender and age. In 2022, breast cancer ranked as the most prevalent cancer among women in 157 out of 185 countries. Notably, breast cancer affects women in every country worldwide. Early detection and diagnosis of breast cancer are essential for minimizing the adverse effects of the disease. On the other hand, cancer prognosis plays a crucial role in designing treatment protocols, which is also of great importance. Cancer prognosis involves estimating the probability of survival within a specific period. A 5-year prognosis of 90% indicates a 90% probability of surviving for 5 years following surgery or diagnosis. Here we formulate the prognosis problem as a classification task, where label information is derived from survival data beyond the prognosis period. For instance, patients who decease before the designated prognosis period are labeled as negative, and vice versa.

In cancer research, cDNA microarrays and high-density oligonucleotide chips were increasingly utilized, presenting numerous excellent yet challenging research opportunities in the field. By simultaneously monitoring the expression levels of tens of thousands of genes in cells, microarray experiments have the potential to enhance our understanding of molecular variations among tumors, thus facilitating more informative classification (Dudoit et al. 2002). Over the last few years, substantial efforts (Nemade and Fegade 2023; deVijver et al. 2002; Veer et al. 2002; vanVilet et al. 2008; Akker et al. 2011) have been made on gene expression profile based classifiers for patient outcome prediction.

Maglogiannis et al. (2009) proposed Support Vector Machines (SVMs) based classifier for the prognosis and diagnosis of breast cancer disease, and was compared with Bayesian classifiers and Artificial Neural Networks. Delen et al. (2005)

H. Jiang and W.-K. Ching, *Kernel Methods for Omics Data Mining*, Intelligent Control and Learning Systems 10, https://doi.org/10.1007/978-981-95-3129-5_4

made comparison on three algorithms for predicting breast cancer survivability. Endo et al. (2008) considered problem of 5-year prognosis in breast cancer, and compared several algorithms on SEER data and results show that decision tree J48 showed the highest sensitivity, ANN had the highest specificity. The data used for model comparisons in Delen et al. (2005); Endo et al. (2008) has characteristics of large n and small p. When dealing with small data sets, SVM-based algorithms often outperform other methods. Chaurasia and Pal (2014) conducted a comparative study of Naive Bayes, SVM with an RBF kernel, RBF neural networks, Decision Trees (J48), and Classification and Regression Trees (CART) to determine the best classifier for breast cancer data sets. In another study, Asri et al. (2016) evaluated the performance of SVM, Decision Tree (C4.5), Naive Bayes, and K-Nearest Neighbors (KNN) on the Wisconsin Breast Cancer Datasets. Their experimental results confirmed that SVM achieved the highest accuracy among the tested algorithms.

In the current perspective, SVM is recognized as a benchmark across various disciplines, particularly for problems involving small sample sizes. The effectiveness of SVMs largely depends on the choice of kernels. In Jiang and Ching (2012), we proposed a novel kernel based on the correlation matrix for cancer diagnosis. Experiments on real-world cancer data sets with gene expression profiles demonstrated that the correlation-based kernel outperformed other classical kernels.

In this chapter, we propose a parsimonious kernel named the Hadamard Kernel for predicting breast cancer outcomes. The chapter is structured as follows: We propose the parsimonious positive semi-definite kernel and provide a theoretical proof of its positive semi-definite property. The performance of the proposed method is then evaluated using publicly available data sets. Concluding remarks are given in the last section.

4.2 Methodology

4.2.1 Preliminaries

The basic SVM considers binary classification problem through building an appropriate model representing data points, mapping them so as to best separate different categories. In a formal setting, if we assume a data set of n data instances with corresponding class annotations:

$$\{(\mathbf{x}_1, y_1), \ldots, (\mathbf{x}_n, y_n)\}$$

where $\mathbf{x}_i \in \mathbf{R}^p$, $y_i \in \{-1, 1\}$. SVM constructs a hyperplane in $\mathbf{R}^p$ to ensure good separation having largest distance from it to the nearest data points in each class category (Cortes and Vapnik 1995). The optimization problem can be formulated as follows:

$$\min \frac{1}{2}\|\mathbf{w}\|^2 \tag{4.1}$$
$$\text{subject to } y_i(\mathbf{w}\cdot\mathbf{x}_i + b) \geq 1 \text{ for any } i \in \{1, 2, \ldots, n\}, \mathbf{w} \in \mathbf{R}^p,$$

where **w** is the normal vector in the hyperplane and b is the bias term.

The dual form of the primal optimization problem is given by:

$$\begin{cases} & \text{Maximize} \sum_{i=1}^{n} \alpha_i - \frac{1}{2}\alpha^T \mathbf{H}\alpha \\ \text{subject to} & \\ & \alpha_i \geq 0 \text{ for any } i \in \{1, 2, \ldots, n\} \\ & \sum_{i=1}^{n} \alpha_i y_i = 0 \end{cases} \tag{4.2}$$

where $\alpha = [\alpha_1, \alpha_2, \ldots, \alpha_n]$,

$$\mathbf{H} = \begin{pmatrix} y_1^2\mathbf{x}_1^T\mathbf{x}_1 & y_1y_2\mathbf{x}_1^T\mathbf{x}_2 & \ldots & y_1y_n\mathbf{x}_1^T\mathbf{x}_n \\ y_2y_1\mathbf{x}_2^T\mathbf{x}_1 & y_2y_3\mathbf{x}_2^T\mathbf{x}_3 & \ldots & y_2y_n\mathbf{x}_2^T\mathbf{x}_n \\ \vdots & \vdots & \ddots & \vdots \\ y_ny_1\mathbf{x}_n^T\mathbf{x}_1 & \ldots & \ldots & y_n^2\mathbf{x}_n^T\mathbf{x}_n \end{pmatrix}.$$

When the data sets are not linearly separable, meaning the classes cannot be separated by a linear hyperplane, one can construct a nonlinear mapping for input vectors $\mathbf{x}_i$ into feature space of higher dimensionality (Aizerman 1964). Different from the previous setting based on inner product of input vectors, kernel matrix is constructed in terms of similarity measure through pairwise comparisons. Given n data instances $\mathbf{X} = \{\mathbf{x}_1, \mathbf{x}_2, \ldots, \mathbf{x}_n\}$, the kernel matrix K is an $n \times n$ matrix, defined elementwise by a kernel function $K(\mathbf{x}_i, \mathbf{x}_j)$ as follows:

$$K_{i,j} = K(\mathbf{x}_i, \mathbf{x}_j), \quad \forall \mathbf{x}_i, \mathbf{x}_j \in \mathbf{X},$$

where the kernel function $K(\cdot, \cdot)$ should be symmetric, i.e.,

$$K(\mathbf{x}, \mathbf{x}') = K(\mathbf{x}', \mathbf{x}).$$

In other words, the notation K indicates the kernel matrix and $K(\cdot, \cdot)$ indicates an element of K.

We can write $K(\mathbf{x_i}, \mathbf{x_j}) = \phi(\mathbf{x_i}) \cdot \phi(\mathbf{x_j})$, where $\mathbf{x_i} \rightarrow \phi(\mathbf{x_i})$ is a mapping from original input space into transformed feature space.

There are a number of popular kernels, the most straightforward one is Linear Kernel:

$$K(\mathbf{x}, \mathbf{x}') = \mathbf{x}^T\mathbf{x}',$$

which is an inner product of $\mathbf{x}$ and $\mathbf{x}'$ in $\mathbf{X}$. In this case, the mapping function can be explicitly as $\phi(\mathbf{x}) = \mathbf{x}$.

Another popularly used kernel matrix is Polynomial Kernel that is expressed as follows:

$$K(\mathbf{x}, \mathbf{x}') = (\mathbf{x}^T \mathbf{x}' + 1)^d.$$

The mapping function in polynomial kernel can still be explicitly expressed and it is of finite dimension. The following example gives an illustration.

Example 4.1 $K(\mathbf{x}, \mathbf{x}') = (\mathbf{x}^T \mathbf{x}' + 1)^2$, $\mathbf{x}, \mathbf{x}' \in R^3$. We can know the mapping function

$$\phi(\mathbf{x}) = (1, \sqrt{2}x_1, \sqrt{2}x_2, \sqrt{2}x_3, {x_1}^2, {x_2}^2, {x_3}^2, \sqrt{2}x_1x_2, \sqrt{2}x_1x_3, \sqrt{2}x_2x_3).$$

Gaussian Radial Basis Function (RBF) kernel is defined as

$$K(\mathbf{x}, \mathbf{x}') = \exp(-d||\mathbf{x} - \mathbf{x}'||^2),$$

where $d > 0$ is parameter. If the distance between $\mathbf{x}$ and $\mathbf{x}'$ is small, the kernel value would be large; on the contrary, if $\mathbf{x}$ is far away from $\mathbf{x}'$ in terms of Euclidean distance, the kernel value would be small. Hence this kernel provides a similarity measure between data points. However in this case, the mapping function $\phi(\mathbf{x})$ is of infinite dimension.

Example 4.2 Assume $\mathbf{x} \in R^1$, then

$$K(\mathbf{x}, \mathbf{x}') = \exp(-d(x - x')^2),$$
$$\phi(\mathbf{x}) = \exp^{(-dx^2)}\left(1, \sqrt{\frac{2d}{1!}}x, \sqrt{\frac{(2d)^2}{2!}}x^2, \sqrt{\frac{(2d)^3}{3!}}x^3, \ldots\right).$$

4.2.2 *Hadamard Kernel*

Kernel trick is useful in the sense that there is no need to calculate $\phi(\mathbf{x})$ explicitly as long as appropriate kernel matrix is constructed. The Positive Semi-Definite (PSD) property (Scholkopf and Smola 2001) of a kernel matrix is required to ensure the existence of a Reproducing Kernel Hilbert Space (RKHS) where a convex optimization formulation can be deduced to yield an optimal solution of the dual problem.

We propose Hadamard Kernel in this way:

$$K_\alpha(\mathbf{x}_i, \mathbf{x}_j) = \sum_{k=1}^{p} \frac{|x_{ik}|^\alpha |x_{jk}|^\alpha}{2(|x_{ik}|^\alpha + |x_{jk}|^\alpha)}, i, j = 1, 2, \ldots, n.$$

Here $\alpha > 0$ is a flexible parameter within the kernel matrix. For some k, if $x_{ik} = 0$, then $\frac{|x_{ik}|^\alpha |x_{jk}|^\alpha}{(|x_{ik}|^\alpha + |x_{jk}|^\alpha)}$ is defined as 0.

Theorem 4.1 *Kernel K_α is positive semi-definite for all data set* $\mathbf{X}$.

The proposed Hadamard Kernel with varying parameter α constitutes a broad range of kernel families which can fit all kinds of data matrix if the theorem holds.

Before we prove the theorem, let's first consider the following kernel:

$$K_0(\mathbf{x}_i, \mathbf{x}_j) = \sum_{k=1}^{p} \frac{x_{ik}x_{jk}}{2(x_{ik} + x_{jk})}, \quad i, j = 1, 2, \ldots, n.$$

For some certain k, if $x_{ik} = 0$, then $\frac{x_{ik}x_{jk}}{x_{ik}+x_{jk}}$ is defined as 0.

This kernel is not generally positive semi-definite. Let's consider the following example.

Example 4.3 Assume $\mathbf{x}_1 = [1, 1 \cdots 1]^T$, $\mathbf{x}_2 = [-1/2, -1/2 \cdots - 1/2]^T$, then the kernel matrix has the following structure:

$$\begin{pmatrix} n & -2n & \cdots \\ -2n & -n/2 & \vdots \\ \vdots & \cdots & \ddots \end{pmatrix}.$$

If $\mathbf{x} = [1, 1, 0, \cdots, 0]^T$, we have

$$\mathbf{x}^T K_0 \mathbf{x} = -7n/2 < 0 \quad \text{when} \quad n \geq 1.$$

If $\mathbf{x} = [-1, 0, \cdots, 0]^T$, we have

$$\mathbf{x}^T K_0 \mathbf{x} = n > 0 \quad \text{when} \quad n \geq 1.$$

However, in our particular case, where all the gene expression values are positive valued, the kernel here is positive semi-definite. We give the proof in the subsequent statement.

Theorem 4.2 *Kernel K_0 is positive semi-definite when that data matrix* $\mathbf{X}$ *is positive valued.*

Proof For a positive matrix $A = (a_{ij})$, we define the Hadamard inverse of A by

$$A^{\circ(-1)} = \left(\frac{1}{a_{ij}}\right).$$

First proved by RB (1988) and reformulated by Reams (1999), we have the following proposition.

Proposition 4.1 *If A is a positive symmetric matrix with only one positive eigenvalue, then $A^{\circ(-1)}$ is positive semi-definite.*

Let $\mathbf{e} = (1, \ldots, 1)$, $\mathbf{X} = \begin{bmatrix} \mathbf{x}_1 \\ \mathbf{x}_2 \\ \vdots \\ \mathbf{x}_n \end{bmatrix} = [\mathbf{w}_1, \mathbf{w}_2, \ldots, \mathbf{w}_p]$, and we define

$$V_{\mathbf{X}}(i, j) = \sum_{r=1}^{p} \frac{1}{\mathbf{X}_{ir} + \mathbf{X}_{jr}}.$$

We therefore have

$$K = \frac{1}{2} V_{\mathbf{X}^{\circ(-1)}}.$$

To show that K is always positive semi-definite is equivalent to showing that $V_{\mathbf{X}}$ is always positive semi-definite.

To show that $V_{\mathbf{X}}$ is PSD, we only need to show that $V_{\mathbf{x}_i e}$ is PSD for any positive column vector $\mathbf{w}_i$ as we have

$$V_{\mathbf{X}} = V_{\mathbf{w}_1 \mathbf{e}} + \cdots V_{\mathbf{w}_p \mathbf{e}}.$$

Suppose $\mathbf{w}_i = (x_{1i}, \ldots, x_{ni})^T$, then we have $V_{\mathbf{w}_i \mathbf{e}} = (\mathbf{w}_i \mathbf{e} + (\mathbf{w}_i \mathbf{e})^T)^{\circ(-1)}$.

Note that $\mathbf{w}_i \mathbf{e} + (\mathbf{w}_i \mathbf{e})^T$ is a positive symmetric matrix of rank 2 and it is not PSD (the determinant of any principal 2×2 submatrix is negative), hence it has exactly one positive eigenvalue. Therefore by the result of Reams, $V_{\mathbf{x}_i \mathbf{e}}$ is PSD.

We can generalize the result to any non-negative matrix $\mathbf{X}$ as well.

Theorem 4.3 *Kernel K_0 is positive semi-definite when data matrix $\mathbf{X}$ is non-negative.*

Proof For $x, y \geq 0$, we define the binary operation

$$x \cdot y = \begin{cases} \frac{x+y}{xy} = \frac{1}{x^{-1}+y^{-1}} & \text{if } xy \neq 0 \\ 0 \quad \text{if } xy = 0 \end{cases}.$$

Here $K = U_{\mathbf{X}} = \frac{1}{2}\left(\sum_{r=1}^{p} \mathbf{X}_{ir} \cdot \mathbf{X}_{jr})\right)$.

Then $U_{\mathbf{X}} = U_{\mathbf{w}_1 \mathbf{e}} + \cdots U_{\mathbf{w}_p \mathbf{e}}$. To show that U_X is positive semi-definite, we only need to show that $U_{\mathbf{we}}$ is PSD for any non-negative column vector $\mathbf{w}$.

Suppose $\mathbf{w}$ has zero entries. Without loss of generality, write $\mathbf{w} = (\mathbf{y}, \mathbf{0})^T$ where $\mathbf{y} > 0$, then

$$U_{\mathbf{we}} = \begin{pmatrix} U_{\mathbf{y}e} & 0 \\ 0 & 0 \end{pmatrix}$$

which is PSD if and only if $U_{\mathbf{ye}}$ is PSD. Hence it suffices to show that $U_{\mathbf{ye}}$ is PSD for any positive column vector $\mathbf{y}$.

Take $\mathbf{y}'$ to be the Hadamard inverse of $\mathbf{y}$, then

$$U_{\mathbf{ye}} = (\mathbf{y}'\mathbf{e} + (\mathbf{y}'\mathbf{e})^T)^{\circ(-1)}.$$

Note that $\mathbf{y}'\mathbf{e} + (\mathbf{y}'\mathbf{e})^T$ is a positive symmetric matrix of rank 2 and it is not PSD (the determinant of any principal 2×2 submatrix is negative), hence it has exactly one positive eigenvalue. Therefore by the result of Reams (1999), $U_{\mathbf{we}}$ is PSD.

We now proceed to prove Theorem 4.1.

Proof For any data sample within matrix $\mathbf{X}$, we can generate a corresponding new matrix $\mathbf{X}_\alpha$ by

$$\mathbf{X}_\alpha(i, j) = |x_{ij}|^\alpha.$$

Then according to Theorem 4.3, we can show the validity of the theorem.

4.2.3 Models for Comparison

In this section, we consider breast cancer outcome predictions based on high dimensional gene expression profiles. Hence the number of samples is relatively small. In the literature, it is shown that SVM is statistically better than other machine learning algorithms. We therefore confine our research in the framework of SVMs and exclude other algorithms from our scope of research. Kernels for comparison are listed below.

- SVM Linear Kernel

$$K(\mathbf{x}, \mathbf{x}') = \mathbf{x}^T\mathbf{x}'.$$

- SVM Quadratic Kernel

$$K(\mathbf{x}, \mathbf{x}') = (\mathbf{x}^T\mathbf{x}' + 1)^2.$$

- SVM RBF Kernel

$$K(\mathbf{x}, \mathbf{x}') = \exp(-\frac{||\mathbf{x} - \mathbf{x}'||^2}{\sigma^2}).$$

- SVM Correlation Kernel
  This kernel construction can be decomposed into three steps.

  Step 1. Based on the correlation matrix of the data set, we first construct a preliminary kernel.

$$K_{CB} = 1 - e^{-\mathrm{corr}(\mathbf{X})},$$

  where X is the data set.

Step 2. We do eigenvalue decomposition for the matrix K_{CB} where V is the orthogonal matrix composed of eigenvectors, P is the diagonal matrix where diagonal entries are eigenvalues. That is,

$$K_{CB} = VPV^T.$$

Step 3. Denoising strategy. If we denote

$$P = \begin{pmatrix} p_1 & 0 & \cdots & 0 \\ 0 & p_2 & \cdots & 0 \\ \vdots & \vdots & \ddots & \vdots \\ 0 & 0 & \cdots & p_n \end{pmatrix}.$$

The denoising strategy is to transform the diagonal matrix P to another diagonal matrix $\tilde{P}$,

$$\tilde{P} = \begin{pmatrix} \tilde{p}_1 & 0 & \cdots & 0 \\ 0 & \tilde{p}_2 & \cdots & 0 \\ \vdots & \vdots & \ddots & \vdots \\ 0 & 0 & \cdots & \tilde{p}_n \end{pmatrix}$$

where

$$\tilde{p}_i = \begin{cases} 0, & p_i < 0; \\ p_i, & p_i \geq 0. \end{cases}, \quad i = 1, 2, \ldots, n.$$

Finally, the kernel matrix becomes

$$K_{DCB} = V\tilde{P}V^T.$$

4.3 Numerical Experiments

4.3.1 Materials

We have selected six real-world data sets from NCBI (National Center for Biotechnology Information (NCBI 2017). The first data set is derived from an N-methyl-N-nitrosourea-induced breast cancer model. It has 35 samples in total, of which 11 are normal. The number of attributes used to describe a sample is 15923. Expression profiles were obtained through Affymetrix Rat Expression 230A Array. The annotation ID for this data set is GSE1872.

Estrogen Receptor-Positive (ER+) and ER- breast cancers tend to show different patterns of metastasis. In this data set where the access number is GSE32394, glycan structure analysed by Custom Affymetrix Glyco v4 GeneChip was conducted to compare the two types of breast cancer. There are 19 samples in total, of which 9 are ER+, the number of attributes is 1259.

The third data set is used to differentiate non-invasive breast cancer and invasive breast cancer, the access number is GSE59246. mRNA, miRNA and DNA copy number profiles are generated to measure the expression of different samples. Arrays consist of 3 normal controls, 46 ductal carcinoma in situ lesions, and 56 small invasive breast cancers. We discard the 3 normal controls, so we have 102 samples in total. In this data set, the number of attributes is 62976.

Studies show that circulating miRNAs have the potential to become biomarkers. This data set involves 78 samples in total, 1205 circulating miRNAs for measurements. 26 of the 78 samples are negative. Identification number for this data set in NCBI is GSE59993.

One more data set is related to breast cancer prognosis, GSE25055 is the identification number. A total number of 310 breast cancer patients is involved. The number of attributes is 22283. This study is conducted with Affymetrix Human Genome U133A Array. It is a neoadjuvant study of HER2-negative breast cancer cases treated with taxane-anthracycline chemotherapy preoperatively and endocrine therapy if ER-positive. Response was assessed at the end of neoadjuvant treatment. Using 5 years as a cutoff, we conduct the outcome prediction.

4.3.2 *Performance Evaluation*

4.3.2.1 5-Fold Cross Validation

Cross validation is a standard way to evaluate the supervised learning model. Every run of the k-fold cross validation is performed as follows: first of all, the training data set $\mathcal{M}$ is randomly divided into k subsets $\mathcal{M}_1, \ldots, \mathcal{M}_k$ of approximately equal size. The prediction model is trained on $k-1$ subsets and the remaining subset is treated as the test set. Repeating this process k times such that each subset is tested once, all the prediction results are recorded for the computation of prediction accuracy. In our case, we conduct fivefold cross validation for model evaluations.

4.3.2.2 Area Under the Receiver Operating Characteristic (ROC) Curve

In the context of classification, suppose the two true classes are P (positive) and N (negative), while the predicted positive and negative classes are P' and N', respectively. This is illustrated by Table 4.1 below. The ROC Curve is a graphical plot of False Positive Rate (FPR) vs. True Positive Rate (TPR) as x and y axes, respectively, for a binary classifier system as its discrimination threshold is varied. FPR and TPR are defined as follow:

Table 4.1 Definitions for true/false positive/negatives

True result	P'	N'
P	True positive (tp)	False negative (fn)
N	False positive (fp)	True negative (tn)

$$\text{FPR} = \frac{fp}{tn + fp} \quad \text{and} \quad \text{TPR} = \frac{tp}{tp + fn}.$$

TPR determines a classifier performance on classifying positive instances correctly among all positive samples available during the test, while FPR measures how many incorrect positive results occur among all negative samples available during the test. Each prediction result represents one point on the ROC curve. The best possible prediction method would yield a point in the upper left corner or coordinate (0, 1) of the ROC space, representing no false negatives and no false positives.

The area under the ROC curve (AUC) (Hanley and McNeil 1983; Mamitsuka 2006) is a widely adopted statistics for assessing the discriminatory capacity of models. It can be interpreted as a measure of aggregated classification performance, and also the tradeoff between specificity and sensitivity (Flach et al. 2011).

4.3.3 Numerical Results

In this section, we will show the performance of the Hadamard Kernel in conjunction with SVM and the other 4 kernels for breast cancer outcome predictions as tested on the five data sets. We employed the AUC measured by running the fivefold cross-validation 10 times to evaluate the performance. All the experiments are conducted using Matlab R2012 under Window 7 Operations System.

In RBF kernel, we have to specify the parameter σ before model training. Therefore, we initially conduct the fivefold cross validation 10 times solely on RBF kernel with $\sigma \in \{10^{-2}, 10^{-1}, 1, 10, 100, 1000\}$. Averaged AUC Values with corresponding standard deviations are shown in Table 4.2. For example, in GSE1872 data set, the performance of RBF kernel is not sensitive to different values of σ. The best σ of RBF kernel for GSE32394 and GSE59246 breast cancer prediction is 1000 whereas the best σ for GSE59993 is 10. Particular case can also arise when RBF kernel is insensitive to values of σ. We can draw the conclusion that there is no optimal σ for all the considered data sets and different data sets may have different best σ.

For Hadamard kernel, we would like to see its performance in relation with the parameter α. Figures 4.1, 4.2, 4.3, 4.4 and 4.5 record the performance of Hadamard Kernel in relation with the parameter α from $(0, 5)$ with step size 0.1 in the six selected data sets. It is observed that the optimal α in Hadamard Kernel varies in different data sets. For example, one can see a steady decrement in performance when $\alpha > 1.3$ in GSE1872 and when $\alpha > 2.8$ in GSE59246. There is no obvious

Table 4.2 Averaged AUC values for determining optimal σ in RBF kernel

Data sets σ	$\sigma = 0.01$	$\sigma = 0.1$	$\sigma = 1$	$\sigma = 10$	$\sigma = 100$	$\sigma = 1000$
GSE1872	0.2379 ± 0.0538	0.2379 ± 0.0538	0.2379 ± 0.0538	0.2379 ± 0.0538	0.2379 ± 0.0538	0.2379 ± 0.0538
GSE32394	0.1811± 0.0707	0.1811± 0.0707	0.2044 ± 0.0845	0.6767 ± 0.1125	0.9456 ± 0.0133	**0.9456 ± 0.0122**
GSE59246	0.4408 ± 0.0446	0.4408 ± 0.0446	0.4408 ± 0.0446	0.4408 ± 0.0446	0.8424 ± 0.0379	**0.8658± 0.0110**
GSE59993	0.3542 ± 0.0283	0.3542 ± 0.0283	0.4305 ± 0.0355	**0.8392 ± 0.0235**	0.6937 ± 0.0340	0.6940 ± 0.0342
GSE25055	0.3651 ± 0.0182	0.3651 ± 0.0182	0.3651 ± 0.0182	0.3651 ± 0.0182	**0.8092 ± 0.0156**	0.7259 ± 0.0127

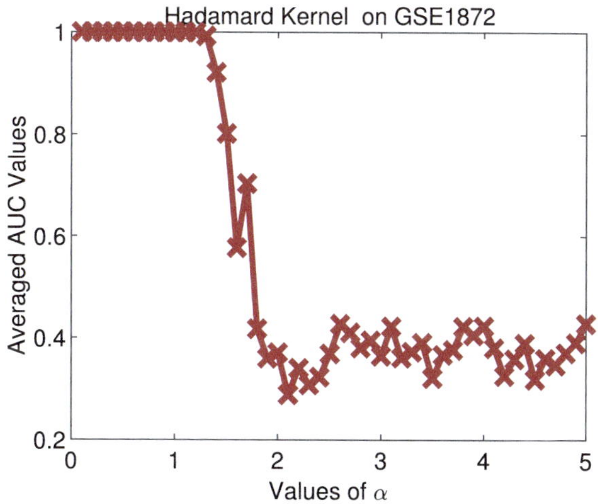

Fig. 4.1 AUC values for hadamard kernel: GSE1872

pattern detected in Fig. 4.2 in GSE32394, the performance is unstable with respect to α. But we can see a tendency of decrement in an overall manner. For GSE59993, the performance increases firstly, achieving the best for $\alpha = 0.5$. The performance then decreases steadily. In GSE25055, the performance of Hadamard kernel stays in a stable range when $\alpha < 2.8$, it then decreases drastically. It can be seen that different data sets may fit for different best α in Hadamard Kernel, the optimal α determination becomes an interesting problem.

Figures 4.6, 4.7, 4.8, 4.9 and 4.10 depict the AUC values of the 5 considered methods in each fivefold cross validations. Dark blue refers to Hadamard Kernel, Linear Kernel is marked in orange, yellow represents Quadratic Kernel, purple stands for RBF Kernel, and green stands for Correlation Kernel. In the x-axis, 1 represents the first fivefold cross-validation. The corresponding values in y axis are the AUC values for the considered 5 methods. For example, in Fig. 4.6 for GSE1872, the best performance is shown in Hadamard Kernel and Correlation Kernel in the first round,

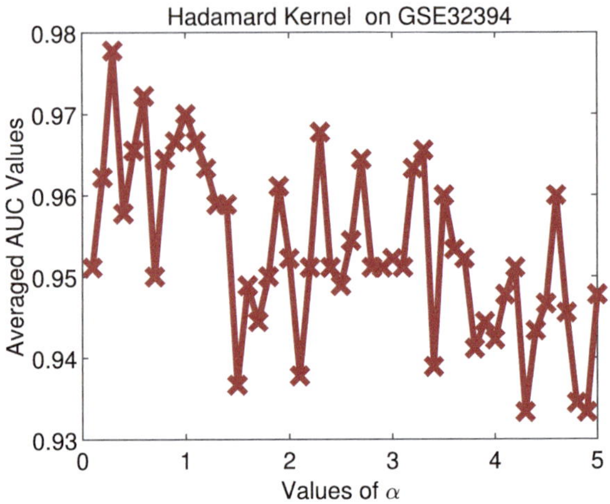

Fig. 4.2 AUC values for hadamard kernel: GSE32394

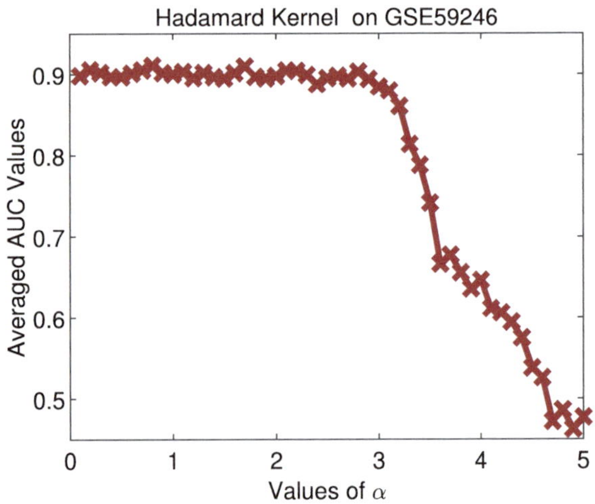

Fig. 4.3 AUC values for hadamard kernel: GSE59246

achieving 100% in accuracy. The performances of Linear Kernel, RBF Kernel and Quadratic Kernel are not satisfactory. RBF Kernel shows the worst performance, the AUC values are below 30%. Similar patterns can be detected in the remaining 9 round fivefold cross-validations. In summary, Hadamard Kernel and Correlation Kernel show the best performance regarding the 10 runs of fivefold cross-validations.

Figure 4.7 shows the performance of different models for data set GSE32394. The best performance is shown in Hadamard Kernel, it is slightly better than Linear Kernel. RBF Kernel and Correlation Kernel show comparable performance, and the worst performance is shown in the Quadratic Kernel.

Figure 4.8 depicts the result for GSE59246 breast cancer outcome prediction. Hadamard Kernel still demonstrates the best performance, the second best performance is shown in Linear Kernel. Overall, RBF Kernel is better than Correlation

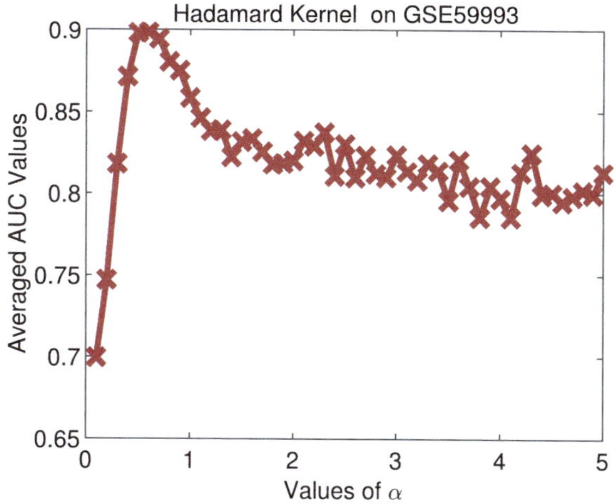

Fig. 4.4 AUC values for hadamard kernel: GSE59993

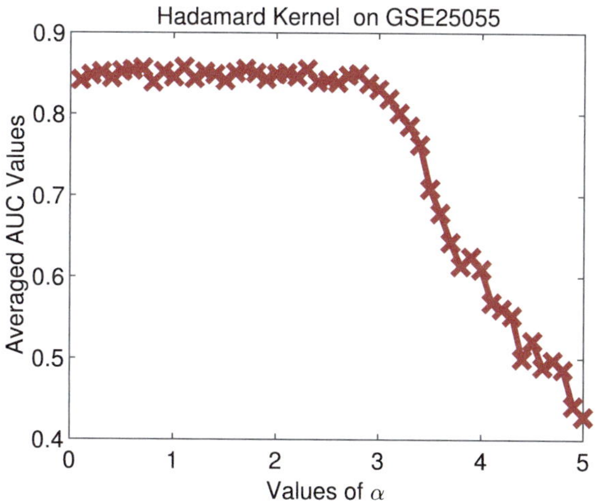

Fig. 4.5 AUC values for hadamard kernel: GSE25055

Kernel. They rank the third the fourth place this time. Quadratic Kernel can only get 50% in AUC values on average.

In GSE59993, Hadamard Kernel is better than the other 4 kernels as shown in Fig. 4.9. RBF Kernel shows the second best in this context. Linear Kernel ranks the third place and Quadratic Kernel shows the worst performance.

Figure 4.10 shows the result for GSE25055 breast cancer outcome prediction. GSE25055 is a data set related to breast cancer prognosis. We formulate the problem into a classification one by labeling patients who survive within 5 years after diagnosis as positive classes. Hadamard Kernel and Linear Kernel reach the top places, yielding around 84% on average in AUC values. The performance of RBF kernel is also acceptable, achieving around 81% in Averaged AUC Values.

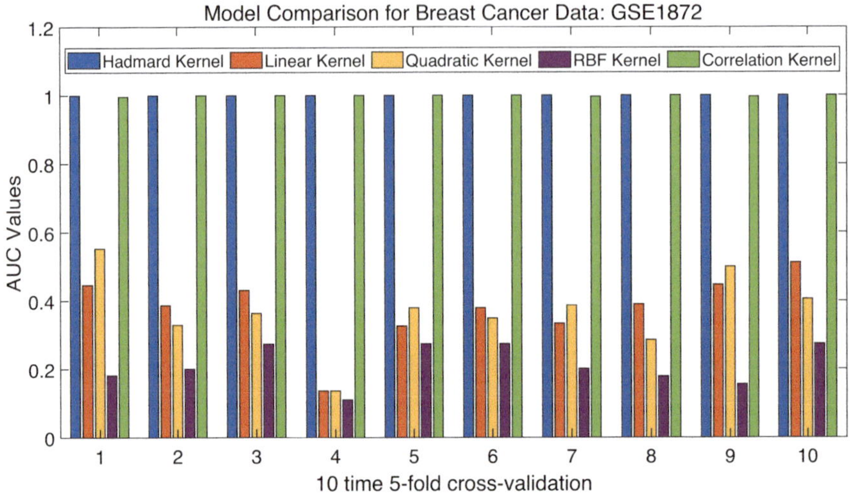

Fig. 4.6 AUC values for comparison of hadamard kernel and other kernels: GSE1872

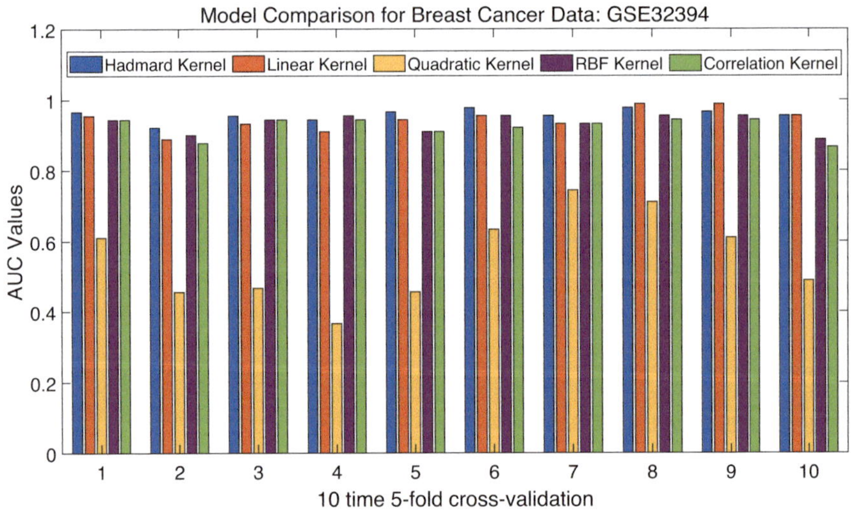

Fig. 4.7 AUC values for comparison of hadamard kernel and other kernels: GSE32394

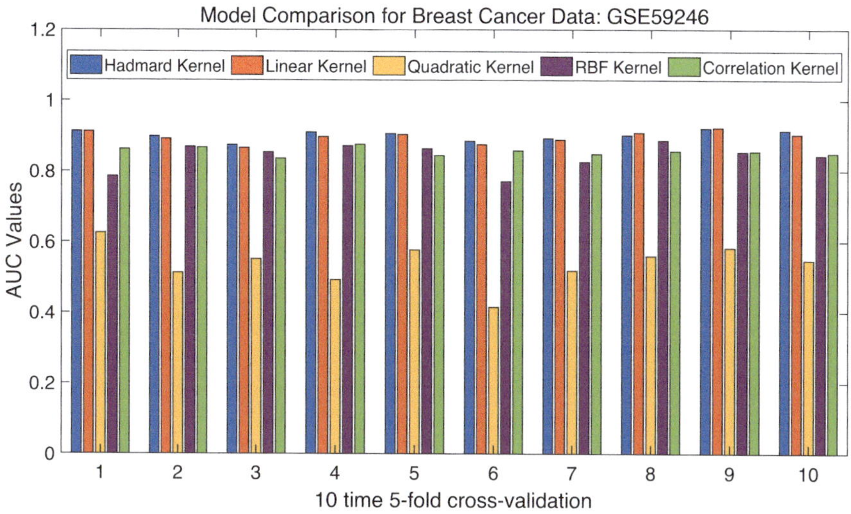

Fig. 4.8 AUC values for comparison of hadamard kernel and other kernels: GSE59246

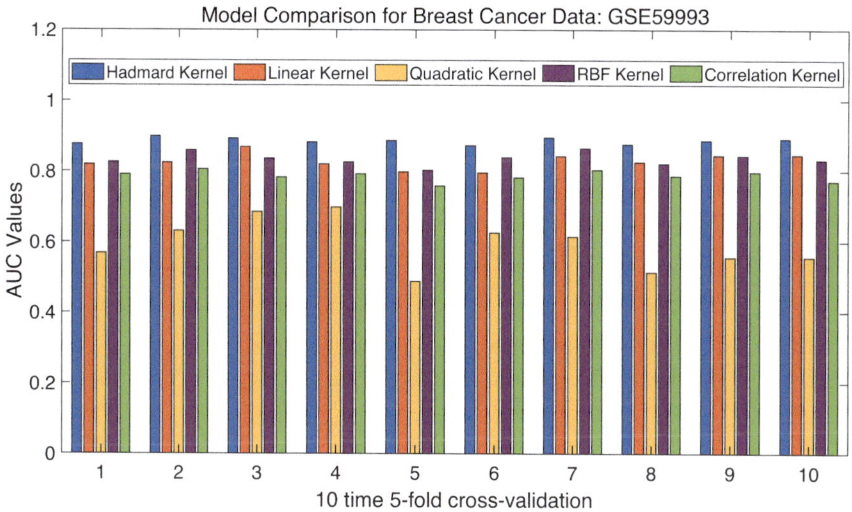

Fig. 4.9 AUC values for comparison of hadamard kernel and other kernels: GSE59993

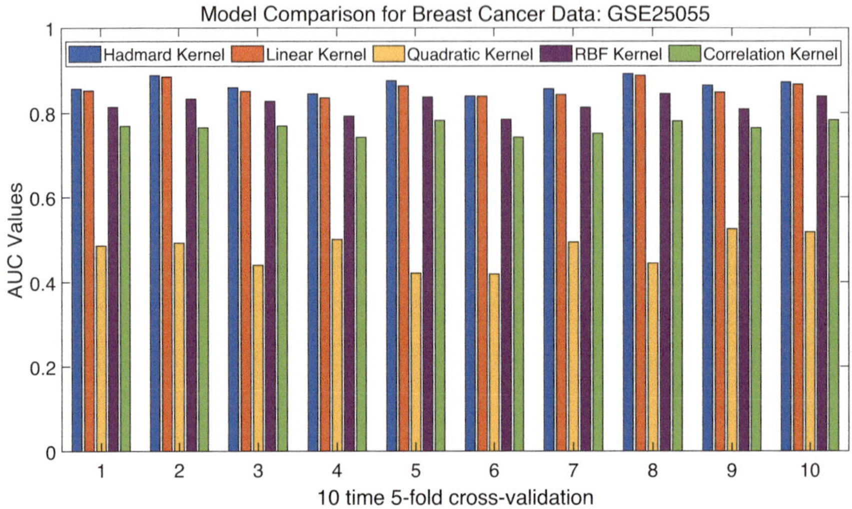

Fig. 4.10 AUC values for comparison of hadamard kernel and other kernels: GSE25055

Table 4.3 illustrates the average AUC value over the 10 runs with standard deviations. The best performance is marked in bold face. It is clear to see that on average Hadamard Kernel shows the best performance on all the considered data sets.

To sum up, Hadamard Kernel is effective and robust in predicting breast cancer outcomes. There is no dominant algorithm for the other 4 considered kernels. Quadratic Kernel always shows the worst performance, implying that Quadratic Kernel may not be a good choice in breast cancer outcome predictions.

Table 4.3 Averaged AUC values for comparison of different methods

Data sets methods	Linear kernel	Quadratic kernel	RBF kernel	Hadamard kernel	Correlation kernel
GSE1872	0.3788 ± 0.1019	0.3686± 0.1136	0.2117±0.0584	**1.000 ± 0.000**	0.9989 ± 0.0018
GSE32394	0.9456±0.0312	0.5544 ± 0.1248	0.9344 ± 0.0254	**0.9589 ± 0.0166**	0.9233 ± 0.0294
GSE59246	0.8977 ± 0.0172	0.5386 ± 0.0579	0.8431 ± 0.0379	**0.9022 ± 0.0145**	0.8562 ± 0.0113
GSE59993	0.8283 ± 0.0226	0.5935 ± 0.0694	0.8347 ± 0.0182	**0.8855 ± 0.0088**	0.7869 ± 0.0144
GSE25055	0.8575 ± 0.0182	0.4743 ± 0.0393	0.8196 ± 0.0203	**0.8653 ± 0.0171**	0.7654 ± 0.0152

4.4 Discussions

In this section, we are going to investigate the effect of normalization strategy on our proposed Hadamard kernel. As most of our data sets are microarray data, we therefore employ "manorm" which is an embedded function in Matlab for microarray data normalization. It scales the values in each column of the microarray data matrix, by dividing by the mean column intensity. Besides, we also include quantile normalization for testing purpose. Quantile normalization is designed for making two distributions identical in statistical properties. We employed the AUC measured by running fivefold cross-validation 10 times to evaluate the performance of Hadamard kernel with and without data normalization. The experimental results are shown below in Figs. 4.11, 4.12, 4.13, 4.14 and 4.15. It can be seen that in general Hadamard kernel after data normalization tend to perform better than the original Hadamard kernel without normalization. Green '∘' represents 'manorm' normalization, red star '⋆' represents Hadamard kernel without normalization, and black square represents 'quantile' normalization. For example, in Fig. 4.11 for GSE1872, after normalization, the performance of Hadamard kernel is approaching 100% in AUC value, while the original Hadamard kernel is relatively unstable. Similar patterns can be detected for GSE32394 and GSE59993 where 'manorm' and 'quantile' normalization with Hadamard kernel perform better than Hadamard kernel without data normalization. In GSE25055, the performance of Hadamard kernel without data normalization is not very stable. When α is relatively large, the performance decreases drastically. When normalization is done on the data, we can see that the performance becomes stable. Besides, 'quantitle' normalization based Hadamard kernel is slightly better than Hadamard kernel without normalization when $\alpha < 3$. In GSE59246, we can see that Hadamard kernel after normalization show comparable performance with Hadamard kernel without normalization when α in relatively small range. When the value of α increases, we can see that Hadamard kernel after normalization is more stable. To sum up, we can see that normalization positively affect the performance of Hadamard kernel.

A new perspective regards Hadamard kernel as a kernel on implicitly normalized data, hence in the following we are going to compare the performance of Hadamard kernel with other kernels under normalization. Similarly we introduce quantile normalization for testing purpose. Since correlation kernel needs to calculate the eigenspace of the correlation matrix, data after normalization sometimes yields unsolvable kernel, hence we use original correlation in this context. We still conduct fivefold cross-validation to test the performance of different methods. In the following Table 4.4, we can see the comparison of Hadamard kernel on raw data and other kernel methods on normalized data. We can find that Hadamard kernel is robust as it performs best for almost all the considered data sets compared to other methods after data normalization. In GSE1872, linear kernel and quadratic kernel after normalization perform significantly better than those without normalization. Almost all kernels can yield 100% averaged AUC value except for RBF kernel. In GSE32394, GSE59246, GSE59993 and GSE25055, quadratic kernel after data normalization

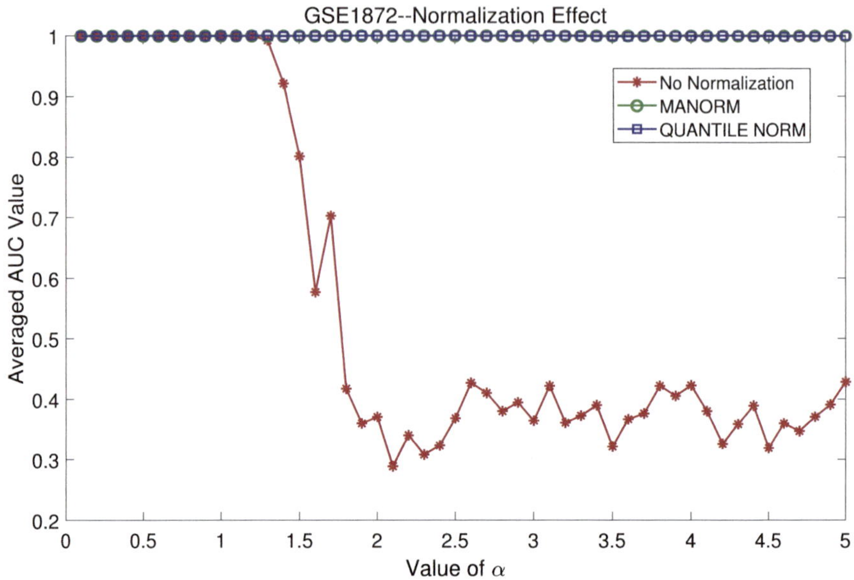

Fig. 4.11 Normalization effect on hadamard kernel: GSE1872

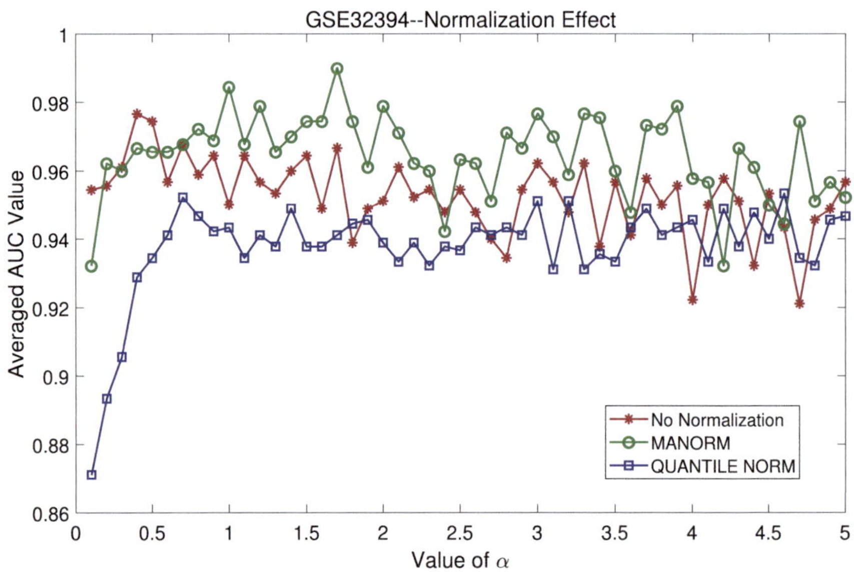

Fig. 4.12 Normalization effect on hadamard kernel: GSE32394

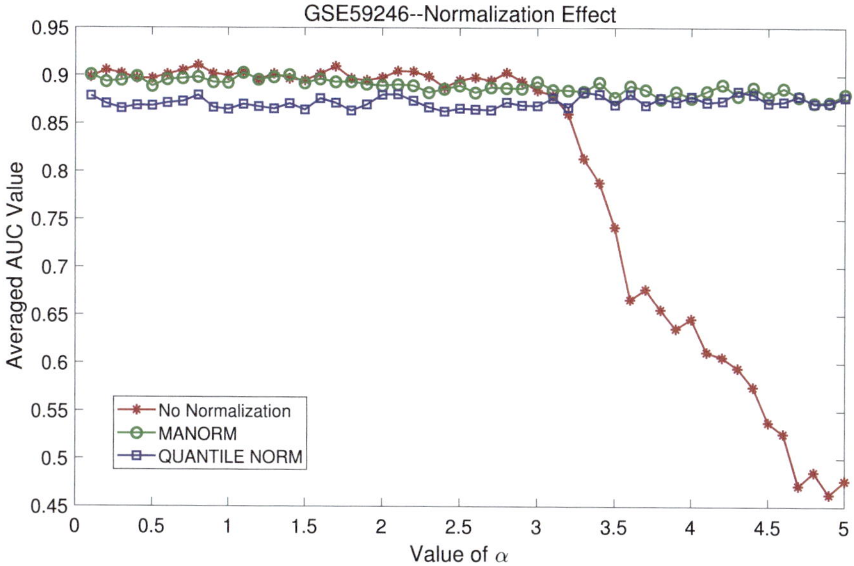

Fig. 4.13 Normalization effect on hadamard kernel: GSE59246

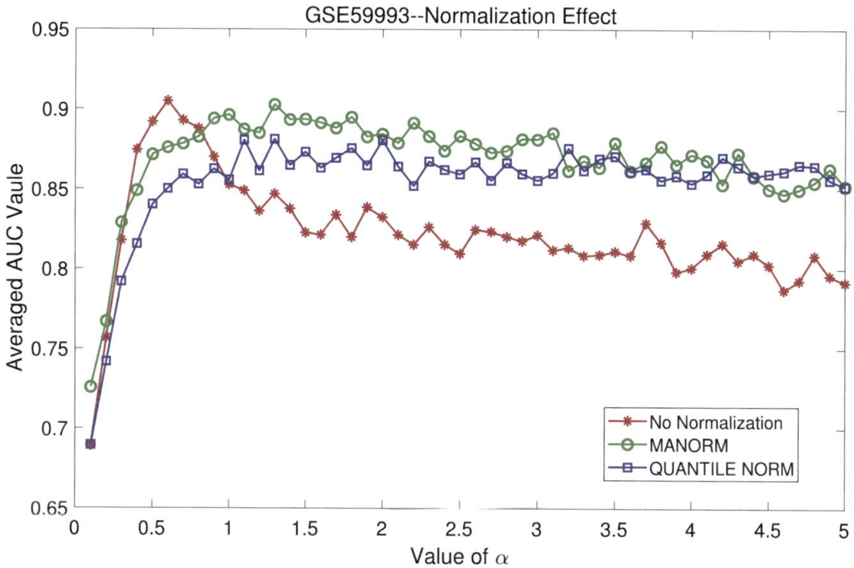

Fig. 4.14 Normalization effect on hadamard kernel: GSE59993

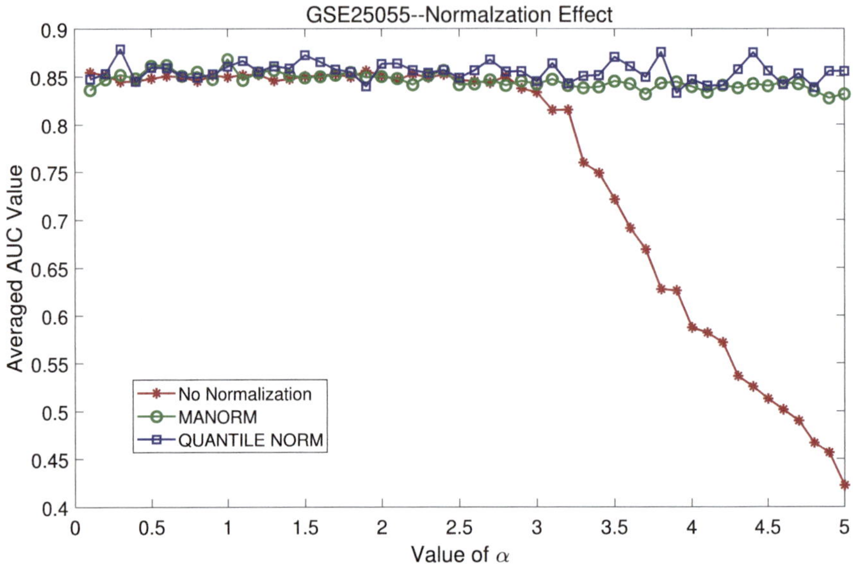

Fig. 4.15 Normalization effect on hadamard kernel: GSE25055

Table 4.4 Comparison of hadamard kernel on raw data and different methods on normalized data

Data sets methods	Linear kernel	Quadratic kernel	RBF kernel	Correlation kernel	Hadamard kernel
GSE1872	1	1	0.2367	0.9962	1
GSE32394	0.9556	0.9556	0.8500	0.9444	**0.9833**
GSE59246	0.8546	0.8546	0.8061	0.8626	**0.8849**
GSE59993	0.8521	0.8476	0.7977	0.8277	**0.8913**
GSE25055	0.8619	0.8615	0.7914	0.7715	**0.8590**

performs significantly better, competing with linear kernel. But Hadamard kernel still demonstrates the best. Normalization effect on linear kernel is demonstrated in GSE1872. We can see that after normalization the performance does improve. For RBF kernel, the performance in some data sets after normalization decreases. Possible reason is that we used the optimal σ selected for data without normalization. When normalization is imposed, perhaps the best σ has changed, and hence the performance in some data sets decreases.

As a generalization ability test on Hadamard kernel, we introduce some RNAseq data sets for validation. The results are illustrated in Table 4.5. One of the test data sets is obtained from NCBI GEO database, the accession number is GSE87517. Gene expression analyses in leukocytes sorted from normal breast tissues, ductal carcinomas in situ (DCIS), and HER2+ and triple negative invasive ductal carcinomas (IDC) were conducted. RNAseq counts are used to measure the expression levels.

Table 4.5 Comparison of hadamard kernel on raw data and different methods on normalized data (RNA)

Data sets methods	Linear kernel	Quadratic kernel	RBF kernel	Correlation kernel	Hadamard kernel
GSE87517	0.6022	0.4562	0.5459	0.7189	**0.9524**
GSE47462	0.7422	0.5322	0.4029	0.7506	**0.8949**
GSE48213	0.9990	0.9982	0.3375	0.9993	**0.9996**

We have 41 samples in total, and the number of attributes is 27011. We focus on differentiating normal samples from breast tumor samples. We conduct experiments on Hadamard kernel without data normalization and imposing quantile normalization on data for other methods. The best σ in RBF kernel and best α in Hadamard kernel are shown to be 0.01 and 0.2, respectively where details are presented in (Table 4.2). We further compare on Hadamard kernel with other kernel methods through fivefold cross-validations. Averaged AUC values are calculated as shown in Table 4.5. It can be seen that Hadamard kernel on raw data shows the best performance, achieving 0.9524 in AUC value. While the best performance in other kernels is achieved in Correlation kernel, yielding only 0.7189 in averaged AUC value.

One of the test data sets is also obtained from NCBI GEO database, the accession number is GSE47462. Raw counts of lncRNAs are used to measure the expression levels. We have 72 samples in total, of which 24 are normal, 25 early neoplasia, 9 carcinoma in situ, and 14 invasive cancer. The number of attributes is 2173. We focus on differentiating normal samples from breast tumor samples. We further compare Hadamard kernel with other kernel methods through 10 runs of fivefold cross-validations. Averaged AUC values are calculated and the results are reported in Table 4.5. It can be shown that Hadamard kernel is robust and can demonstrate satisfactory performance compared to other kernels even with data normalization. The average AUC value in Hadamard kernel is 0.8949 while in linear kernel 0.7422. The performance in RBF kernel is not satisfactory, achieving only 0.4029 in averaged AUC value.

The third data set is under accession number GSE48213. 56 breast cancer cell lines were profiled to identify patterns of gene expression associated with subtype and response to therapeutic compounds using RNAseq technology. There are 4 unknown cell lines, with 27 samples related to Luminal, 14 samples related to Basal like breast cancer, 5 normal samples and 6 samples of Claudin-low subtype. Subtype Luminal constitutes the majority of all the considered subtypes, hence we try to differentiate Luminal from others by removing the 4 unknown samples. Hadamard kernel on raw data can yield 0.9996 in average AUC value. The performance in other kernels after data normalization is also comparable except in RBF kernel. In addition, we also record the performance of the 4 compared kernels on considered RNAseq data sets without data normalization in Table 4.5.

In a word, we can see that Hadamard kernel is robust for dealing with expression data in general.

4.5 Conclusions

In this chapter, we propose Hadamard Kernel for breast cancer outcome predictions. It is a valid and effective kernel for dealing with high dimensional gene expression data when they are positive valued. In particular, we have given theoretical verification on the positive semi-definiteness of the kernel matrix for all kinds of data. Through comparison with classical kernels in SVM and correlation kernel that is good at cancer predictions, we show the superiority of Hadamard Kernel. The Hadamard kernel is flexible in varying the parameter α, the determination of optimal α can be devoted to our future work. We hope Hadamard kernel as a novel class of kernels can enrich kernel communities in SVM and contribute to the wider biological problems.

References

Aizerman MA (1964) Theoretical foundations of the potential function method in pattern recognition learning. Autom Remote Control 25:821–837

Asri H, Mousannif H, Moatassime HA, Noel T (2016) Using machine learning algorithms for breast cancer risk prediction and diagnosis. Procedia Comput Sci 83:1064–1069. The 7th international conference on ambient systems, networks and technologies (ANT 2016)/The 6th international conference on sustainable energy information technology (SEIT-2016)/Affiliated workshops

Bapat RB (1988) Multinomial probabilities, permanents and a conjecture of Karlin and Rinott. Proc Am Math Soc 102:467–472

Chaurasia V, Pal S (2014) Data mining techniques: to predict and resolve breast cancer survivability. Int J Comput Sci Mob Comput 3:10–22

Cortes C, Vapnik VN (1995) Support-vector networks. Mach Learn 20:273–297

Delen D, Walker G, Kadam A (2005) Predicting breast cancer survivability: a comparison of three data mining methods. Artif Intell Med 34(2):113–27

DeSantis CE, Siegel RL, Bandi P, Jemal A (2011) Breast cancer statistics. CA: A Cancer J Clin 61

Dudoit S, Fridlyand J, Speed TP (2002) Comparison of discrimination methods for the classification of tumors using gene expression data. J Am Stat Assoc 97:77–87

Endo A, Shibata T, Tanaka H (2008) Comparison of seven algorithms to predict breast cancer survival(contribution to 21 century intelligent technologies and bioinformatics). Biomed Fuzzy Hum Sci Off J Biomed Fuzzy Syst Assoc 13:11–16

Flach PA, Hernández-Orallo J, Ferri C (2011) A coherent interpretation of AUC as a measure of aggregated classification performance. In: International conference on machine learning

Hanley JA, McNeil BJ (1983) A method of comparing the areas under receiver operating characteristic curves derived from the same cases. Radiology 148:839–43

Jiang H, Ching WK (2012) Correlation kernels for support vector machines classification with applications in cancer data. Comput Math Methods Med 2012

Maglogiannis I, Zafiropoulos EP, Anagnostopoulos I (2009) An intelligent system for automated breast cancer diagnosis and prognosis using SVM based classifiers. Appl Intell 30:24–36

Mamitsuka H (2006) Selecting features in microarray classification using roc curves. Pattern Recognit

NCBI (National Center of Biotechnology Information) GEO (Gene Expression Omnibus) Repository. https://www.ncbi.nlm.nih.gov/gds/. Accessed 2 Mar 2017

Nemade V, Fegade V (2023) Machine learning techniques for breast cancer prediction. Procedia Comput Sci 218:1314–1320. https://doi.org/10.1016/j.procs.2023.01.110. https://www.sciencedirect.com/science/article/pii/S1877050923001102. International conference on machine learning and data engineering

Reams R (1999) Hadamard inverses, square roots and products of almost semidefinite matrices. Linear Algebra Appl 288:35–43

Scholkopf B, Smola A (2001) Learning with kernels: support vector machines, regularization, optimization, and beyond. In: Adaptive computation and machine learning series

van den Akker E, Verbruggen B, Heijmans BT, Beekman M, Kok JN, Slagboom E, Reinders MJT (2011) Integrating protein-protein interaction networks with gene- gene co-expression networks improves gene signatures for classifying breast cancer metastasis. J Integr Bioinform 8:222–238

van Vliet MH, Reyal F, Horlings HM, van de Vijver MJ, Reinders MJT, Wessels LFA (2008) Pooling breast cancer datasets has a synergetic effect on classification performance and improves signature stability. BMC Genomics 9:375

van de Vijver MJ, He Y, van t Veer LJ, Dai H, Hart AAM, Voskuil DW, Schreiber GJ, Peterse JL, Roberts CJ, Marton MJ, Parrish ML, Atsma DE, Witteveen AT, Glas AM, Delahaye LJ, van der Velde T, Bartelink H, Rodenhuis S, Rutgers EJ, Friend SH, Bernards R (2002) A gene-expression signature as a predictor of survival in breast cancer. N Engl J Med 347(25):1999–2009

van't Veer LJ, Dai H, van de Vijver MJ, He Y, Hart AAM, Mao M, Peterse HL, van der Kooy K, Marton MJ, Witteveen AT, Schreiber GJ, Kerkhoven RM, Roberts CJ, Linsley PS, Bernards R, Friend SH (2002) Gene expression profiling predicts clinical outcome of breast cancer. Nature 415:530–536

Chapter 5
Regularized Multiple Kernel Learning Framework

5.1 Introduction

Kernel methods have attracted considerable attention in machine learning area, such as pattern recognition (Smola and Schlkopf 1998; Sun et al. 2012), regression estimation (Wang 2003; Gautam et al. 2019; Tehrani 2021), function approximation (Pillonetto et al. 2014), owing to their capability of working not only with linear inference models, but also to identify nonlinear relationships among input patterns (Scholkopf et al. 1998; Cristianini and Shawe-Taylor 2007; Tang et al. 2019). The modelling of nonlinear relationships between input patterns has always been a critical task in machine learning, where kernel methods not only provide the possibility in a natural way, but also are largely founded on solid mathematics. In particular, the kernel methods (Zhang and Cao 2011) embed data into an Euclidean space of higher or infinite dimensions, and provide the flexibility of modelling the complex relationship among data samples without explicitly computing a huge number of and potentially infinite dimensional feature vector.

Kernels model the data relationships through kernel functions, where different data fit into different types of kernel functions. There are a number of well-known kernel functions in applications and theory. Among these kernels, the linear kernel (Chang and Lin 2006; Kim et al. 2015) and radial basis function (RBF) kernel (Chung et al. 2003; Ring and Eskofier 2016) are the most popular representatives. Polynomial kernel is also widely used (Meijering and Zuiderveld 1999; Zhou and Jetter 2006). For examples, Meijering and Zuiderveld (1999) developed symmetrical piecewise nth-order polynomial kernel functions to approximate sine-function in image reconstruction and Zhou and Jetter (2006) provided an error analysis for classification algorithms. Other promising kernels include sigmoid kernel (Lin and Lin 2003), generalized histogram kernel (Boughorbel et al. 2005), chi-square kernel (Daliri 2013) etc.

As a newly proposed kernel function, Hadamard kernel has been successfully applied in omics-data mining problems recently (Jiang et al. 2017). The Hadamard

H. Jiang and W.-K. Ching, *Kernel Methods for Omics Data Mining*, Intelligent Control and Learning Systems 10, https://doi.org/10.1007/978-981-95-3129-5_5

kernel is flexible in varying the kernel parameter. Theoretical verification has been given on the validity of the kernel for modelling all kinds of data (Jiang et al. 2017). Experiments showed its effectiveness in dealing with high dimensional gene expression data. Through comparison with classical kernels including linear kernel, quadratic kernel, RBF kernel and correlation kernel, Hadamard kernel can demonstrate superiority to achieve the best performance. However, it is yet unresolved how to select an appropriate kernel parameter for optimizing the performance of Hadamard kernels.

The selection of the kernel parameter in Support Vector Machines (SVMs) does not have a set of mature theory. Traditional SVM kernel parameter optimization methods obtain better kernel parameters through repeated experiments, but this method often results in high computational cost. Here we investigate the problem of kernel parameter optimization in Hadamard kernel SVMs, aiming to make full use of the superiority of Hadamard kernel in modeling relationships for complex data, while optimizing the performance of Hadamard kernels through effective optimization strategies.

5.2 Related Works

The selection of parameters plays an critical role to achieve the optimal performance (Tian and Wang 2012; Yin and Yin 2016). Various metaheuristics approaches have been employed to solve the parameter selection problem. In Huang (2009), an ant colony optimization approach was developed to optimize the kernel parameters and feature subset selections simultaneously. In Aydin et al. (2011), a multi-objective artificial immune algorithm was proposed for parameter optimization. In Huang and Wang (2006), the genetic algorithm was employed. In Lin and Chien (2009), the cat swarm optimization (CSO) approach was adopted for kernel parameter optimization. In Kolomvatsos and Hadjieftymiades (2014), the kernel SVM is combined with the particle swarm optimization (PSO) technique to generate an optimal design of synchronous reluctance motor, which is superior to the conventional PSO.

An alternative direction for optimizing kernel parameters is to derive closed formulas (Tian and Wang 2012; Xu et al. 2009; Jiang et al. 2017). In Tian and Wang (2012), kernel parameter optimization with the Gaussian kernel for binary-class problems was achieved using centered kernel polarization. In Xu et al. (2009), a direct setting formula was proposed for the kernel parameters by a multi-objective artificial immune algorithm, inspired by theoretical immune system. Successful applications to fault diagnosis of induction motors and anomaly detection problems have verified the proposed scheme.

In Chap. 2, the optimal kernel parameter was derived by the Bregman matrix divergence theory, and we proposed LogDet divergence and perturbed von-Neumann divergence to measure kernel relationships. Consequently, we found the suggested optimal parameter in the projection method using unconstrained optimization in kernel learning. The superiority has been verified by several experimental validations.

Kernel-based learning methods realize parameter optimization in a new perspective. Many powerful kernel-based learning methods have been developed such as SVMs (Cortes and Vapnik 1995; Informatik and Scholkopf 2000; Zheng et al. 2021; Li et al. 2021), kernel Fisher discriminant (KFD) (Roth and Steinhage 2000; Baudat and Anouar 2000) using kernel tricks representing dot products by kernel functions, and kernel Principal Component Analysis (KPCA) (Mika et al. 1999; Scholkopf et al. 1999; Qaraei et al. 2021). By optimizing a linear combination of base kernels, the Multiple Kernel Learning (MKL) offers an important technique in kernel learning (Guo et al. 2021). It was initially introduced in Lanckriet et al. (2002), where the kernel matrix is learned through semi-definite programming. L_1-MKL has been shown effective in identifying the appropriate combination of data sources over heterogeneous data fusion in real-world applications (Lanckriet et al. 2004; Ratsch et al. 2005), where the framework establishes a sparse linear combination of candidate kernels. However, L_1-MKL may be inappropriate when a simplex solution space may discard critical information (Xu et al. 2021). Non-sparse MKL alternatively provides a new way to optimize kernel combinations. For example, L_2-MKL introduced a L_2-regularization to allow for non-sparse kernel mixtures (Kloft et al. 2008). L_p-norm regularized MKL was proposed in Kloft et al. (2009), where two efficient optimization strategies for $p > 1$ were developed. The L_p-MKL help achieve accuracies that go beyond the existing method (Lv and Zhou 2015). A mixed norm setting to learn multiple kernel classifiers is given in Kowalski et al. (2009), which can be applied to indefinite kernels while guaranteeing the sparsity structure. As a generalized version of L_1-MKL and L_2-MKL, an elastic-net-type constraint was considered to seek the optimal kernel combination weights for generating a favorable MKL model. The generalized MKL framework enjoys the favorable sparsity property on the solution and facilitates the grouping effect (Yang et al. 2011). The optimal kernel learning is studied in Shiju et al. (2017) for the linear combination of composite kernel functions. The matrix regularized MKL (Han et al. 2018), an extension of the above-mentioned MKL frameworks, has been proposed to explore the interactions of kernels. Theoretical guarantee based on Rademacher complexity bound was provided on the superiority of L_p-MKL in non-sparse scenario. Besides, experiments show the high-order regularization framework tend to be more favorable.

In general, L_p $(p > 1)$ space form an important class of Banach spaces that are separable, reflexive, and uniform convex. In particular, L_4-norm demonstrates a number of intriguing properties. The L_4-norm objective is smooth that is amenable for better optimization. It has been long used spherical harmonics, and the Stanton-Weinstein Theorem (Stanton and Weinstein 1981) showed that L_4-norm is locally maximized by the 'highest-weight' function among all the L_2-normalized spherical harmonics of a given degree. Independent component analysis also made full use of the 4th-order statistical cumulants. Besides, the understanding and usage of L_4-norm can also be justified in terms of sum of squares (Zhai et al. 2020). It quite fits into the framework of multiple kernel learning with a number of parameters for optimization.

In this chapter, we focus on the Hadamard kernel to introduce our main idea. Inspired by MKL technique for optimizing the kernel combination and the nice properties that L_4-norm possesses, we propose an $L_4L_p(p > 1)$ norm-product regularized MKL framework of Hadamard kernel functions over a number of candidate parameters, where the concrete best parameter is no need to explicitly specified but the linear combination coefficients are optimized. Three loss functions, i.e., hinge loss, log loss and square loss, are employed in the proposed MKL framework and then the dual optimization problems are derived according to the duality theory. Extensive experiments have been conducted to show the superiority of the proposed MKL framework by comparing with single Hadamard kernel technique with different kernel parameters and other kernel SVMs. Results demonstrate that our L_4L_p-MKL framework achieve the best performance by optimizing the linear combination of a limited number of Hadamard kernel candidates. This framework provides a novel effective way to obtain SVMs of high performance.

The rest of this chapter is arranged as follows. Section 5.3 presents the L_4L_p-MKL framework and specifies the optimization problem under the three aforementioned loss functions. Section 5.4 shows experiments on L_4L_p-MKL framework over a number of data sets and demonstrates the superiority of the high-order multiple kernel learning framework over various kernels with single parameter including Hadamard kernel, linear kernel and RBF kernel. Discussions on the capability of L_4L_p-MKL framework for optimizing parameterized kernels like RBF kernel are also provided. Section 5.5 concludes the chapter.

5.3 Method

5.3.1 Hadamard Kernel

Assume we have a data set $\mathbb{D}$ of n labeled data instances with corresponding class annotations:

$$\{(\mathbf{x}_1, y_1), \ldots, (\mathbf{x}_n, y_n)\}$$

where $\mathbf{x}_i \in \mathbf{R}^p$, $y_i \in \{-1, 1\}$, $i = 1, 2, \ldots, n$. The definition for Hadamard kernel function on the given data set is shown as follows (Jiang et al. 2017):

$$K_\alpha(\mathbf{x}_i, \mathbf{x}_j) = \sum_{k=1}^{p} \frac{|x_{ik}|^\alpha |x_{jk}|^\alpha}{2(|x_{ik}|^\alpha + |x_{jk}|^\alpha)}, \qquad i, j = 1, 2, \ldots, n.$$

Here $\alpha \neq 0$ is a flexible parameter within the kernel matrix. For some k, if $x_{ik} = 0$, then $\frac{|x_{ik}|^\alpha |x_{jk}|^\alpha}{(|x_{ik}|^\alpha + |x_{jk}|^\alpha)}$ is defined as 0. It has been shown in Jiang et al. (2017) that Hadamard kernel K_α is semi-positive definite for any data matrix $\mathbb{D}$.

The Hadamard kernels with varying parameters α constitute a broad range of kernel families which can fit all kinds of data matrix. Hence, it is critical to select an appropriate parameter α for the Hadamard kernel in applications. For more details of the Hadamard kernel, the readers can refer to Chap. 4.

5.3.2 Hadamard-MKL

The Hadamard MKL framework considers learning a linear combination of Hadamard kernels K_{α_i}, where α_i are nonzero kernel parameters, $i = 1, 2, \ldots, m$. The optimized MKL K can be represented as follows:

$$K = \sum_{i=1}^{m} \mu_i K_{\alpha_i}, \tag{5.1}$$

where μ_i are the non-negative kernel weights, $i = 1, 2, \ldots, m$.

The primal optimization problem with $L_4 L_p$-norm product regularization can be expressed as:

$$\begin{aligned} \min_{\mathbf{w},b,\mathbf{t},\mu} \quad & C\sum_{i=1}^{n} l(t_i, y_i) + \frac{1}{2}\sum_{i=1}^{m}\frac{||\mathbf{w}_i||_{H_i}^2}{\mu_i} \\ \text{s.t.} \quad & \sum_{i=1}^{m} < \mathbf{w}_i, \phi_i(\mathbf{x}_j) >_{H_i} +b = t_j, \\ & \qquad j = 1, 2, \ldots, n \\ & \|\mu\|_4 ||\mu||_p \leq 1, \quad \mu \geq 0, \end{aligned} \tag{5.2}$$

where $\mu = (\mu_1, \mu_2, \ldots, \mu_m)$, $|| \cdot ||_4$ is the L_4 norm, $|| \cdot ||_p$ is L_p norm, and $|| \cdot ||_{H_i}$ denotes the Hilbertian norm of H_i. Furthermore, C is the regularization parameter, $l(t_i, y_i)$ is the loss function between t_i and y_i, and $\mathbf{w}$ is a parameter vector.

We derive the dual problem through the Lagrange multiplier method. To this end, we first obtain the Lagrangian $\mathbb{L}$ of the above problem:

$$\begin{aligned} \mathbb{L} = & \, C\sum_{i=1}^{n} l(t_i, y_i) + \frac{1}{2}\sum_{i=1}^{m}\frac{||\mathbf{w}_i||_{H_i}^2}{\mu_i} \\ & - \sum_{j=1}^{n}\gamma_j\left(\sum_{i=1}^{m} < \mathbf{w}_i, \phi_i(\mathbf{x}_j) >_{H_i} +b - t_j\right) \\ & + \lambda\left(\frac{1}{2}\|\mu\|_4||\mu||_p - \frac{1}{2}\right) - \eta^{\mathbf{T}}\mu, \end{aligned} \tag{5.3}$$

where $\gamma \in \mathbf{R}^n$, $\lambda \in \mathbf{R}^+$, and $\eta \in \mathbf{R}^m$ are the Lagrange multipliers.

Setting the partial derivatives of $\mathbb{L}$ with respect to $\mathbf{w}$ and b to zero, we get

$$\begin{aligned} & \mathbf{w}_j = \mu_j \sum_{i=1}^{n} \gamma_i \phi_j(\mathbf{x}_i), \ \ j = 1, 2, \ldots, n \\ & \gamma^T \mathbf{1} = 0. \end{aligned}$$

Hence, the Lagrangian problem can be rewritten as follows:

$$\max_{\substack{\gamma,\lambda,\eta,\\ \gamma^T\mathbf{1}=0,\\ \lambda\geq 0,\eta\geq 0}} \min_{\mathbf{t},\mu} \Bigg\{ C\sum_{i=1}^{n}(l(t_i, y_i) + \frac{\mu_i t_i}{C}) + \frac{1}{2}\sum_{i=1}^{m}\mu_i\gamma^T K_{\alpha_i}\gamma + \lambda(\frac{1}{2}\|\mu\|_4\|\mu\|_p - \frac{1}{2}) - \eta^{\mathbf{T}}\mu \Bigg\},$$

which is equivalent to

$$\max_{\substack{\gamma,\lambda,\eta,\\ \gamma^T\mathbf{1}=0,\\ \lambda\geq 0,\eta\geq 0}} \Bigg\{ -C\sum_{i=1}^{n}\max_{t_i}\Big\{-l(t_i, y_i) - \frac{\mu_i t_i}{C}\Big\} - \lambda\max_{\mu}\Big\{\frac{1}{\lambda}\sum_{i=1}^{m}\mu_i(\frac{1}{2}\gamma^T K_{\alpha_i}\gamma + \eta_i) - \frac{1}{2}\|\mu\|_4\|\mu\|_p\Big\} - \frac{\lambda}{2}\Bigg\}.$$

Based on Fenchel duality theory, we can derive the Lagrangian as

$$\max_{\substack{\gamma,\lambda,\eta,\\ \gamma^T\mathbf{1}=0,\\ \lambda\geq 0,\eta\geq 0}} \Bigg\{ -C\sum_{i=1}^{n} l^*(-\frac{\gamma_i}{C}, y_i) - \frac{1}{\lambda}\|G\|_s\|G\|_q - \frac{\lambda}{2}\Bigg\}, \tag{5.4}$$

where $G = (\frac{1}{2}\gamma^T K_{\alpha_i}\gamma + \eta_i)_{i=1}^m \in \mathbf{R}^m$ and $l^*(\cdot)$ denotes the dual loss.

Plugging $\lambda^* = \|G\|_{\frac{4}{3}}^{\frac{1}{2}}\|G\|_q^{\frac{1}{2}}$, where $p^{-1} + q^{-1} = 1$, into the optimization problem (5.4), we obtain

$$\max_{\substack{\gamma,\eta,\\ \gamma^T\mathbf{1}=0,\\ \eta\geq 0}} \Bigg\{ -C\sum_{i=1}^{n} l^*(-\frac{\gamma_i}{C}, y_i) - \|G\|_{\frac{4}{3}}^{\frac{1}{2}}\|G\|_q^{\frac{1}{2}}\Bigg\}. \tag{5.5}$$

Therefore, the final dual problem would be different when different loss functions are considered. To this end, we hereby present three specific loss functions, namely, hinge loss, log loss, and square loss, in detail. The results are given in the following proposition.

Proposition 5.1 *For the final dual problem* (5.5), *the derivations are given below.*

(1) Dual Problem under Hinge Loss:
Consider the hinge loss

$$l_{hinge}(t, y) = \max(0, 1 - ty).$$

Then, the dual loss becomes

$$l^*_{hinge}(t, y) = \begin{cases} \frac{t}{y}, & if\ -1 \le \frac{t}{y} \le 0, \\ \infty, & elsewise. \end{cases}$$

Therefore, we have

$$-1 \le -\frac{\gamma_i}{C y_i} \le 0 \to 0 \le \frac{\gamma_i}{y_i} \le C.$$

The final dual problem ($\eta^* = 0$) becomes

$$\begin{aligned} &\max_{\gamma} \ \ \mathbf{1}^T \gamma - \|G\|_{\frac{4}{3}}^{\frac{1}{2}} \|G\|_q^{\frac{1}{2}} \\ &s.t. \ \ \mathbf{y}^T \gamma = 0 \ \ and \ \ \mathbf{0} \le \gamma \le C\mathbf{1} \end{aligned}$$

where $G = (\frac{1}{2}(\gamma \otimes \mathbf{y})^T K_{\alpha_i} (\gamma \otimes \mathbf{y}))_{i=1}^m \in R^m$ and $\otimes$ denotes the element-wise product.

(2) Dual Problem under Log Loss:
Consider the log loss

$$l_{\log}(t, y) = \log(1 + \exp(-ty)).$$

Then, the dual loss becomes

$$l^*_{log}(t, y) = \begin{cases} -\frac{t}{y} \log(-\frac{t}{y}) + (1 + \frac{t}{y}) \log(1 + \frac{t}{y}), & if\ -1 \le \frac{t}{y} \le 0 \\ \infty, & elsewise. \end{cases}$$

The final dual problem ($\eta^* = 0$) becomes

$$\begin{aligned} &\max_{\gamma} \ \ \left\{ \mathbf{1}^T (\gamma \otimes \log \frac{\gamma}{C} + (C - \gamma) \otimes \log(1 - \frac{\gamma}{C})) - \|G\|_{\frac{4}{3}}^{\frac{1}{2}} \|G\|_q^{\frac{1}{2}} \right\} \\ &s.t. \ \ \mathbf{y}^T \gamma = 0 \ \ and \ \ \mathbf{0} \le \gamma \le C\mathbf{1} \end{aligned}$$

where

$$G = \left(\frac{1}{2} (\gamma \otimes \mathbf{y})^T K_{\alpha_i} (\gamma \otimes \mathbf{y}) \right)_{i=1}^m \in \boldsymbol{R}^m.$$

(3) Dual Problem under Square Loss:
Consider the square loss

$$l_{square}(t, y) = \frac{1}{2}(1 - ty)^2.$$

Then, the dual loss becomes

$$l^*_{square}(t, y) = \begin{cases} \frac{t}{y} + \frac{1}{2}\frac{t^2}{y^2}, & if \ \frac{t}{y} \le 0 \\ \infty, & elsewise. \end{cases}$$

The final dual problem ($\eta^* = 0$) becomes

$$\begin{aligned} \max_{\gamma} \ & \mathbf{1}^T(\gamma + \frac{1}{2C}\gamma \otimes \gamma) - \|G\|_{\frac{4}{3}}^{\frac{1}{2}} \|G\|_{q}^{\frac{1}{2}} \\ s.t. \ & \mathbf{y}^T\gamma = 0 \ \ and \ \ \mathbf{0} \le \gamma \end{aligned}$$

where

$$G = (\frac{1}{2}(\gamma \otimes \mathbf{y})^T K_{\alpha_i}(\gamma \otimes \mathbf{y}))_{i=1}^m \in \boldsymbol{R}^m.$$

5.3.3 Optimizing Strategy

In the proposed Hadamard MKL framework, we try to optimize

$$\begin{aligned} \min_{\mathbf{w}, b, \mu, \epsilon \ge 0} \ & C \sum_{i=1}^{n} \epsilon_i + \frac{1}{2} \sum_{i=1}^{m} \frac{||\mathbf{w}_i||^2_{H_i}}{\mu_i} \\ \text{s.t.} \ & \sum_{i=1}^{m} < \mathbf{w}_i, \phi_i(\mathbf{x}_j) >_{H_i} + b \ge 1 - \epsilon_i, \\ & \qquad j = 1, 2, \ldots, n, \\ & \|\mu\|_4 ||\mu||_p \le 1, \quad \mu \ge 0. \end{aligned}$$

The framework differs from the traditional multiple kernel learning frameworks as the extra constraint $\|\mu\|_4||\mu||_p \le 1$ is imposed. This constraint denotes the L_4L_p-norm product regulation term help fit into the framework of multiple kernel learning with a number of parameters for optimization.

This optimization problem can be equivalently written as follows:

$$\begin{aligned} \min_{\substack{\mathbf{w}, b, \mu, \\ \boldsymbol{\mu} \ge 0}} \ & \left\{ C \sum_{j=1}^{n} l \left(\sum_{i=1}^{m} < \mathbf{w}_i, \phi_i(\mathbf{x}_j) >_{H_i} + b, y_j \right) \right. \\ & \left. + \frac{\rho}{2} \|\mu\|_4 ||\boldsymbol{\mu}||_p + \frac{1}{2} \sum_{i=1}^{m} \frac{||\mathbf{w}_i||^2_{H_i}}{\mu_i} \right\}. \end{aligned} \tag{5.6}$$

We can employ alternating optimization strategy (Han et al. 2018) to update the parameters in the optimization framework. The specific procedure is given as follows:

1. Fixing μ, Optimizing $(\mathbf{w}, b)$:

$$||\mathbf{w}_i||_{H_i}^2 = \mu_i^2(\gamma \otimes \mathbf{y})^T K_{\alpha_i}(\gamma \otimes \mathbf{y}). \tag{5.7}$$

2. Fixing $(\mathbf{w}, b)$, Optimizing μ: Differentiating on μ, we obtain

$$\mu_i = \frac{\frac{||\mathbf{w}_{\mu_i}||_{H_i}^2}{\left(\frac{\mu_i}{||\mu||_4}\right)^4 + \left(\frac{\mu_i}{||\mu||_p}\right)^p}}{\sum_{i=1}^m || \left(\mathbf{w}_{\mu_i}||_{H_i}^{2p}\right)^{\frac{1}{2p}} \cdot \sum_{i=1}^m || \left(\mathbf{w}_{\mu_i}||_{H_i}^8\right)^{\frac{1}{8}}}. \tag{5.8}$$

5.4 Numerical Experiments

In this section, we show experimental results of the proposed Hadamard-MKL framework and its compared partners over a number of publicly available data sets as well as simulation data sets.

5.4.1 *Materials*

We have incorporated a number of publicly available data sets and two simulated datasets into results evaluation. The details are given below.

- **Heart**
  Heart data is extracted from UCI Machine Learning Repository (UCI 2025) that contains 270 data instances, each data instance is described by 13 attributes including age, sex, blood pressure etc. The label information is indicated by the absence or presence of heart disease. There are 120 heart disease instances and the remaining 150 are healthy controls.
- **Diabetes**
  The Diabetes data set was created by National Institute of Diabetes and Digestive Kidney Diseases, and it was downloaded from UCI machine learning repository (UCI 2025). It contains 768 instances where each instance was described by 8 variables: 'Pregnancies', 'Glucose', 'BloodPressure', 'SkinThickness', 'Insulin', 'BMI', 'DiabetesPedigreeFunction', 'Age'.
- **Credit Approval**
  This data set describes credit card applications (UCI 2025). It is an interesting data set as it is a good mix of attributes: continuous, nominal with small numbers

of values, and nominal with larger numbers of values. The data set contains 690 instances with 15 attributes. There are 307 positive applicants and 383 are negative applications.

- **Colon Cancer**
  This data set was obtained from NCBI GEO database (NCBI GEO DataBase 2025), the accession number is GSE49246. It was microRNA profiling of colon tumor tissues vs adjacent normal tissues, containing 40 tumor samples and 40 normal samples. The top 100 differentially expressed microRNA attributes were selected for performance evaluation.
- **Prostate Cancer**
  This data set was obtained from NCBI GEO database (NCBI GEO DataBase 2025), the accession number is GSE76260. In this dataset, miRNA expression profiles were evaluated in a series of 64 prostate clinical specimens, including 32 cancer and 32 non-neoplastic tissues. The top 100 differentially expressed microRNA attributes were selected for performance evaluation.
- **Simulation_Uniform**
  A (0, 1) uniformly distributed data matrix $A_0 \in \mathbf{R}^{100\times 5}$ is generated, denoting a 100 samples characterized by 5 different features, and the 100 samples are denoted as negative class. For control purpose, we perturb each entry $A_0(i, j)$ to be $A_0(i, j) + 0.1$ and denote the corresponding 100 samples as positive class.
- **Simulation_Beta**
  Data matrix $A_0 \in \mathbf{R}^{100\times 5}$ with beta distribution of shape parameters $(1, 2)$ is generated, and the 100 samples are denoted as negative class. For control purpose, we perturb each entry $A_0(i, j)$ to be $A_0(i, j) + 0.1$ and denote the corresponding 100 samples as positive class.

5.4.2 *Performance Evaluation*

5.4.2.1 5-Fold Cross Validation

Cross validation is a standard way to evaluate the supervised learning model. The 5-fold cross validation is performed, where the training data set $\mathcal{M}$ is randomly divided into 5 subsets $\mathcal{M}_1, \ldots, \mathcal{M}_5$ of approximately equal size. The prediction model is trained on 4 subsets and the remaining subset is treated as the test set. Repeat this process 5 times such that each subset is tested once. All the prediction results are recorded for the computation of prediction accuracy.

5.4.2.2 Area Under the Receiver Operating Characteristic (ROC) Curve

The ROC curve is a graphical plot of False Positive Rate (FPR) vs. True Positive Rate (TPR) as x and y axes, respectively, for a binary classifier system as its discrimination threshold is varied. FPR and TPR are defined as follows:

$$\text{FPR} = \frac{fp}{tn + fp} \quad \text{and} \quad \text{TPR} = \frac{tp}{tp + fn}.$$

TPR determines the classifier's performance on classifying positive instances correctly among all positive samples available during the test, while FPR defines how many incorrect positive results occur among all negative samples available during the test. Each prediction result represents one point on the ROC curve. The area under the ROC curve (AUC) (Hanley and Mcneil 1983; Mamitsuka 2006) is a widely adopted statistics for assessing the discriminatory capacity of models. It can be interpreted as a measure of aggregated classification performance, and also the tradeoff between specificity and sensitivity (Flach et al. 2011).

5.4.3 Compared Partners

To evaluate the performance of the proposed Hadamard MKL method under L_4L_p regularization, we conduct experimental comparisons from multiple perspectives.

1. **Comparison with Different MKL Methods**
   The proposed Hadamard MKL framework under L_4L_p regularization, where $p = 3, 4$, is first compared with MKL methods with L_1, L_2, L_3, and L_4 regularization: L_1-MKL, L_2-MKL and L_p-MKL. In addition, the results are compared with MKL framework under norm-product L_iL_j regularization, $i \neq j, 1 \leq i, j \leq 4$.
2. **Comparison with Different Kernel SVMs**
   Apart from MKL framework comparisons, the proposed framework is also compared with SVM methods in conjunction with Hadamard kernels under different parameters (Hadamard-SVM). The purpose is to check whether the MKL idea can help guarantee a robust and reliable performance. Besides, we also compare the proposed Hadamard MKL method with RBF kernel SVM (RBF-SVM) and linear SVMs (Linear SVM). In other words, our purpose is to check whether the Hadamard kernel has advantages in evaluating data relationships.
3. **Comparison in Loss Functions**
   We also evaluate the performance of the proposed Hadamard MKL framework under three different loss functions: hinge loss, log loss, and square loss.

5.4.4 Computational Results

In this subsection, we will show the performance of the Hadamard-MKL with $L_4L_p(p = 3, 4)$ and the other comparative methods as tested on real-world data sets and simulation data sets. We employed the AUC measured by running 10 times the fivefold cross-validation to evaluate their performance. All the experiments are conducted using Matlab R2017b under Window 7 Operations System.

In the initial stage, we determine the optimal C^* for each data set in the training phase where C is set to 1 and 10 individually. The determined optimal Cs for each data set is marked by star.

5.4.4.1 Results on Multiple Kernel Learning Comparisons

Table 5.1 shows the averaged AUC values for different MKL algorithms on the considered datasets. In Table 5.1 and throughout the rest of our discussion, HMKL is short for the Hadamard MKL. We can see that most of the MKL algorithms perform in a similar manner, expect for the MKL algorithm with regularization term including L_1 norm. In the colon cancer data set, when $C = 1$, L_1-MKL algorithm can only achieve an average AUC value 0.850, showing the worst performance among all the MKL algorithms. Besides, MKL-L_1L_2 (with average AUC value 0.868) and MKL-L_1L_3 (with average AUC value 0.886) are also among the worst algorithms in accuracy evaluation perspective. In prostate cancer data, when $C = 1$, L_1-MKL algorithm still shows the worst performance with averaged AUC value 0.851. But when $C = 10$, we can see that L_1-MKL algorithm demonstrates the best performance. Hence the performance of L_1-MKL algorithm is relatively unstable. Considering our proposed high order norm-product MKL methods, they tend to perform in a relatively robust manner where they achieve most of the best AUC values on the considered datasets. From the above observations, we can conclude that it is better to choose high-order norm-product MKL algorithm for its robustness in performance on both real-world datasets as well as simulation data sets.

5.4.4.2 Results on Kernel SVMs

- **Results on Hadamard Kernel SVM**

  Figures 5.1, 5.2, 5.3, 5.4, 5.5, 5.6 and 5.7 show the comparison results on Hadamard kernel SVM under different parameters. In each figure, we plot on the left-hand side the averaged AUC values for Hadamard kernel SVM when kernel parameter ranges from 0.05 to 2 with step-size 0.05. On the right-hand side of the figure, we show the averaged AUC values obtained by our proposed high order norm-product Hadamard MKL: HMKL-L_3L_4 and HMKL-L_4L_4. In our Hadamard MKL framework, we consider 10 candidate kernels under the kernel parameters 0.05 to 0.5 with step-size 0.05 for final optimal kernel construction.

  Figure 5.1 shows the averaged AUC values on Hadamard kernel SVM under different parameters in heart data. We find that Hadamard kernel SVM cannot converge when kernel parameter is greater than 1.4, meaning that the kernel parameter setting needs to be properly estimated, large kernel parameter may make the problem divergent. For kernel parameters in [0.05, 1.3], the averaged AUC values on heart data is steadily increasing and become stable. In comparison, the averaged AUC values obtained by HMKL-L_3L_4 and HMKL-L_4L_4: 0.909 are near optimal

Table 5.1 Performance comparison on multiple kernel learning algorithms under hinge loss

Datasets	HMKL-L_4L_3	HMKL-L_4^2	L_1-HMKL	L_2-HMKL	L_3-HMKL	HMKL-L_1L_2	HMKL-L_1L_3	HMKL-L_1L_4	HMKL-L_2L_3	HMKL-L_2L_4
Heart C^*=1	0.909	0.909	0.909	0.909	0.909	0.909	0.908	**0.909**	0.909	0.909
Heart C=10	0.902	0.902	0.909	0.905	0.903	0.905	0.903	0.902	0.903	0.902
Diabetes C=1	0.834	0.835	0.827	0.832	0.834	0.828	0.830	0.832	0.834	0.834
Diabetes C^*=10	**0.837**	**0.837**	0.836	0.836	0.837	0.836	0.836	0.836	0.836	0.836
Credit C=1	0.922	0.922	0.922	0.921	0.922	0.922	0.921	0.922	0.922	0.922
Credit C^*=10	**0.926**	**0.926**	0.923	0.925	0.926	0.924	0.925	0.925	0.925	0.925
Colon C=1	0.909	0.913	0.850	0.889	0.905	0.868	0.886	0.895	0.899	0.906
Colon C^*=10	**0.994**	**0.994**	0.990	0.993	0.994	0.992	0.993	0.994	0.994	0.994
Prostate C^*=1	0.861	0.861	0.851	0.860	0.864	0.860	0.864	0.861	0.864	0.861
Prostate C=10	0.843	0.843	0.855	0.853	0.847	0.853	0.847	0.843	0.847	0.843
Simulation-uniform C=1	0.726	0.726	0.720	0.723	0.725	0.723	0.725	0.726	0.725	0.726
Simulation-uniform C^*=10	**0.733**	**0.733**	0.732	0.731	0.731	0.731	0.731	0.733	0.731	0.733
Simulation-beta C^*=1	0.806	0.806	0.798	0.801	0.806	0.801	0.804	0.806	0.804	0.806
Simulation-beta C=10	**0.807**	**0.807**	0.806	0.807	0.807	0.807	0.807	0.807	0.807	0.807

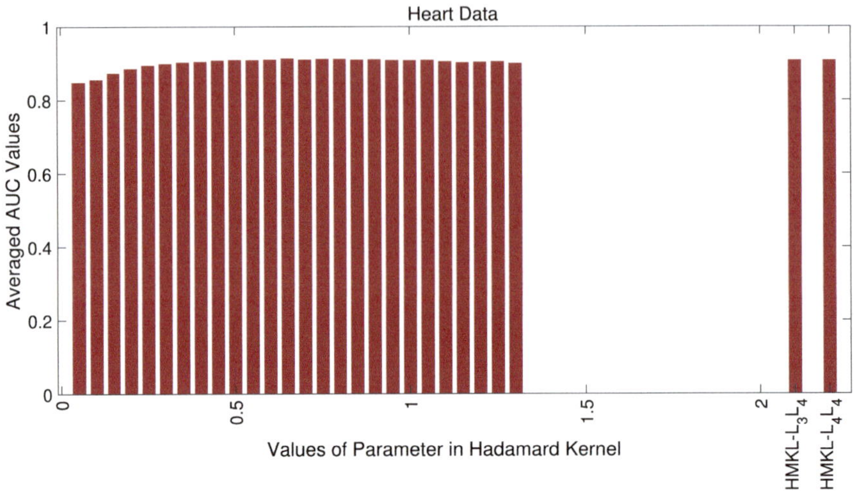

Fig. 5.1 AUC comparisons with Hadamard Kernel SVM under different parameters in heart data

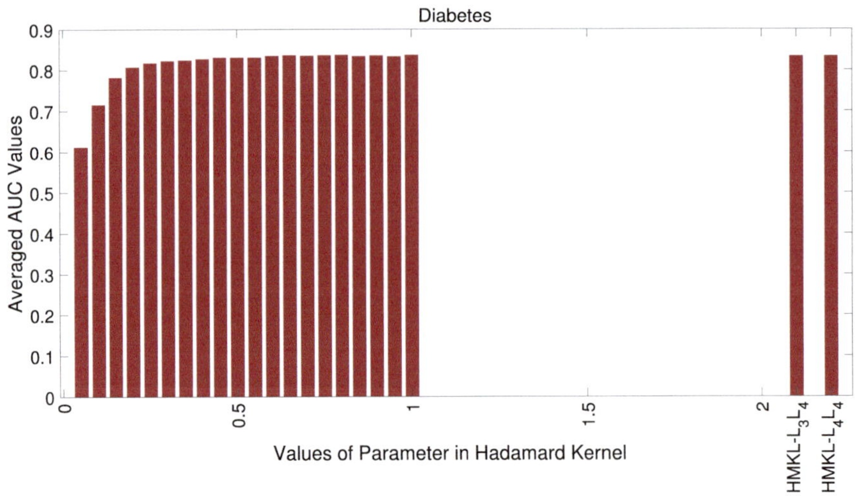

Fig. 5.2 AUC comparisons with Hadamard kernel SVM under different parameters in diabetes data

compared to Hadamard kernel SVM on all possible parameters whose optimal AUC value is 0.910.

Figure 5.2 shows the averaged AUC values on Hadamard kernel SVM under different parameters in diabetes data. We find that Hadamard kernel SVM cannot converge when kernel parameter was greater than 1. When kernel parameter is very small, say 0.05, the performance of Hadamard kernel SVM is not satisfactory, achieving only 0.62 in averaged AUC value. For kernel parameters in

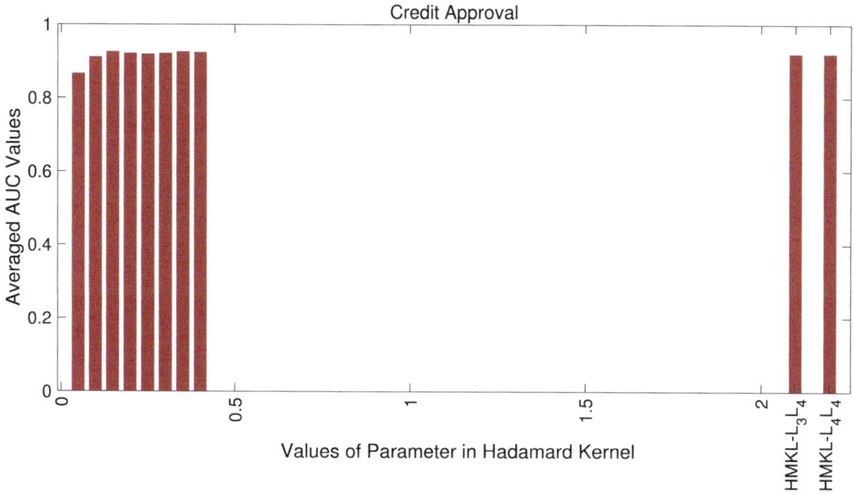

Fig. 5.3 AUC comparisons with Hadamard kernel SVM under different parameters in credit data

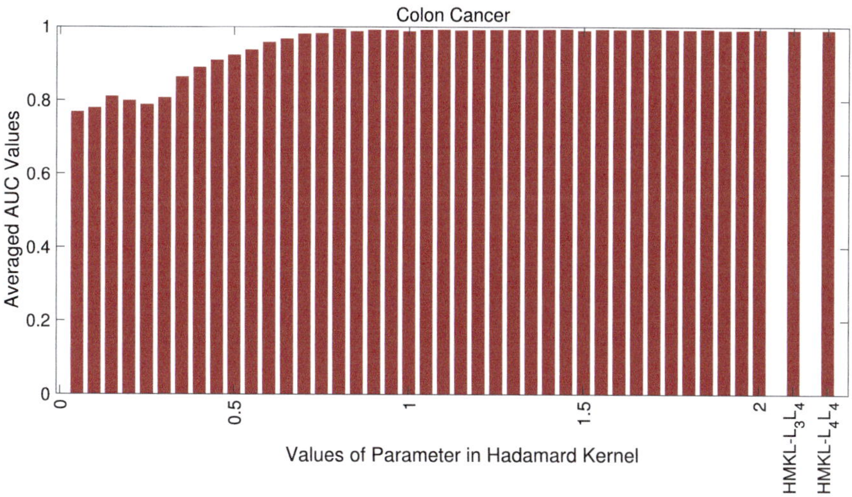

Fig. 5.4 AUC comparisons with Hadamard kernel SVM under different parameters in colon data

[0.05, 1], the averaged AUC value on diabetes data was steadily increasing and become stable. In comparison, the averaged AUC values obtained by HMKL-L_3L_4 and HMKL-L_4L_4: 0.84 are optimal compared to Hadamard kernel SVM on all possible parameters whose optimal averaged AUC value is 0.84 as well.

Figure 5.3 shows the averaged AUC values on Hadamard kernel SVM under different parameters in credit approval data. When kernel parameter is 0.05, Hadamard kernel SVM achieves the averaged AUC value 0.87. When kernel parameter is 0.1, Hadamard kernel SVM achieves the averaged AUC value 0.91. We find that

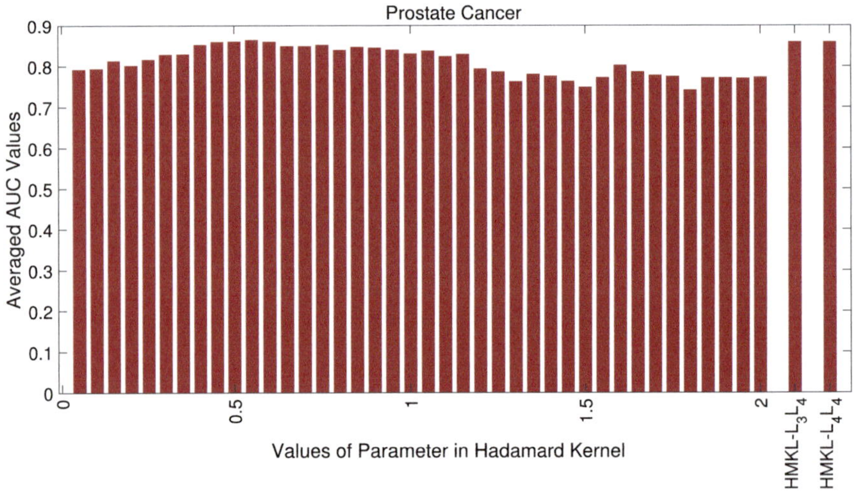

Fig. 5.5 AUC comparisons with Hadamard kernel SVM under different parameters in prostate cancer data

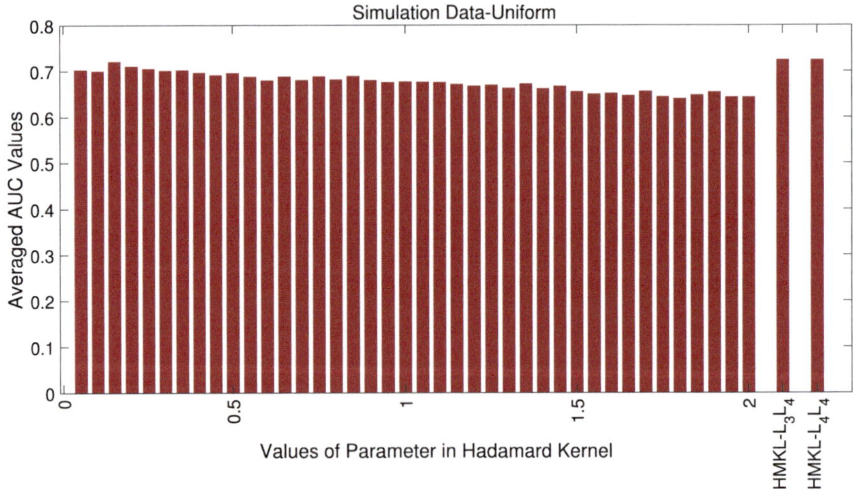

Fig. 5.6 AUC comparisons with Hadamard kernel SVM under different parameters in uniformly distributed simulation data

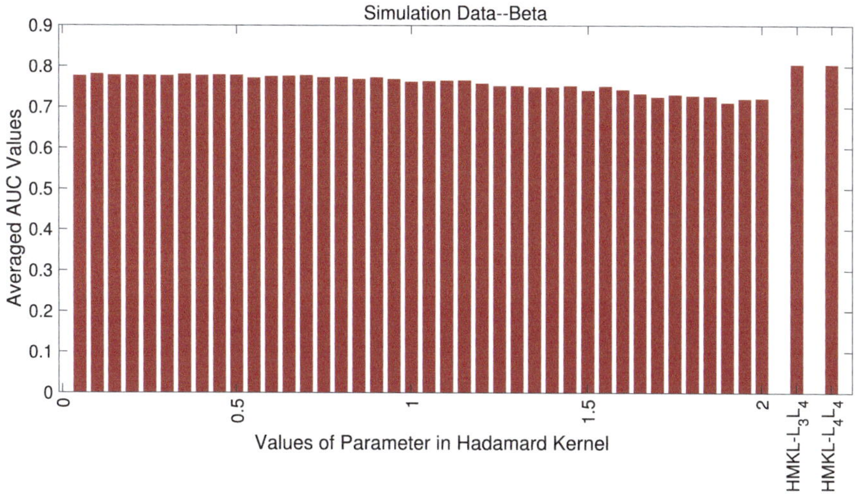

Fig. 5.7 AUC comparisons with Hadamard kernel SVM under different parameters in beta distributed simulation data

Hadamard kernel SVM cannot converge when kernel parameter was greater than 0.4. The averaged AUC value on heart data is stable in an overall manner. In comparison, the averaged AUC values obtained by HMKL-L_3L_4 and HMKL-L_4L_4: 0.92 are optimal compared to Hadamard kernel SVM on all possible parameters whose optimal averaged AUC value is 0.92 as well.

Figure 5.4 shows the averaged AUC values on Hadamard kernel SVM under different parameters in colon cancer data. Hadamard kernel SVM can converge for all the kernel parameters in [0.05, 2]. When kernel parameter is in [0.05, 0.5], Hadamard kernel SVM is not stable, the averaged AUC value is decreasing first and then increasing, when the maximum averaged AUC value 0.92 is achieved when the kernel parameter is 0.5. It is interesting to see that the maximum averaged AUC value 0.99 is achieved when kernel parameter is greater than 0.8. For HMKL-L_3L_4 and HMKL-L_4L_4, though we only considered 10 Hadamard kernels where kernel parameters were 0.05, 0.1, 0.15, 0.2, 0.25, 0.3, 0.35, 0.4, 0.45, 0.5, the performance of multiple kernel learning using these 10 kernels is optimal, achieving 0.99, superior to the performance of Hadamard kernel SVM in each single kernel SVM under parameters in [0.05, 0.5]. This shows that MKL using the linear combination of Hadamard kernels outperforms single Hadamard kernel SVMs.

Figure 5.5 shows the averaged AUC values on Hadamard kernel SVM under different parameters in prostate cancer data. The output of Hadamard kernel SVM can converge for all the kernel parameters in [0.05, 2]. The performance of Hadamard kernel SVM fluctuates, and the averaged AUC values are around 0.8. It is interesting to see that the maximum averaged AUC value 0.87 is achieved when kernel parameter is 0.55. Then we can detect the performance has a decreasing tendency.

For HMKL-L_3L_4 and HMKL-L_4L_4, though we only consider 10 Hadamard kernels where kernel parameters are 0.05, 0.1, 0.15, 0.2, 0.25, 0.3, 0.35, 0.4, 0.45, 0.5, the performance of MKL using these 10 kernels is optimal, achieving 0.86 when $C = 1$, equivalent to the best performance of Hadamard kernel SVM in each single kernel SVM under parameters in [0.05, 0.5]. This shows that MKL using the linear combination of Hadamard kernels helps guarantee the best performance over single Hadamard kernel SVMs under parameters in [0.05, 0.5].

Figures 5.6 and 5.7 show the performance of Hadamard kernel SVM on two simulated data sets. In both data sets, Hadamard kernel SVM training converges to an optimal solution on all the considered kernel parameters in [0.05, 2]. The optimal performance for Hadamard kernel SVM on simulated data in beta distribution was achieved when kernel parameter is 0.1, with the averaged AUC value 0.78. For HMKL-L_3L_4 and HMKL-L_4L_4, the averaged AUC value was 0.8, though we only consider 10 Hadamard kernels where kernel parameters are 0.05, 0.1, 0.15, 0.2, 0.25, 0.3, 0.35, 0.4, 0.45, 0.5, the performance of multiple kernel learning using these 10 kernels is optimal, outperforming Hadamard kernel SVMs on all the kernel parameters. The optimal performance for Hadamard kernel SVM on simulated data in uniform distribution was achieved when kernel parameter is 0.15, with the averaged AUC value 0.72. For HMKL-L_3L_4 and HMKL-L_4L_4, the averaged AUC value was 0.73, though we only consider 10 Hadamard kernels where kernel parameters are 0.05, 0.1, 0.15, 0.2, 0.25, 0.3, 0.35, 0.4, 0.45, 0.5, the performance of multiple kernel learning using these 10 kernels is optimal, outperforming Hadamard kernel SVMs on all the kernel parameters.

- **Results on RBF Kernel SVM**

  Table 5.2 shows the averaged AUC values obtained by RBF kernel SVM with different kernel parameter values. The performance of RBF kernel SVM is very sensitive to the kernel parameter σ in many data sets. Hence the selection of kernel parameter is a critical problem. In heart data, the best averaged AUC value was obtained when $\sigma = 10$ and in colon cancer data, the best averaged AUC value was obtained when $\sigma = 1$. In simulation data sets, the performance of RBF kernel SVM is less sensitive to the kernel parameter and the performance is very stable though unsatisfactory, staying around 0.35 in the averaged AUC value for both data sets. When we further compared RBF kernel SVM with Hadamard multiple kernel learning algorithms, we find that, for all the data sets, even the best averaged AUC value by RBF kernel SVM still cannot compete with our Hadamard MKL algorithm. We can make conclusions that our Hadamard MKL algorithm elegantly avoids the problem of parameter selection while at the meantime optimizes the performance through MKL framework incorporating kernels with different kernel parameters.

- **Results on Linear SVM**

  Figure 5.8 shows the performance of linear SVM on considered data sets. For each data set, we conduct 10 runs of cross-validations with linear SVM to calculate the averaged AUC values in each run. For heart data, diabetes data and credit approval data, linear SVM cannot converge. For colon cancer data, linear SVM performs in a

Table 5.2 Performance of RBF Kernel SVM on considered datasets

	Heart	Diabetes	Credit	Colon	Prostate	Simulation-uniform	Simulation-Beta
$\sigma = 1$	0.69	0.72	0.75	**0.95**	**0.83**	**0.34**	**0.35**
$\sigma = 10$	**0.74**	**0.81**	**0.81**	0.81	0.67	0.33	**0.35**
$\sigma = 10^2$	0.70	0.73	0.75	0.80	0.69	0.33	**0.35**
$\sigma = 10^3$	0.70	0.61	0.70	0.81	0.67	0.33	0.32

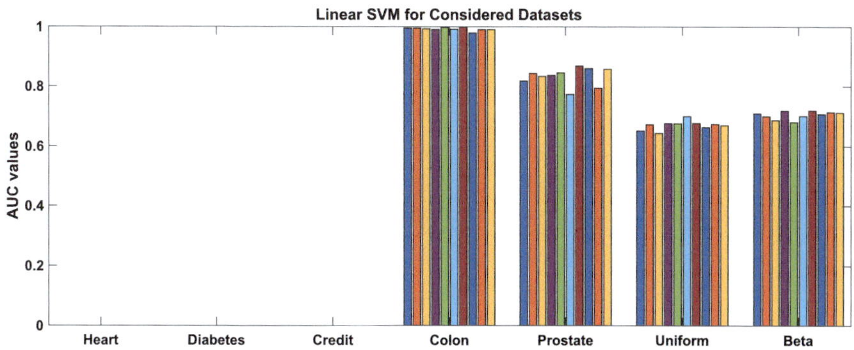

Fig. 5.8 AUC values by linear SVM on considered data sets

satisfactory way, the AUC values are all around 0.99, and the averaged AUC values are 0.99. For prostate cancer data, linear SVM performs in a relatively satisfactory way, the AUC values are all around 0.80, and the averaged AUC values are 0.83, which is equivalent to the best performance obtained in RBF kernel SVM ($\sigma = 1$). However, they both still cannot compete with our HMKL-L_3L_4 or HMKL-L_4L_4 framework. For the simulation data with uniform distribution, both HMKL-L_3L_4 and HMKL-L_4L_4 can achieve averaged AUC values around 0.73, linear SVM can only achieve 0.67 in AUC value on average. For the simulation data with beta distribution, both HMKL-L_3L_4 and HMKL-L_4L_4 can achieve averaged AUC values around 0.80, linear SVM can only achieve 0.71 in AUC value on average. The results further support the effectiveness of the HMKL framework in dealing with supervised learning problems on the considered data sets.

- **Comparison of HMKL Framework with Different Loss Functions**
  We also compared HMKL algorithms under different loss functions: Hinge loss, Log loss, and Square loss. The corresponding results are illustrated in Tables 5.1, 5.3 and 5.4. They perform in a similar way where HMKL with L_1 regularization is less stable, HMKL-L_3L_4 and HMKL-L_4L_4 tend to be more robust.

Table 5.3 Performance comparison on multiple kernel learning algorithms under square loss

Datasets	HMKL-L_4L_3	HMKL-L_4^2	L_1-HMKL	L_2-HMKL	L_3-HMKL	HMKL-L_1L_2	HMKL-L_1L_3	HMKL-L_1L_4	HMKL-L_2L_3	HMKL-L_2L_4
Heart $C^*=1$	**0.911**	**0.911**	0.911	0.911	0.911	0.911	0.911	0.911	0.911	0.911
Heart $C=10$	0.901	0.901	0.908	0.904	0.902	0.904	0.902	0.901	0.902	0.901
Diabetes $C=1$	0.832	0.832	0.827	0.830	0.832	0.830	0.832	0.832	0.832	0.832
Diabetes $C^*=10$	**0.838**	**0.838**	0.837	0.838	0.838	0.837	0.838	0.838	0.838	0.838
Credit $C=1$	0.922	0.922	0.923	0.922	0.922	0.922	0.922	0.922	0.922	0.922
Credit $C^*=10$	**0.930**	**0.930**	0.928	0.929	0.930	0.929	0.930	0.930	0.930	0.930
Colon $C=1$	0.918	0.918	0.839	0.891	0.908	0.891	0.908	0.918	0.908	0.918
Colon $C^*=10$	**0.993**	**0.993**	0.988	0.993	0.993	0.993	0.993	0.993	0.993	0.993
Prostate $C^*=1$	0.848	0.848	0.841	0.849	0.849	0.849	0.849	0.848	0.849	0.848
Prostate $C=10$	0.828	0.828	0.843	0.839	0.833	0.839	0.833	0.828	0.833	0.828
Simulation-uniform $C=1$	0.730	0.730	0.724	0.729	0.730	0.729	0.730	0.730	0.730	0.730
Simulation-uniform $C^*=10$	**0.734**	**0.734**	0.734	0.734	0.734	0.734	0.734	0.734	0.734	0.734
Simulation-beta $C^*=1$	**0.806**	**0.806**	0.801	0.804	0.806	0.804	0.806	0.806	0.806	0.806
Simulation-beta $C=10$	**0.806**	**0.806**	0.806	0.806	0.806	0.806	0.806	0.806	0.806	0.806

Table 5.4 Performance comparison on multiple kernel learning algorithms under log loss

Datasets	HMKL-L_4L_3	HMKL-L_4^2	L_1-HMKL	L_2-HMKL	L_3-HMKL	HMKL-L_1L_2	HMKL-L_1L_3	HMKL-L_1L_4	HMKL-L_2L_3	HMKL-L_2L_4
Heart $C^*=1$	0.910	0.910	0.910	0.910	0.910	0.910	**0.911**	**0.911**	0.910	0.910
Heart $C=10$	0.906	0.906	**0.911**	0.908	0.906	0.910	0.908	0.907	0.907	0.906
Diabetes $C=1$	0.834	0.835	0.827	0.832	0.834	0.828	0.830	0.832	0.834	0.834
Diabetes $C^*=10$	**0.837**	**0.837**	0.836	0.836	0.837	0.836	0.836	0.836	0.836	0.836
Credit $C=1$	0.922	0.922	0.921	0.922	0.922	0.922	0.921	0.922	0.922	0.922
Credit $C^*=10$	**0.926**	**0.926**	0.923	0.925	0.926	0.924	0.925	0.925	0.925	0.925
Colon $C=1$	0.909	0.913	0.850	0.889	0.905	0.868	0.886	0.895	0.899	0.906
Colon $C^*=10$	**0.994**	**0.994**	0.990	0.993	0.994	0.992	0.993	0.994	0.994	0.994
Prostate $C^*=1$	**0.856**	**0.856**	0.848	0.855	0.856	0.852	0.855	0.856	0.856	0.856
Prostate $C=10$	0.837	0.835	0.844	0.842	0.838	0.844	0.843	0.841	0.840	0.838
Simulation-uniform $C=1$	0.730	0.730	0.725	0.729	0.730	0.728	0.729	0.730	0.730	0.730
Simulation-uniform $C^*=10$	0.734	**0.735**	0.731	0.732	0.734	0.731	0.732	0.732	0.733	0.734
Simulation-beta $C^*=1$	**0.804**	**0.804**	0.798	0.802	0.804	0.800	0.802	0.803	0.803	0.804
Simulation-beta$C=10$	0.802	0.802	0.803	0.803	0.802	0.803	0.803	0.802	0.802	0.802

5.4.4.3 Applications in RBF Multiple Kernel Learning

From the previous subsections we can conclude that MKL-$L_4 L_p$ can effectively optimize the performance of Hadamard kernel when involving a number of kernel parameters for multiple kernel learning. The high order multiple kernel learning framework can also outperform several single kernels in SVMs. In this subsection, we aim to test the application capability of MKL-$L_4 L_p$ in optimizing performance of other kernels. We here consider MKL for RBF kernel, one of the most frequently used kernel in SVM, with different kernel parameters. In our RBF MKL framework, we consider 10 candidate kernels under the kernel parameters starting from 2^{-2} with scale size 2:$\{2^{-2}, 2^{-1}, 2^0, 2^1, 2^2, 2^3, 2^4, 2^5, 2^6, 2^7\}$ for final optimal kernel construction. RBFMKL-$L_4 L_p (p \geq 3)$ cannot compete with HMKL-$L_4 L_p (p \geq 3)$ for the considered datasets, as can be seen in Table 5.5; however, RBFMKL-$L_4 L_p (p \geq 3)$ showed the best performance when compared to L_1-MKL, L_2-MKL, L_p-MKL frameworks. From another perspective, when we consider the comparisons to RBF kernel with single parameter $\sigma = 1, 10, 10^2, 10^3$ respectively shown in Table 5.2, we can still show the superiority of MKL framework. The 10 kernel MKL framework can help achieve optimal performance or at least near optimal performance compared to RBF kernel with $\sigma = 1, 10, 10^2, 10^3$ respectively. In particular, for Simulation_Uniform data, RBF kernel with $\sigma = 1, 10, 10^2, 10^3$ respectively can best achieve 0.34 in averaged AUC value. However, RBFMKL-$L_4 L_p (p \geq 3)$ helps guarantee 0.5051 ($C = 1$) in averaged AUC value, outperforms all the single kernels considered. For Simulation_Beta data, RBF kernel with $\sigma = 1, 10, 10^2, 10^3$ respectively can best achieve 0.35 in averaged AUC value. However, RBFMKL-$L_4 L_p (p \geq 3)$ helps guarantee 0.6716 ($C = 1$) in averaged AUC value, outperforms all the single kernels considered.

5.5 Conclusions

In this chapter, we have proposed a MKL framework to optimize the performance of Hadamard kernel SVM under different kernel parameters. It implicitly avoids the parameter specification problem by optimizing the linear combination of Hadamard kernel functions over different kernel parameters. The Hadamard MKL framework with $L_4 L_p$ norm-product regularization has shown robust performance compared to MKL framework with L_1, L_2, and L_p regularization. For future research, it is of great significance to investigate the quantitative performance of the proposed Hadamard MKL framework as well as its efficient training scheme.

Table 5.5 RBF multiple kernel learning results

Datasets	RBFMKL-L_4L_3	RBFMKL-L_4^2	L_1-RBFMKL	L_2-RBFMKL	L_3-RBFMKL	RBFMKL-L_1L_2	RBFMKL-L_1L_3	RBFMKL-L_1L_4	RBFMKL-L_2L_3	RBFMKL-L_2L_4
Heart $C=1$	**0.7250**	**0.7250**	0.7124	0.7216	0.7237	0.7217	0.7237	0.7250	0.7237	0.7250
Heart $C^*=10$	**0.7321**	**0.7321**	0.7142	0.7286	0.7309	0.7286	0.7309	0.7321	0.7309	0.7321
Diabetes $C^*=1$	**0.8034**	**0.8034**	0.8007	0.8031	0.8034	0.8030	0.8034	0.8034	0.8034	0.8034
Diabetes $C=10$	**0.8012**	**0.8012**	0.7991	0.8009	0.8011	0.8007	0.8011	0.8012	0.8011	0.8012
Credit $C^*=1$	**0.8326**	**0.8326**	0.8186	0.8288	0.8314	0.8289	0.8314	0.8326	0.8314	0.8326
Credit $C=10$	**0.8316**	**0.8316**	0.8186	0.8278	0.8304	0.8280	0.8304	0.8316	0.8304	0.8316
Colon $C=1$	**0.9393**	**0.9393**	0.9333	0.9362	0.9382	0.9366	0.9382	0.9393	0.9382	0.9393
Colon $C^*=10$	**0.9450**	**0.9450**	0.9423	0.9425	0.9439	0.9426	0.9439	0.9450	0.9439	0.9450
Prostate $C=1$	**0.8041**	**0.8041**	0.7633	0.7956	0.8018	0.7965	0.8019	0.8041	0.8019	0.8041
Prostate $C^*=10$	**0.8159**	**0.8159**	0.7804	0.8094	0.8138	0.8097	0.8138	0.8159	0.8138	0.8159
Simulation-uniform $C=1$	**0.5051**	**0.5051**	0.3917	0.4736	0.4959	0.4743	0.4959	0.5051	0.4959	0.5051
Simulation-uniform $C^*=10$	**0.5229**	**0.5229**	0.4197	0.4948	0.5146	0.4953	0.5146	0.5229	0.5146	0.5229
Simulation-beta $C^*=1$	**0.6716**	**0.6716**	0.6242	0.6544	0.6663	0.6553	0.6663	0.6716	0.6663	0.6716
Simulation-beta $C=10$	**0.6695**	**0.6695**	0.6233	0.6523	0.6642	0.6529	0.6642	0.6695	0.6642	0.6695

References

Aydin I, Karakose M, Akin E (2011) A multi-objective artificial immune algorithm for parameter optimization in support vector machine. Appl Soft Comput 11(1):120–129

Baudat G, Anouar F (2000) Generalized discriminant analysis using a kernel approach. Neural Comput

Boughorbel S, Tarel J, Boujemaa N (2005) Generalized histogram intersection kernel for image recognition. In: IEEE International conference on image processing, 2005. ICIP 2005

Chang YW, Lin CJ (2006) Feature ranking using linear SVM 2:47–57

Chung K, Kao W, Sun C, Wang L, Lin C (2003) Radius margin bounds for support vector machines with the RBF kernel. Neural Comput 15(11):2643–2681

Cortes C, Vapnik V (1995) Support-vector networks. Mach Learn 20(3):273–297

Cristianini N, Shawe-Taylor J (2007) Support vector and kernel methods

Daliri M (2013) Chi-square distance kernel of the gaits for the diagnosis of Parkinson's disease. Biomed Signal Process Control 8(1):66–70

Flach P, Hernandez-Orallo J, Ferri C (2011) A coherent interpretation of AUC as a measure of aggregated classification performance 657–664

Gautam C, Tiwari A, Tanveer M (2019) KOC+: kernel ridge regression based one-class classification using privileged information. Inf Sci 504:324–333

Guo L, Zhang X, Liu Z, Xue X, Wang Q, Zheng S (2021) Robust subspace clustering based on automatic weighted multiple kernel learning. Inf Sci 573:453–474

Hanley JA, Mcneil BJ (1983) A method of comparing the areas under receiver operating characteristic curves derived from the same cases. Radiology 148(3):839–843

Han Y, Yang Y, Li X, Liu Q, Ma Y (2018) Matrix-regularized multiple kernel learning via (R, P) norms. IEEE Trans Neural Netw Learn Syst 1–11

Huang C (2009) ACO-based hybrid classification system with feature subset selection and model parameters optimization. Neurocomputing 73(1):438–448

Huang C, Wang C (2006) A ga-based feature selection and parameters optimization for support vector machines. Expert Syst Appl 31(2):231–240

Informatik V, Scholkopf B (2000) Support vector learning

Jiang H, Ching W, Cheung W, Hou W, Yin H (2017) Hadamard kernel SVM with applications for breast cancer outcome predictions. BMC Syst Biol 11(S7):138

Jiang H, Ching WK, Qiu Y, Cheng XQ (2017) Optimal projection method determination by Logdet divergence and perturbed von-Neumann divergence. BMC Syst Biol 11(S6):115

Kim E, Langer A, Paul C, Reidl F, Rossmanith P, Sau I, Sikdar S (2015) Linear kernels and single-exponential algorithms via protrusion decompositions. ACM Trans Algorithms 12(2):1–41

Kloft M, Brefeld U, Laskov P (2008) Non-sparse multiple kernel learning. In: NIPS 08 workshop: kernel learning automatic selection of optimal kernels

Kloft M, Brefeld U, Laskov P, Muller K, Zien A, Sonnenburg S (2009) Efficient and accurate LP-norm multiple kernel learning. In: Advances in neural information processing systems, pp 997–1005

Kolomvatsos K, Hadjieftymiades S (2014) On the use of particle swarm optimization and kernel density estimator in concurrent negotiations. Inf Sci 262:99–116

Kowalski M, Szafranski M, Ralaivola L (2009) Multiple indefinite kernel learning with mixed norm regularization. In: Proceedings of the 26th international conference of machine learning. https://doi.org/10.1145/1553374.1553445

Lanckriet G, Cristianini N, Bartlett P, Ghaoui L, Jordan M (2002) Learning the kernel matrix with semidefinite programming. J Mach Learn Res 5(1):27–72

Lanckriet G, De Bie T, Cristianini N, Jordan M, Noble W (2004) A statistical framework for genomic data fusion. Bioinformatics 20(16):2626–2635

Li Y, Sun H, Yan W, Cui Q (2021) R-CTSVM+: robust capped L1-norm twin support vector machine with privileged information. Inf Sci 574:12–32

Lin KC, Chien HY (2009) CSO-based feature selection and parameter optimization for support vector machine. In: 2009 joint conferences on pervasive computing (JCPC), pp 783–788
Lin H, Lin C (2003) A study on sigmoid kernels for SVM and the training of non-PSD kernels by SMO-type methods. Submitt Neural Comput
Lv S, Zhou F (2015) Optimal learning rates of LP-type multiple kernel learning under general conditions. Inf Sci 294:255–268. Innov Appl Artif Neural Netw Eng
Mamitsuka H (2006) Selecting features in microarray classification using roc curves. Pattern Recognit
Meijering E, Zuiderveld K (1999) Image reconstruction by convolution with symmetrical piecewise nth-order polynomial kernels. IEEE Trans Image Process 8(2):192–201
Mika S, Schölkopf B, Smola A, Müller, K., Scholz, M., Rätsch. G (1999) Kernel PCA and de-noising in feature spaces. Adv Neural Inf Process Syst 11:536–542
NCBI GEO DataBase (2025). https://www.ncbi.nlm.nih.gov/geo/
Pillonetto G, Dinuzzo F, Chen T, De Nicolao G, Ljung L (2014) Kernel methods in system identification, machine learning and function estimation: a survey. Automatica 50(3):657–682
Qaraei M, Abbaasi S, Ghiasi-Shirazi K (2021) Randomized non-linear PCA networks. Inf Sci 545:241–253
Ratsch G, Sonnenburg S, Schafer C (2005) Learning interpretable SVMs for biological sequence classification. In: Proceedings of the 9th annual international conference on research in computational molecular biology
Ring M, Eskofier B (2016) An approximation of the gaussian RBF kernel for efficient classification with SVMs. Pattern Recognit Lett
Roth V, Steinhage V (2000) Nonlinear discriminant analysis using kernel functions. Adv Neural Inf Process Syst 12
Scholkopf B, Mika S, Burges C, Knirsch P, Muller K, Ratsch G, Smola A (1999) Input space versus feature space in kernel-based methods. IEEE Trans Neural Networks 10(5):1000–1017
Scholkopf B, Burges C, Smola A (1998) Advances in kernel methods: Support vector machine
Shiju S, Asif S, Sumitra S (2017) Multiple kernel learning using composite kernel functions. Eng Appl Artif Intell 64:391–400
Smola A, Schlkopf B (1998) On a kernel-based method for pattern recognition, regression, approximation, and operator inversion. Algorithmica 22(1):211–231
Stanton RJ, Weinstein A (1981) On the L4 norm of spherical harmonics. Math Proc Cambridge Philos Soc 89(2):343–358
Sun J, Li X, Yang Y, Luo J, Bai Y (2012) Scaling the kernel function based on the separating boundary in input space: a data-dependent way for improving the performance of kernel methods. Inf Sci 184(1):140–154
Tang J, Tian Y, Liu D, Kou G (2019) Coupling privileged kernel method for multi-view learning. Inf Sci 481:110–127
Tehrani AF (2021) The choquet kernel on the use of regression problem. Inf Sci 56:256–272
Tian M, Wang W (2012) A global-local optimization approach to parameter estimation of RBF-type models. Inf Sci 197:144–160
UCI machine learning repository (2025). https://archive.ics.uci.edu/ml/datasets.php
Wang N (2003) Marginal nonparametric kernel regression accounting for within-subject correlation. Biometrika 1:43–52
Xu K, Zhang Y, Xiong Z (2021) Iterative rank-one matrix completion via singular value decomposition and nuclear norm regularization. Inf Sci 578:574–591
Xu Z, Dai M, Meng D (2009) Fast and efficient strategies for model selection of gaussian support vector machine. IEEE Trans Syst, Man, Cybern, Part B (Cybernetics) 39(5):1292–1307
Yang H, Xu Z, Ye J, King I, Lyu M (2011) Efficient sparse generalized multiple kernel learning. IEEE Trans Neural Netw 22(3):433–446
Yin S, Yin J (2016) Tuning kernel parameters for SVM based on expected square distance ratio. Inf Sci 370–371:92–102

Zhai X, Yang Z, Liao Z, Wright J, Ma Y (2020) Complete dictionary learning via L4-norm maximization over the orthogonal group. J Mach Learn Res 21(1):1–68
Zhang L, Cao Q (2011) A novel ant-based clustering algorithm using the kernel method. Inf Sci 181(20):4658–4672. Special Issue on Interpretable Fuzzy Systems
Zheng X, Zhang L, Yan L (2021) CTSVM: a robust twin support vector machine with correntropy-induced loss function for binary classification problems. Inf Sci 559:22–45
Zhou D, Jetter K (2006) Approximation with polynomial kernels and SVM classifiers. Adv Comput Math 25(1–3):323–344

Chapter 6
Correlation Kernels for SVM Classification

6.1 Introduction

High dimensional bioinformatics data sets provide an excellent and challenging research problem in machine learning area. In particular, DNA microarrays generated gene expression data are of high dimension with significant level of noise. Supervised kernel learning with an Support Vector Machine (SVM) classifier has been successfully applied in biomedical diagnosis such as discriminating different kinds of tumor tissues. Correlation Kernel has been recently applied to classification problems with SVMs. In this chapter, we develop a novel and parsimonious positive semi-definite kernel. The proposed kernel is shown experimentally to have better performance when compared to the usual correlation kernel. In addition, we propose a new kernel based on the correlation matrix incorporating techniques dealing with indefinite kernel. The resulting kernel is shown to be positive-semi-definite and it exhibits superior performance to the two kernels mentioned above. We then apply the proposed method to some cancer data in discriminating different tumor tissues, providing information for diagnosis of diseases. Numerical experiments indicate that our method outperforms the existing methods such as the decision tree method and KNN method.

This chapter is structured as follows. In Sect. 6.2, we propose the parsimonious positive-semi-definite kernel. We then introduce the construction of usual correlation kernel as well as the novel kernel after *denoising* on an indefinite kernel having the same indefinite property with the usual correlation kernel. Theoretical proof on the positive semi-definite property of parsimonious kernel was provided. We also give explanations for indefinite property of related kernels. In Sect. 6.3, publicly available data sets are utilized to check the performance of the proposed method and compare to some existing methods such as the KNN (k-nearest neighbors) method and the decision tree method. A discussion on the results obtained is given in Sect. 6.4. Finally concluding remarks are in Sect. 6.5.

H. Jiang and W.-K. Ching, *Kernel Methods for Omics Data Mining*, Intelligent Control and Learning Systems 10, https://doi.org/10.1007/978-981-95-3129-5_6

6.2 The Proposed Parsimonious Positive-Semi-Definite Kernel Method

In this section, we first introduce the usual correlation kernel. Based on the indefinite property of the usual correlation kernel, we then propose a parsimonious Positive Semi-Definite (PSD) kernel. Apart from that, our novel kernel, namely Denoised Correlation Based (DCB) kernel will also be presented.

6.2.1 A Parsimonious Correlation Kernel

In this subsection, we assume that there are n data instances in the data set. The number of features used to describe a data instance is p. Then the data matrix can be expressed as a $p \times n$ matrix which we denote as follows:

$$X = [X_1, X_2, \ldots, X_n] \quad \text{where} \quad X_i = [x_{1i}, x_{2i}, \ldots, x_{pi}]^T, \; i = 1, 2, \ldots, n.$$

It is straightforward to obtain the correlation matrix of X:

$$\text{corr}(X) = \begin{bmatrix} \text{corr}(X_1, X_1) & \text{corr}(X_1, X_2) & \cdots & \text{corr}(X_1, X_n) \\ \text{corr}(X_2, X_1) & \text{corr}(X_2, X_2) & \cdots & \text{corr}(X_2, X_n) \\ \vdots & \vdots & \ddots & \vdots \\ \text{corr}(X_n, X_1) & \text{corr}(X_n, X_2) & \cdots & \text{corr}(X_n, X_n) \end{bmatrix}$$

where

$$\text{corr}(X_i, X_j) = \frac{(X_i - \bar{X})^T (X_j - \bar{X})}{\sqrt{(X_i - \bar{X})^T (X_i - \bar{X})} \sqrt{(X_j - \bar{X})^T (X_j - \bar{X})}} \tag{6.1}$$

and $\bar{X}$ is the sample mean of data matrix X.

To deal with the positive-semi-definite requirement of a kernel matrix, in this subsection we propose a parsimonious kernel which is simply the correlation matrix $K_P = \text{corr}(X)$. The proposition below shows that the proposed kernel is PSD.

Proposition 6.1 *The matrix $K_P = corr(X)$ is a positive semi-definite matrix.*

Proof From Eq. (6.1), we know that the *ij*th entry of $\text{corr}(X)$ is given by

$$K_P(i, j) = \frac{(X_i - \bar{X})^T (X_j - \bar{X})}{\sqrt{(X_i - \bar{X})^T (X_i - \bar{X})} \sqrt{(X_j - \bar{X})^T (X_j - \bar{X})}}.$$

Alternatively, we may write

$$K_P(i,j) = \left\langle \frac{(X_i - \bar{X})}{\sqrt{(X_i - \bar{X})^T(X_i - \bar{X})}}, \frac{(X_j - \bar{X})}{\sqrt{(X_j - \bar{X})^T(X_j - \bar{X})}} \right\rangle.$$

If we denote

$$Q = \left[\frac{(X_1 - \bar{X})}{\sqrt{(X_1 - \bar{X})^T(X_1 - \bar{X})}}, \ldots, \frac{(X_n - \bar{X})}{\sqrt{(X_n - \bar{X})^T(X_n - \bar{X})}} \right],$$

we can re-writte $K_P = Q^T \cdot Q$. Then for any

$$Y = [y_1, y_2, \ldots, y_n]^T \in R^n$$

we have

$$Y^T K_P Y = (TY)^T (TY)$$

If we further set

$$Z = TY = [z_1, z_2, \ldots, z_n]^T$$

then

$$Y^T K_P Y = Z^T Z = \sum_{i=1}^{n} z_i^2 \geq 0.$$

This demonstrates that $K_P = \text{corr}(X)$ itself is PSD. □

Therefore, K_P can be employed as a kernel matrix for training classifiers in machine learning framework. This further proves the PSD of the usual correlation matrix.

6.2.2 The Usual Correlation Kernel

Correlation is a mean-centered distance metric that is not common for kernel constructions. However, it is an important metric and it is problem-specific. The usual correlation kernel is constructed based on the correlation matrix defined above, and the kernel value between X_i and X_j is

$$K(X_i, X_j) = e^{-\gamma(1-\text{corr}(X_i, X_j))}.$$

This kernel definition intuitively describes the similarity between two data instances. It is straightforward to see the symmetric property of the kernel matrix as well. To have a better understanding of the usual kernel matrix, we can describe it as follows:

$$K = \begin{bmatrix} 1 & k_{12} & \cdots & k_{1n} \\ k_{21} & 1 & \cdots & k_{2n} \\ \vdots & \vdots & \ddots & \vdots \\ k_{n1} & k_{n2} & \cdots & 1 \end{bmatrix}$$

where $k_{ij} = K(X_i, X_j)$ and $0 < k_{ij} \leq 1,\ i, j = 1, 2, \ldots, n$. The following proposition presents relationship with corr(X).

Proposition 6.2 *The usual correlation kernel is positive-semi-definite if corr(X) is positive-semi-definite.*

Proof The correlation kernel is symmetric and we have $k_{ij} = k_{ji},\ i, j = 1, 2, \ldots, n$. On the other hand, one can write

$$K = e^{(-\gamma)} e^{(\gamma * \mathrm{corr}(X))}.$$

Because $\gamma > 0$, we have $e^{(-\gamma)} > 0$. What's more, $e^{(\gamma \cdot \mathrm{corr}(X))}$ has the same definiteness property with $e^{\mathrm{corr}(X)}$. Using kernel trick in machine learning area (Smola and Schölkopf 1998), we can see that if corr(X) is PSD, then usual correlation kernel is also PSD. □

6.2.3 *Denoised Correlation Based Kernel*

From the successful experience of the usual correlation kernel in Raman spectra classification (Kyriakides et al. 2011), we construct a novel kernel utilizing the advantage of the usual correlation kernel: the Denoised Correlation Based kernel construction involves two steps. First, we formulate an indefinite kernel matrix sharing similar property of the usual correlation kernel. Second, *denoising* techniques are applied in order to construct a PSD kernel matrix. The above ideas can be summarized in the following two steps.

6.2.3.1 Step 1: A New Kernel

Here we propose a new kernel having equivalent indefinite property with the usual correlation kernel. It it defined as follows:

$$K_{CB} = 1 - e^{-\mathrm{corr}(X)}$$

and we can write it in another way as

$$K_{CB} = (1 - e^{-1}) K1_{CB}$$

where

$$K1_{CB} = \begin{bmatrix} 1 & \frac{1-e^{-\mathrm{corr}(X_1,X_2)}}{1-e^{-1}} & \cdots & \frac{1-e^{-\mathrm{corr}(X_1,X_n)}}{1-e^{-1}} \\ \frac{1-e^{-\mathrm{corr}(X_2,X_1)}}{1-e^{-1}} & 1 & \cdots & \frac{1-e^{-\mathrm{corr}(X_2,X_n)}}{1-e^{-1}} \\ \vdots & \vdots & \ddots & \vdots \\ \frac{1-e^{-\mathrm{corr}(X_n,X_1)}}{1-e^{-1}} & \frac{1-e^{-\mathrm{corr}(X_n,X_2)}}{1-e^{-1}} & \cdots & 1 \end{bmatrix}$$

has similar expression with the usual correlation kernel.

6.2.3.2 Step 2: The Denoising Strategy

Since the kernel matrix K_{CB} may not be PSD, we incorporate *denoising* strategy in the kernel construction. Because $K_{CB} = VPV^T$ where V is the orthogonal matrix composed of all the eigenvectors of the matrix K_{CB} and P is a diagonal matrix where the diagonal entries are the eigenvalues of the matrix K_{CB}. Let us write

$$P = \begin{bmatrix} p_1 & 0 & \cdots & 0 \\ 0 & p_2 & \cdots & 0 \\ \vdots & \vdots & \ddots & \vdots \\ 0 & 0 & \cdots & p_n \end{bmatrix}.$$

The *denoising* strategy is to transform the diagonal matrix P to another diagonal matrix $\tilde{P}$,

$$\tilde{P} = \begin{bmatrix} \tilde{p}_1 & 0 & \cdots & 0 \\ 0 & \tilde{p}_2 & \cdots & 0 \\ \vdots & \vdots & \ddots & \vdots \\ 0 & 0 & \cdots & \tilde{p}_n \end{bmatrix}$$

where

$$\tilde{p}_i = \begin{cases} 0, & p_i < 0; \\ p_i, & p_i \geq 0. \end{cases}, \; i = 1, 2, \ldots, n.$$

Finally, $K_{DCB} = V\tilde{P}V^T$ is a positive-semi-definite kernel matrix.

6.3 Numerical Experiments

6.3.1 Materials

We prepared three publicly available data sets from libsvm (Libsvm data set 2025) related to three types of cancers.

The first data set is related to colon cancer. In this data set, there are 22 normal and 40 tumor colon tissues. Each tissue is characterized by intensities of 2000 genes with highest minimal intensity through the samples (Alon et al. 1999). The data preprocessing process has been done through instance-wise normalization to standard normal distribution. Then feature-wise normalization was performed to the standard normal distribution as well. In total there are 62 data instance with 2000 features, and there are 40 positive data which means 40 exhibiting colon-cancer while 22 are normal.

The second data set is related to breast cancer. Similar to the first data set, the same preprocessing technique has been applied to normalize the data. Initially, there are 49 tumor samples. They are derived from the Duke Breast Cancer SPORE tissue resource. And they are divided into two groups: estrogen receptor-positive and estrogen receptor-negative, via immunohistochemistry (West et al. 2001). However, the classification results using immunohistochemistry and protein immunoblotting assay conflicted so that 5 of them were then removed. Therefore, there are 44 data instances in total, 21 are negative and 23 are positive. The number of genes used to describe the tumor sample is 7129.

The third data set is related to leukemia cancer. Preprocessing procedure for this data set is exactly the same as the previous two data sets. The data set is composed of 38 bone marrow samples, 27 of them are acute myeloid leukemia and the remaining 11 are acute lymphoblastic leukemia (Golub et al. 1999). Expression levels of 7129 genes are used to measure each data.

We compare our proposed methods with the following three existing methods.

(1) **Decision Tree**: Decision tree learning is a method commonly used in data mining. It employs a decision tree as a predictive model which maps observations about an item to conclusions about the item's target value. In these tree structures, leaves represent classifications and branches represent conjunctions of features that lead to those classifications.
(2) **K-Nearest Neighborhood (KNN)**: The K-nearest neighbor algorithm is the simplest method among all machine learning algorithms. An object is classified by a majority vote of its neighbors, with the object being assigned to the class most common amongst its K nearest neighbors. K is a positive integer, typically small. In the experiments, the KNN method with $K = 1, 5, 10$ is examined. If $K = 1$, then the object is simply assigned to the class of its nearest neighbor.
(3) **Support Vector Machines (SVMs)**: A support vector machine constructs a hyperplane or set of hyperplanes in a high- or infinite-dimensional space, which can be used for classification. A good separation is achieved by the hyperplane that has the largest functional margin that is the distance to the nearest training data points of any class. In the experiments, we employ SVMs with the aforementioned three correlation kernels.

In this study, we employed the Decision Tree algorithm and the KNN method for comparison with our proposed Parsimonious Correlation Kernel and Denoised Correlation Based kernel with SVM. The aim is to demonstrate superiority of our proposed kernels to the usual correlation kernel.

Tables 6.1, 6.2 and 6.3 present the prediction accuracy comparison in different algorithms. We employed the fivefold cross-validation setting in the study. To obtain

Table 6.1 Prediction accuracy comparison among different algorithms for colon cancer

D.T.	U.C.			P.C.	D.C.B	K.N.N.		
	$\gamma = 0.1$	$\gamma = 1$	$\gamma = 10$			$K = 1$	$K = 5$	$K = 10$
0.6945	0.6623	0.8059	0.6459	0.8490	**0.8599**	0.7244	0.7519	0.7404

Here D.T. means Decision Tree Algorithm, U.C. means the usual Correlation Kernel, P.C. stands for the Parsimonious Correlation we proposed, D.C.B. is the novel kernel proposed by us representing Denoised Correlation Based Kernel and K.N.N. is the K Nearest Neighborhood Algorithm

Table 6.2 Prediction accuracy comparison among different algorithms for breast cancer

D.T.	U.C.			P.C.	D.C.B	K.N.N.		
	$\gamma = 0.1$	$\gamma = 1$	$\gamma = 10$			$K = 1$	$K = 5$	$K = 10$
0.7653	0.6642	0.7914	0.4114	0.8075	**0.8278**	0.7447	0.7147	0.6872

Here D.T. means Decision Tree Algorithm, U.C. means the usual Correlation Kernel, P.C. stands for the Parsimonious Correlation we proposed, D.C.B. is the novel kernel proposed by us representing Denoised Correlation Based Kernel and K.N.N. is the K Nearest Neighborhood Algorithm

Table 6.3 Prediction accuracy comparison among different algorithms for Leukemia cancer

D.T.	U.C.			P.C.	D.C.B	K.N.N.		
	$\gamma = 0.1$	$\gamma = 1$	$\gamma = 10$			$K = 1$	$K = 5$	$K = 10$
0.8189	0.7111	0.7868	0.7111	0.9150	**0.9257**	0.8443	0.8557	0.8082

Here D.T. means Decision Tree Algorithm, U.C. means the usual Correlation Kernel, P.C. stands for the Parsimonious Correlation we proposed, D.C.B. is the novel kernel proposed by us representing Denoised Correlation Based Kernel and K.N.N. is the K Nearest Neighborhood Algorithm

relatively stable results, fivefold cross-validation was performed 10 times and the accuracy was measured as the averaged accuracy over the 10 runs. The best performance is marked in bold size in the tables, where the accuracy is measured through the averaged AUC value.

For the colon cancer data set, decision tree method exhibited inferior performance compared to KNN algorithm. However, both decision tree method and the KNN algorithm could not do better than the usual correlation kernel when $\gamma = 1$. For different values of γ, the performance of the usual correlation kernel differed widely. The best performance was achieved when $\gamma = 1$ was adopted. But when $\gamma = 0.1$ or 10, only around 0.65 accuracy was obtained.

For the breast cancer data, decision tree method performed better than KNN algorithm. The accuracy for decision tree method was 0.7653, but for the KNN algorithm, the best result obtained was 0.7447 when $K = 1$ which was significantly <0.7653. But still they could not catch up with the usual correlation kernel when $\gamma = 1$ that was 0.7914. Similar to colon cancer data set, when $\gamma = 0.1$ and 10, the usual correlation kernel demonstrated poorly, the accuracies were only 0.6642 and 0.4114 respectively. As a whole, the parsimonious correlation kernel and the denoised correlation based kernel were the best two.

Finally for the leukemia data set, the accuracies of the decision tree method and the KNN algorithm were higher than usual correlation kernel. They were all over 0.8000

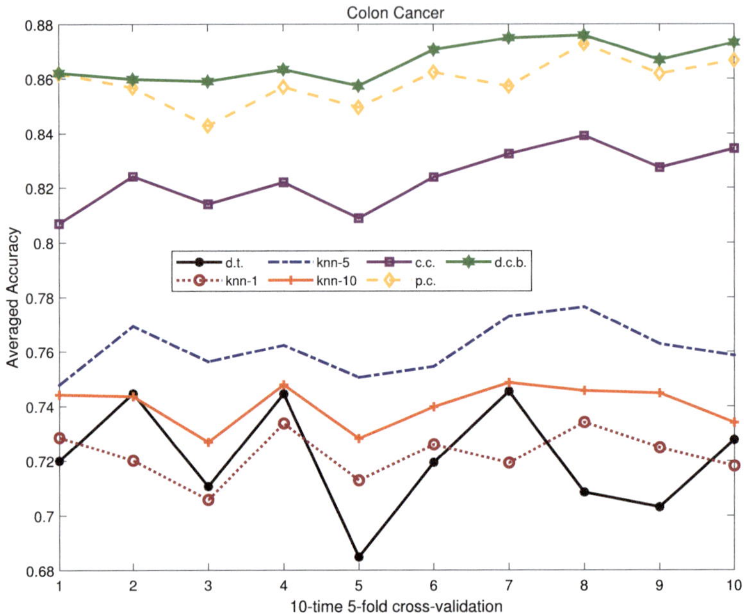

Fig. 6.1 10 runs 10-time fivefold cross-validation for colon cancer data. Solid line with black '*' with legend d.t. is the Decision Tree Method, dashed line with red 'o' marked 'knn-1' means K Nearest Neighborhood when $K = 1$, dash-dot line with blue point marked 'knn-5' means K Nearest Neighborhood when $K = 5$, solid line with '+' in orange labeling 'knn-10' is the K Nearest Neighborhood when $K = 10$, solid line with purple '□' is the usual Correlation Kernel, diamond yellow line represents the Parsimonious Correlation Kernel and hexagram green line is the denoised correlation based kernel

while the best performance of the usual correlation kernel was 0.7868 when $\gamma = 1$, <0.8. However, both parsimonious correlation kernel and denoised correlation based kernel could achieve over 0.9000 accuracy.

As we could conclude that for the usual correlation kernel, $\gamma = 1$ ensured the best performance. Hence we chose $\gamma = 1$ in the following studies. Figures 6.1, 6.2 and 6.3 show the performance of 10 runs of 10-time fivefold cross-validation for the 3 data sets. Value i in the X-label means the ith run while Y-label means the averaged accuracy of each 10-time fivefold cross-validation. We compare the decision tree method, the KNN algorithm, the usual correlation kernel and the 2 proposed PSD kernels: parsimonious correlation kernel and denoised correlation based kernel. The figures clearly demonstrate the superiority of our 2 proposed Kernels (as presented in starred green and diamond yellow in the figures) over all the other algorithms compared.

Table 6.4 presents the dominant eigenvalues in parsimonious correlation kernel and denoised correlation based kernel. We observe that the dominant eigenvalues for parsimonious correlation kernel and denoised correlation based kernel are very close to each other, with a gap of only 0.0168. This explain why the two algorithms

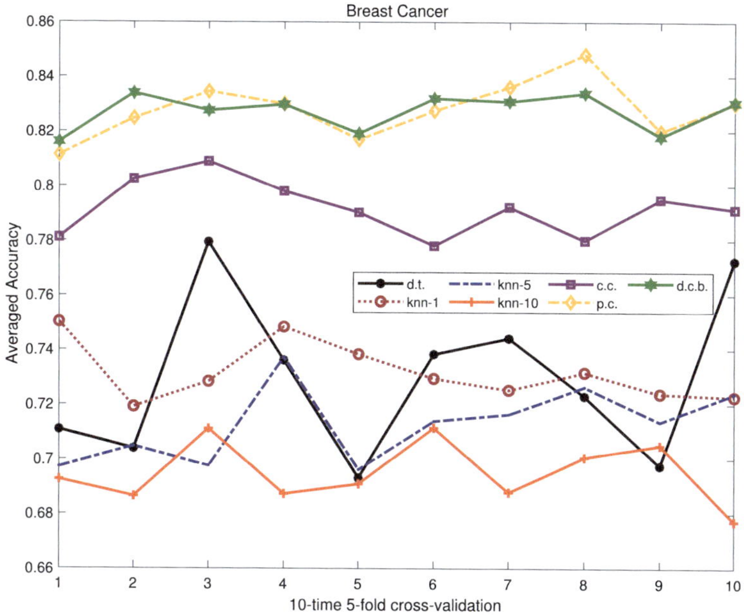

Fig. 6.2 10 runs 10-time fivefold cross-validation for breast cancer data. Solid line with black '*' with legend d.t. is the Decision Tree Method, dashed line with red 'o' marked 'knn-1' means K Nearest Neighborhood when $K = 1$, dash-dot line with blue point marked 'knn-5' means K Nearest Neighborhood when $K = 5$, solid line with '+' in orange labeling 'knn-10' is the K Nearest Neighborhood when $K = 10$, solid line with purple '□' is the usual Correlation Kernel, diamond yellow line represents the Parsimonious Correlation Kernel and hexagram green line is the denoised correlation based kernel

exhibit similar performance. And for the colon cancer data set, the difference in dominant eigenvalues is 0.1421. While for the leukemia data set, the difference is the largest: 0.3048. One can see that the performance difference is also the largest, the superiority of denoised correlation based kernel over parsimonious correlation kernel is the clearest. The difference in the dominant eigenvalues is consistent with the difference in performance in classification. The larger the difference in dominant eigenvalues, the larger the difference in classification performance will be.

6.4 Discussions

From the tables, one can see the consistent superiority of the denoised correlation based kernel for classification. All of them can achieve the best for the 3 tested data sets. And the PSD parsimonious correlation kernel is the second best among all the algorithms compared. Moreover, we observe no dominant superiority for decision tree or KNN algorithm over the other.

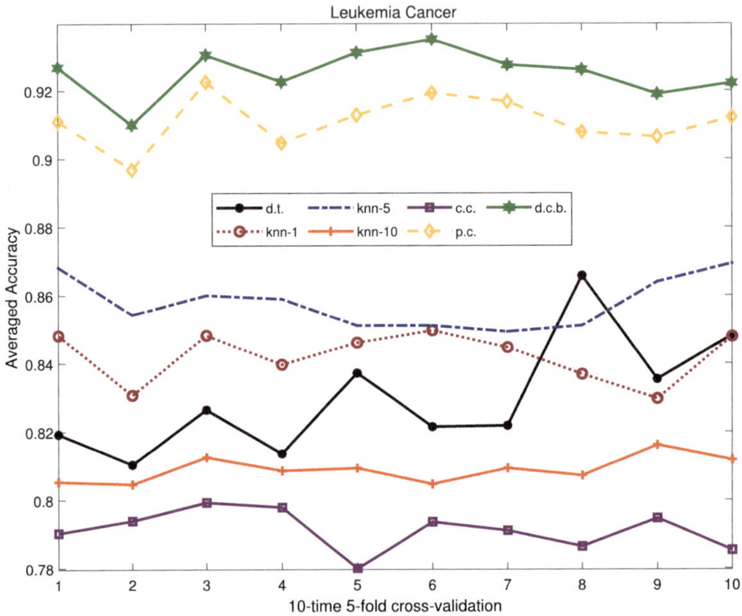

Fig. 6.3 10 runs 10-time fivefold cross-validation for leukemia cancer data. Solid line with black '*' with legend d.t. is the Decision Tree Method, dashed line with red 'o' marked 'knn-1' means K Nearest Neighborhood when $K = 1$, dash-dot line with blue point marked 'knn-5' means K Nearest Neighborhood when $K = 5$, solid line with '+' in orange labeling 'knn-10' is the K Nearest Neighborhood when $K = 10$, solid line with purple '□' is the usual Correlation Kernel, diamond yellow line represents the Parsimonious Correlation kernel and hexagram green line is the denoised correlation based kernel

Table 6.4 Dominant eigenvalues for parsimonious correlation kernel and denoised correlation based kernel

	Colon cancer	Breast cancer	Leukemia cancer
P.C.	8.9108	8.7721	5.2066
D.C.B.	9.0529	8.7889	5.5114

Here P.C. stands for the Parsimonious correlation we proposed, D.C.B. is the novel kernel proposed by us representing denoised correlation based kernel

From the perspective of the usual correlation kernel, in the colon cancer data, it is better compared to decision tree and KNN algorithm, the average accuracy is located around 0.8000 while decision tree and KNN algorithm cannot exceed 0.7500 in general. In the breast cancer data, similar conclusions can be drawn for the usual correlation kernel. Second to our proposed parsimonious correlation kernel and denoised correlation based kernel, it ranks 3 in all the investigated methods. But in the leukemia data set, usual correlation kernel is the lowest in accuracy. It cannot compete with all the other methods presented. This concludes that there is also no dominant advantage of the usual correlation kernel over the decision tree method and the KNN algorithm.

If we focus on the comparison of the 2 proposed PSD kernels: parsimonious correlation kernel and denoised correlation based kernel, we can also reach some conclusions. For breast cancer data, the two kernels show comparable performance. But for colon cancer data and leukemia data, denoised correlation based kernel demonstrates its superiority. The superiority is much clearer in leukemia data set. The reasons explaining the difference can be possibly given by the dominant eigenvalue theory. In finance, the largest eigenvalue gives a rough idea on the largest possible risk of the investment in the market (Couillet and Debbah 2011). The dominant eigenvalue is the one provides the most valuable information about the dynamics from which the matrix came from Goh et al. (2006).

6.5 Conclusions

In this chapter, two PSD which we call parsimonious correlation kernel and denoised correlation based kernel have been proposed in discriminating different tumor tissues, offering diagnostic suggestions. We have provided theoretical illustrations on the PSD property of the usual correlation kernel. Taking into consideration of the PSD of correlation matrix, we have proposed two PSD kernels. The robustness of the two proposed kernels in conjunction with SVM has been demonstrated through three publicly available data sets related to cancer in tumor discrimination. Comparisons with the existing methods like the decision tree method and the KNN algorithm have been made. Investigation on the performance analysis for the two proposed PSD kernels was conducted with eigenvalue theory support. The proposed kernels highlight the importance of positive-semi-definiteness in kernel construction. As novel kernels using distance-metric for kernel construction that are not common in machine learning framework, the proposed kernels are expected to be applicable in a wider range of areas.

References

Alon U, Barkai N, Notterman D, Gish K, Ybarra S, Mack D, Levine A (1999) Broad patterns of gene expression revealed by clustering analysis of tumor and normal colon tissues probed by oligonucleotide arrays. Proc Natl Acad Sci 96(12):6745

Couillet R, Debbah M (2011) Random matrix methods for wireless communications. Cambridge University Press

Goh K, Cusick M, Valle D, Childs B, Vidal M, Barabási A (2006) Determination of the dominant eigenvalue using the trace method. IEEE Multidisc Eng Educ Mag 1(1):1–2

Golub T, Slonim D, Tamayo P, Huard C, Gaasenbeek M, Mesirov J, Coller H, Loh M, Downing J, Caligiuri M et al (1999) Molecular classification of cancer: class discovery and class prediction by gene expression monitoring. Science 286(5439):531–537

Kyriakides A, Kastanos E, Hadjigeorgiou K, Pitris C (2011) Classification of Raman spectra using the correlation kernel. J Raman Spectrosc 42(5):904–909
Libsvm data set. http://www.csie.ntu.edu.tw/~cjlin/libsvmtools/datasets/binary.html
Smola AJ, Schölkopf B (1998) Learning with Kernels, vol 4. Citeseer
West M, Blanchette C, Dressman H, Huang E, Ishida S, Spang R, Zuzan H, Olson J, Marks J, Nevins J (2001) Predicting the clinical status of human breast cancer by using gene expression profiles. Proc Natl Acad Sci 98(20):11,462

Chapter 7
Weighted GTS Kernel and Applications in Drug Side-Effect Profiles Prediction

7.1 Introduction

In the realm of drug development, pinpointing potential side-effects for promising medications is a pivotal phase. However, a significant and formidable obstacle emerges from the expensive and time-intensive nature of unraveling drug adverse effects. Traditional drug design, often fixated on individual target genes, tends to overlook broader systemic impacts, thereby hindering drug efficacy. Recent research on drug side-effect prediction has shifted towards methodical examinations of drug side-effect profiles. There is now a pressing need to streamline the side-effect identification process and devise efficient evaluation strategies in drug development. Traditional methodologies typically align with two main categories: the ligand-based approach and the docking approach.

However, the effectiveness of machine learning methods in predicting the binding of a candidate ligand using Quantitative Structure-Activity Relationship (QSAR) tends to diminish as the number of ligands available for target proteins decreases (Butina et al. 2002; Byvatov 2003), whereas docking approach is not applicable to proteins with unknown 3D structures (Rarey 1996).

Drug-therapy networks, which have been constructed to investigate the interactions between drugs and human therapies, shed light on strategies for future drug development by associating known drugs with their corresponding therapies (Nacher and Schwartz 2008). Apart from this, drug-target networks (Edda et al. 2010; Ma'ayan et al. 2007; Yildirim et al. 2007) also provide novel information on vast databases of drugs and drug targets. In silico prediction of drug-target interactions is increasingly supported in various tasks in the process of drug discovery, see for instance (Edda et al. 2010; Yamanishi et al. 2010). However, the endeavors devoted to network construction have not led to a significant expansion of novel targets. Drugs are initially designed to intervene a particular pathway or a target gene. Nevertheless, due to the existence of complex cellular mechanisms, other pathways might be activated, resulting in undesirable side-effects. A novel method has been

H. Jiang and W.-K. Ching, *Kernel Methods for Omics Data Mining*, Intelligent Control and Learning Systems 10, https://doi.org/10.1007/978-981-95-3129-5_7

developed in Fukuzaki et al. (2009) to enumerate cooperative pathways, which is limited to the observed gene expression data under drug perturbations. Previous studies of in silico pharmacology mainly concern the prediction of single adverse effects such as hERG inhibition (Pearlstein et al. 2003; Roche et al. 2002), blockage of P450 subtypes (Zuegge et al. 2002), or PXR nuclear hormone receptor binding (Ekins 2004). For independent analysis on a specific side-effect, one can employ the Linear Discriminant Analysis (LDA) where a classification function is built for each side-effect (Cruz-Monteagudo et al. 2006). However, the performance of the method is difficult to assess.

Drugs might probably form a structural network (Scheiber et al. 2009), but there is no integrated framework to predict side-effects for a drug. A method combining the chemical structures for predicting side-effects information was developed in Yamanishi et al. (2010), and was used to infer drug-target interactions. However, it was limited to the prediction of high-dimensional side-effect profiles. Systematic approaches for drug side-effects prediction have been discussed in Atias and Sharan (2011). In Yen et al. (2011), prediction of serious adverse drug reactions is realized by artificial neural network models. Taking into account the information on other drugs and their side-effects, a combination of Canonical Correlation Analysis (CCA) and network-based diffusion method has been applied to predict the side-effects of a drug. Motivated by the technique of CCA, Sparse Canonical Correlation Analysis (SCCA) based model was constructed to predict drug side-effects profiles (Pauwels et al. 2011).

Phenotypic effects of drugs have been examined based on drug-target interaction networks called "pharmacogenomic features". However, the underlying molecular mechanisms are too complicated to be completely described. To resolve this, Iwata et al. (2013) turned to protein domains instead of the protein itself, and applied logistic regression as a binary classifier to detect drug side-effects-protein domains pairs in the drug-target interactions. They proposed four methods to infer pharmacogenomic features. Then the prediction of a larger interaction network of all drugs and proteins according to pharmacogenomic features obtained can be achieved. However, the performance of their proposed methods relies heavily on the data profile (Chen et al. 2009; Consortium 2010; The pfam protein families database 2008; Kuhn et al. 2010).

Recently, some significant works have been done. For example, Liu et al. (2012) built an Adverse Drug Reaction (ADR) prediction model by using logistic regression, naive Bayes, KNN, random forest and SVM; and found that SVM with RBF kernel improves the ADR prediction significantly to combine different types of information (phenotypic, chemical, and biological information) at the different stages of drug surveillance. However, the parameter embedded in RBF kernel needs to be carefully predefined as the results are sensitive to parameter setting, besides the model training with RBF kernel sometimes show over-fitting phenomenon and lacks generalization ability. Later, Bresso et al. (2013) integrated decision-trees and inductive-logic programming to explicitly characterize drug side-effects associations in several drugs; but inductive-logic programming and decision trees are both time-consuming, for example, the bounded ILP-consistency problem is $\sum_2^p$ hard. Then in Zhang et al.'s study (2015), they proposed a Feature Selection-based Multi-Label K-Nearest

Neighbor method (FS-MLKNN) to achieve feature dimensions reduction and high-accuracy prediction of side-effects, and further adopted weighted scoring to ensemble individual feature-based FS-MLKNN models. In Drug side effect prediction (2016), authors further proposed using linear neighborhood representation and data integration to improve drug side-effect profiles prediction accuracy. The methods were very promising in similarity construction and integration, the importance of regularization was also pointed out. But different side-effect profiles may rely on different similarity measure.

Inspired by the similarity measure construction framework and taking into consideration that different side-effect profiles may need different similarity measures, we propose model in terms of hyperplane separation named as Weighted Generalized T-Student (WGTS) kernel SVM. It allows different hyperplanes separating different side-effects by constructing an appropriate kernel for sample relationship evaluation, and the computational complexity is acceptable. The measures in revealing the potential mechanism between structures and side-effects are satisfactory. It is therefore very efficient to predict the drug side-effect profiles with our proposed models.

7.2 Preliminaries

7.2.1 NR and RR Models

We assume that there are n drugs and the number of side-effects is m. For each drug, the chemical structure representation is postulated to a $1 \times p$ vector which means each drug is described by p attributes. This will generate a drug attribute matrix of size $n \times p$ and a drug side-effect association matrix of size $n \times m$.

We denote the chemical structure representation for drug j, $j = 1, 2, \ldots, n$, by

$$\mathbf{x}_j = (x_{j1}, x_{j2}, \ldots, x_{jp}), \ j = 1, 2, \ldots, n,$$

and the ground truth profile representation for drug j by

$$\mathbf{y}_j = (y_{j1}, y_{j2}, \ldots, y_{jm}), \ j = 1, 2, \ldots, n.$$

A naive intuitive is to minimize the distance between the $n \times p$ attribute matrix X and the $n \times m$ ground truth profile matrix Y where the distance between two matrices is measured by the Frobenius norm. Thus, we have the following Naive Regression (NR) minimization problem:

$$\min_{B} \{\| XB - Y \|_F\}$$

where the $p \times m$ matrix B gives the relation between the attribute matrix and the ground truth profile matrix of the drugs. Here

$$||M||_F := \sqrt{\sum_{i=1}^{m}\sum_{j=1}^{n} M_{ij}^2}$$

is the Frobenius norm of the $m \times n$ matrix M. Define the objective function as follows:

$$f(B) = \| XB - Y \|_F,$$

which is a function of the variable B, and its gradient is given by

$$\frac{\partial f}{\partial B} = \frac{X^T XB - X^T Y}{f(B)}.$$

In this formulation, $X^T X$ is a $p \times p$ positive semi-definite (PSD) matrix. If the matrix $X^T X$ is nonsingular, one can directly deduce that f is minimized when

$$B = \{X^T X\}^{-1} X^T Y. \tag{7.1}$$

If $X^T X$ is singular, then we can replace $X^T X$ by its pseudo-inverse (Golub and Loan 1996). This is the first step in our prediction method. Secondly, with the obtained model parameters, one can predict drug side-effect profiles. If $\tilde{X}$ is the testing attribute matrix, and we have $\tilde{Y} = B\tilde{X}$. Here $\tilde{Y}$ is not a binary matrix, the final ground truth profile determination can be achieved by the following:

$$\tilde{Y}(\tilde{Y} > 0.5) = 1 \quad \text{and} \quad \tilde{Y}(\tilde{Y} \leq 0.5) = 0,$$

which represents having side-effects and no side-effects, respectively. The obtained drug side-effects profiles are then compared with the ground truth profile for performance evaluation.

In practice, the matrix X is usually rank-deficient, so that the matrix $X^T X$ is singular. Instead of replacing $(X^T X)^{-1}$ simply by its pseudo-inverse, we overcome the previous problem by introducing a regularized term for the objective function. In the following, we will propose regularized regression (RR) model. Define the objective function as follows:

$$\min_B \{\| XB - Y \|_F + \lambda \| B \|_F\}$$

where $\lambda > 0$. Then the gradient becomes

$$\frac{\partial f}{\partial B} = 2((X^T X + \lambda I)B - X^T Y).$$

It is straightforward to show that $(X^T X + \lambda I)$ is a symmetric positive definite matrix. With the eigenvalue decomposition formula, we have $X^T X = UPU^T$ where P is the diagonal matrix containing all eigenvalues, and U is the corresponding orthogonal eigenvector matrix corresponding to the eigenvalues. Since the identity matrix can have the trivial decomposition $I = UIU^T$, we have

$$X^T X + \lambda I = U(P + \lambda I)U^T. \tag{7.2}$$

Because of the positive semi-definiteness property of the matrix $X^T X$, we know that all the eigenvalues of $X^T X$ are non-negative. This validates the positive-definiteness of the matrix $(X^T X + \lambda I)$. Therefore, the matrix B solving the objective function can be obtained as follows:

$$B = \{X^T X + \lambda I\}^{-1} X^T Y.$$

When λ is a relatively small positive number, the solution would be close to the actual one. Finally, performance evaluation is conducted as in the NR model.

7.2.2 Materials

Information on drugs and their recorded side-effects are extracted from the SIDER database, see for instance (Kuhn et al. 2010). In the database, there are 888 approved drugs, each of which is represented by a 1385 dimensional side-effect binary profile encoding for the presence or absence of the known side-effects. Chemical structure representations for drugs are encoded using fingerprints corresponding to chemical substructures in PubChem database, in which descriptions of the chemical structures are available at the PubChem website (Chen et al. 2009). PubChem is an open chemistry database at the National Institutes of Health (NIH). In this context, each drug is represented by a binary vector with 1 representing the presence of corresponding substructure, and 0 for the absence.

7.2.3 Performance Evaluation Metrics

Cross-validation is a technique for assessing the generalization ability of a statistical analysis. It is mainly used to estimate the accuracy of a predictive model in practice. One round of cross-validation involves partitioning the data into two complementary subsets, namely, the training set and the testing set. The training set is the one used for analysis, and the testing set is used for validating the analysis. Multiple rounds of cross-validation are performed with different partitions, and the validation results are obtained by taking average over the results of all rounds.

7.2.3.1 5-Fold Cross-Validation

The performance of the classification model is measured through 5-fold cross-validation. In this model evaluation method, the original set of samples is randomly partitioned into 5 subsets. Among the 5 subsets, one subset is retained as the validation data for testing the model, and the remaining 4 subsets are used as training data. The cross-validation process is then repeated for 5 times (folds), results of which are then averaged (or combined) to produce a test statistics. The accuracy of the learning performance is assessed as follows:

$$\text{Accuracy} = \frac{\text{TP} + \text{TN}}{\text{TP} + \text{TN} + \text{FP} + \text{FN}}$$

where TP is the number of true positive instances, TN is the number of true negative instances, FP is the number of false positive instances and FN is the number of false negative instances. We note that the accuracy is actually the ratio of the number of correctly predicted items to the total number of data instances.

7.2.4 Results

We present the performance comparison among the NR method, our proposed method RR, and other three existing methods including Decision Tree algorithm (DT), K-Nearest Neighbors algorithm (KNN) and Support Vector Machines (SVM). The Central Processing Unit (CPU) time and accuracy of different methods are compared. For the KNN algorithm, we utilized the same parameter $K = 50$ as suggested in Pauwels et al. (2011). Support vector machines were then performed with the Radial Basis Function Kernel and the parameter σ was set to be 0.2. For the other three methods, the learning schemes were performed 1385 times as they can only conduct classification for one ground truth at each time.

Table 7.1 presents the CPU time comparison among NR, DT, KNN and SVM. The elapsed time in each fold is recorded during the 5-fold cross validation. Significant differences can be observed between our method NR and the other three methods. For example, in the first cross-validation, our method requires 0.68 seconds, whereas it takes 1470.98, 281.74 and 243.59 s for DT, KNN, and SVM, respectively. This evidently highlights the superiority of our proposed method in fulfilling the task of prediction rapidly. DT needs around 60000 s to finish the whole 5-fold cross-validation process, and KNN and SVM show similar performance, requiring about 1000 s in total. Overall, it takes around 5 s for our method NR to finish the whole 5-fold cross-validation process, while other three methods take hundreds or thousands of seconds. Therefore, NR method drastically saves computational cost from the perspective of efficiency.

Table 7.2, on the other hand, depicts the accuracy of all five methods: NR, RR, DT, KNN and SVM. Results were obtained by taking the average over the 5 rounds.

Table 7.1 Comparison on CPU time (ET: elapsed time)

Methods	ET				
	Fold 1 (s)	Fold 2 (s)	Fold 3 (s)	Fold 4 (s)	Fold 5 (s)
DT	1470.98	1447.66	1507.90	1570.54	1463.33
KNN	281.74	277.35	272.22	273.69	274.63
SVM	243.59	252.31	245.32	240.78	230.97
NR	0.68	0.66	0.75	1.05	0.69

Table 7.2 Comparison on prediction accuracy (Min_AC: minimum accuracy, Mean_AC: averaged accuracy)

Methods	Min_AC (%)	Mean_AC (%)
DT	52.59	93.95
KNN	52.48	95.37
SVM	16.44	95.03
NR	51.92	89.18
RR	54.73	94.35

The minimum and the averaged accuracy of the predictions of the 1385 side-effects among the four methods were compared. Concerning the minimum accuracy, NR is comparable to the DT and KNN. In the worst situation, it can still achieve an accuracy of around 52%. The minimum accuracy of SVM is the lowest, yielding 16%. Hence SVM is not favorable, even though its averaged accuracy attains 95%. Taking into consideration the averaged accuracy, the performance of NR, with an accuracy of 89%, is comparable with that of DT and KNN method, reaching 94% and 95%, respectively. Apart from that, NR outshines other methods in terms of computation pace. Note that the input matrix is positive semi-definiteness, so there is room for improvement in prediction accuracy.

The regularized minimization framework overcomes the positive semi-definiteness of the matrix $X^T X$ in Eq. (7.1). As can be seen from Table 7.2, the minimum accuracy of NR increases from 52 to 55%, and the averaged accuracy goes up from 89% to 94%. This kind of performance is comparable to, if not better than, other three methods. Thus, experimental results show the necessity of incorporating the regularized term in model construction.

Table 7.3 presents the CPU time of our original method NR and the regularized one RR for the 5-Fold cross validation. We have observed from Table 7.1 that the computational cost of NR is much less than the other three methods. The RR model, however, exhibits superior efficiency. The execution time was decreased, for example, from 0.75 to 0.39 s in the first round. Such decrease was observed in each fold. Therefore, as anticipated, not only the speed but also the prediction accuracy has been improved after NR being improved to RR.

Table 7.3 Comparison on CPU time: NR and RR (ET: elapsed time)

Methods	ET				
	Fold 1 (s)	Fold 2 (s)	Fold 3 (s)	Fold 4 (s)	Fold 5 (s)
RR	0.39	0.39	0.43	0.45	0.38
NR	0.75	0.87	0.89	0.85	0.99

Figure 7.1 depicts the accuracy distribution achieved by all the five methods: NR, RR, DT, KNN and SVM. Y-axis represents the averaged accuracy values for different side-effects, while X-axis indicates the corresponding methods. As in Tables 7.2 and 7.3, the regularized parameter λ in RR methods has been set to be 1. The first important message this figure delivers is that SVM is of relatively low reliability. Although it achieves an averaged accuracy of 95.03% (described in Table 7.2), it reaches very low accuracy for predicting many of the side-effects. We can see from the figure that many scatter points are located below 0.5, while some are even lower than 0.2. In addition, the minimum accuracy for DT and KNN methods are around 53%, whereas that of our method NR is around 53%. This shows the comparability of our method with the existing methods. After the regularization, the minimum

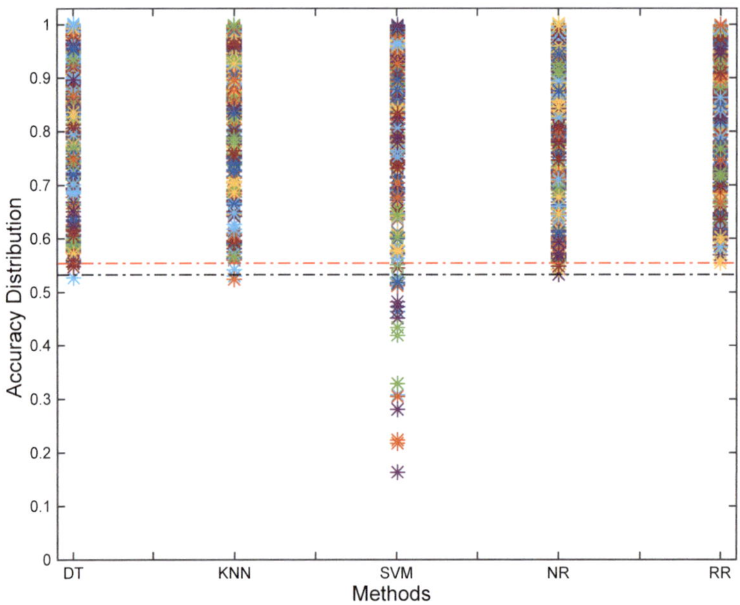

Fig. 7.1 Distribution of accuracy achieved by five methods on 1385 drug side-effects prediction. DT, KNN, SVM, NR and RR are short forms of Decision Tree algorithm, K-nearest Neighbors algorithm, Naive Regression, and Regularized Regression

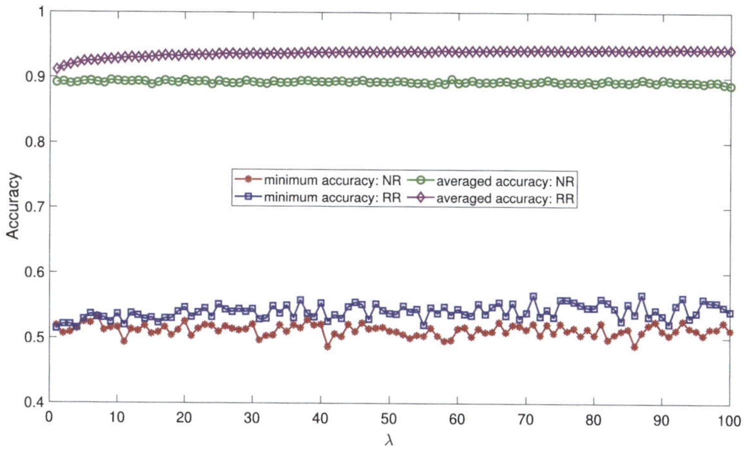

Fig. 7.2 Comparison of minimum and averaged accuracy achieved by NR and RR methods

accuracy of RR is increased to around 55%, which is consistent with the description in Table 7.1.

Furthermore, as λ can be varied in (0, 1], we display in Fig. 7.2 the comparison between the RR method with the original NR in terms of both minimum accuracy and averaged accuracy. Y-axis shows the values of λ, while X-axis indicates the values of accuracy. From Fig. 7.2, the curves of averaged (minimum) accuracy of both NR and RR methods overlap a little bit when $\lambda \in (0, 1]$, and at some points NR even performs better than RR. The reason is that when λ is relatively small, say, <0.05, the superiority of RR is not obvious as the perturbation to the original solution is too small to be effective. When λ is larger than 0.05, the superiority of RR becomes remarkable. We can observe a general increase in averaged accuracy for drug profile prediction in regularized method with the increase of λ.

In the following, we discuss the selection of the parameter λ in the regularized term of the RR method. We claim that when λ is not very large, the effect is trivial. From Eq. (7.2), we know that the eigenvalues of the n-by-n matrix $(X^T X + \lambda I)$ are given by

$$P_{ii} + \lambda, \qquad i = 1, 2, \ldots, n$$

where P_{ii} $(i = 1, 2, \ldots, n)$ are the eigenvalues of $X^T X$. In this situation, the eigenvalues of the matrix $(X^T X + \lambda I)^{-1}$ are given by

$$\frac{1}{(P_{ii} + \lambda)}, \qquad i = 1, 2, \ldots, n.$$

Note that P_{ii} $(i = 1, 2, \ldots, n)$ are all non-negative and λ is positive. Assume that $\lambda_{\max}$ and $\lambda_{\min}$ are the maximum and minimum eigenvalues for P, then the largest distance between any two eigenvalues of $(X^T X + \lambda I)^{-1}$ is bounded above by

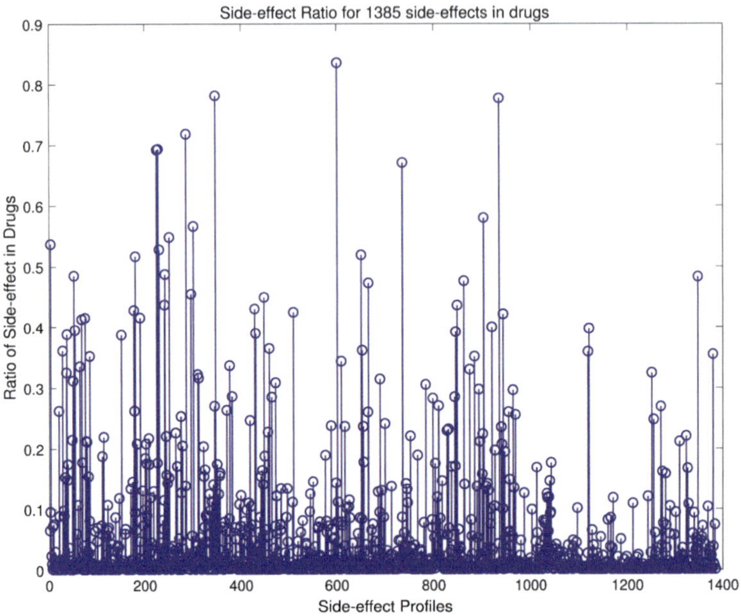

Fig. 7.3 Side-effect ratio of drug side-effect profiles. For 1385 side-effect profiles, the ratio (the percentage of the number of drugs having side-effect over all the number of drugs investigated) for each side-effect is plotted

$$\frac{\lambda_{\max} - \lambda_{\min}}{(\lambda_{\max} + \lambda)(\lambda_{\min} + \lambda)}.$$

As λ increases, the range of the eigenvalues of $(X^T X + \lambda I)^{-1}$ decreases, making the eigenvalues closer to each other. Alternatively, if the side-effect profiles are dominant in negative or positive ground-truth for the majority of drug candidates, then the similarity in eigenvalues will in general contribute to the improvement of the averaged prediction accuracy. With regard to this, we further plot Fig. 7.3.

Figure 7.3 shows the ratio of the presence of each side-effect in all drug candidates. Y-axis indicates the ratio of a side-effect, while X-axis indicates the side-effects from the first to the 1385th one. From Fig. 7.3, one can see that actually most of the side-effects profiles are with negative dominance. From the statistical point of view, the majority of the drug side-effect profiles are <0.2 in side-effects ratio, providing further support for the above claim in the improvement of prediction accuracy.

7.3 Discussions

Taking into the fact that each drug on average has 68.8 side-effects where the number of side-effects for a given drug is 1385, we would like to further adopt measures such as AUC to measure the performance of our proposed method. Though the averaged accuracy and minimum accuracy in RR method is relatively acceptable, the AUC value is not satisfying. Hence, inspired by SVM in single side-effect based model construction, we propose the following weighted Generalized T-Student Kernel (GTS) model, which has been proven to be a Mercer kernel, thus having a positive semi-definite kernel matrix (Boughorbel et al. 2004). It is given by

$$K(\vec{x}, \vec{y}) = \frac{1}{1 + ||\vec{x} - \vec{y}||^d}.$$

We propose a weighted GTS kernel in the following formula:

$$K(\vec{x}, \vec{y}) = \frac{1}{1 + [(\vec{x} - \vec{y})^T W (\vec{x} - \vec{y})]^d}$$

where

$$W = \begin{Bmatrix} \frac{\max(\text{std(A)})}{\text{std}(A_1)} & \cdots & 0 \\ 0 & \ddots & 0 \\ 0 & \cdots & \frac{\max(\text{std(A)})}{\text{std}(A_n)} \end{Bmatrix}$$

is a diagonal matrix $A_i, i = 1, 2, \ldots, p$, represents the ith column (attribute) of data matrix A, and $\max(\text{std(A)}) \triangleq \max_{1 \le i \le n}(\text{std}(A_i))$. The reason for proposing weighted GTS kernel is that, the data matrix A is very sparse where each drug has 120.8 substructures on average. Therefore, the distribution of attributes is quite uneven. We regard the attribute with higher standard deviation more important.

It can be proved that

$$K(\vec{x}, \vec{y}) = \frac{1}{1 + [(\vec{x} - \vec{y})^T W (\vec{x} - \vec{y})]^d}$$

is a Mercer kernel as shown below.

Proof It is clear that W as a diagonal matrix can be decomposed as follows:

$$W = \begin{pmatrix} \sqrt{\frac{\max(\text{std(A)})}{\text{std}(A_1)}} & \cdots & 0 \\ 0 & \ddots & 0 \\ 0 & \cdots & \sqrt{\frac{\max(\text{std(A)})}{\text{std}(A_n)}} \end{pmatrix}^2$$

Denote $A' = AW^{\frac{1}{2}}$ where

$$W^{\frac{1}{2}} = \begin{pmatrix} \sqrt{\frac{\max(\mathrm{std(A)})}{\mathrm{std}(A_1)}} & \cdots & 0 \\ 0 & \ddots & 0 \\ 0 & \cdots & \sqrt{\frac{\max(\mathrm{std(A)})}{\mathrm{std}(A_n)}} \end{pmatrix}$$

and

$$\vec{x'} = \vec{x} * W^{\frac{1}{2}}, \vec{y'} = \vec{y} * W^{\frac{1}{2}},$$

then we have

$$K(\vec{x}, \vec{y}) = \frac{1}{1 + [(\vec{x'} - \vec{y'})^T(\vec{x'} - \vec{y'})]^d} = \frac{1}{1 + ||\vec{x'} - \vec{y'}||^{2d}}.$$

Therefore the kernel matrix can be regarded as a GTS kernel with degree $2d$ for data matrix A'.

The most recent proposed method in drug side-effect prediction: Linear Neighborhood Similarity Method (LNSM) Drug side effect prediction (2016) shows excellent performance in AUC as well as other types of measures for multi-label classification tasks. The main objective function in the model deals with linear combination for data point X_i by its neighborhoods.

$$\min \quad \varepsilon_i = ||X_i - \sum_{i,j,x_{i_j} \in N(x_i)} w_{i,i_j} X_{i_j}||^2 + \lambda|||\boldsymbol{w}_i||^2,$$

$$\text{s.t.} \quad ||X_i - \sum_{i,j,x_{i_j} \in N(x_i)} w_{i,i_j} X_{i_j}||^2| \leq p.$$

Here, $\boldsymbol{w}_i = [w_{i,1}, w_{i,2}, \ldots, w_{i,n}]^T$. The method has been applied to the 888 approved drugs with chemical and side-effects information. And it was shown that the AUC value under fivefold cross validation was 0.8941 (Drug side effect prediction 2016). In the following, we present the performance of weighted GTS kernel in conjunction with SVM for drug side-effect profiles prediction. We also introduced the same measures in Drug side effect prediction (2016) for evaluation purpose. Firstly, two most popular metrics: AUC and the Area Under the Precision-Recall curve (AUPR) were used. Secondly, multi-label learning evaluation metrics were also used as the problem we considered can be formulated as a multi-label classification task. Hamming loss corresponds to the Hamming distance between predicted labels and true labels which is equivalent to the fraction of the wrong labels to the total number of labels. The one-error evaluates the fraction of instances whose top-ranked label is not in the relevant label set. The Coverage evaluates how many steps are needed, on average, to move down the ranked label list so as to cover all the relevant labels of the instance. Ranking loss evaluates the average fraction of label pairs that are reversely ordered for the instance. The average precision evaluates the average fraction of relevant labels ranked higher than a particular label.

Table 7.4 Comparison on CPU time: GTS Kernel SVM and RR (ET: elapsed time)

Methods	ET				
	Fold 1 (s)	Fold 2 (s)	Fold 3 (s)	Fold 4 (s)	Fold 5 (s)
RR	0.33	0.33	0.33	0.33	0.30
GTS	114.32	113.49	114.43	117.79	101.99

Table 7.5 Performances of GTS Kernel SVM and RR model

Method	AUC	AUPR	Hamming loss	Ranking loss	One-error	Coverage	Average precision
RR model	0.7506	0.3015	0.0565	0.2136	0.3694	1.2348×10^3	0.3607
GTS Kernel	0.9052	0.4176	0.0454	0.0707	0.1622	782.6532	0.5077

Table 7.6 Performances of GTS Kernel SVM and WGTS Kernel SVM

Method	AUC	AUPR	Hamming loss	Ranking loss	One-error	Coverage	Average precision
GTS model	0.9054	0.4180	0.0454	0.0709	0.1734	781.1622	0.5037
WGTS Kernel	0.9054	0.4187	0.0453	0.0708	0.1667	781.0597	0.5045

We first compared the performance of GTS kernel with RR model through fivefold cross-validations. In regard to the computational time, we can obtain an obvious conclusion that GTS kernel cannot compete with RR model. Because from Table 7.1, we know that RBF-SVM needs roughly 250 s in one round while RR only needs about 0.33 s. Though GTS kernel SVM is more efficient than RBF-SVM in terms of computational time as shown in Table 7.4, and it still cannot compete with RR model. Regarding the other measures as shown in Table 7.5, we can see that Hamming Loss that represents classification error is larger in RR model. Therefore, GTS kernel is superior to RR model in this perspective. Apart from that, GTS kernel outperforms RR model in the remaining 6 measures. For example, the AUC value in GTS kernel is 0.9052 while in RR model, the AUC value can only achieve 0.7506.

In the next stage, we are going to compare the performance of WGTS kernel with GTS kernel. Here, we use the same degree parameter $d = 1$. In Table 7.6, we can find the performance of WGTS kernel is slightly better than GTS kernel. It can be seen that one-error in GTS kernel is clearly inferior to WGTS kernel. Besides, WGTS kernel is slightly better than GTS kernel in other considered measures such as Hamming Loss, Ranking Loss etc. The AUC value in both kernels are the same.

The WGTS kernel performs similarly when $\lambda = 0.6, 0.7, 0.8$. Hence, we choose $\lambda = 0.8$ to compare with the most recent LNSM method through fivefold cross-validations for its relative superiority in obtaining smaller one-error. In Table 7.7, we can see that WGTS Kernel is comparable to LNSM Method. WGTS Kernel is superior

Table 7.7 Performances of WGTS Kernel SVM and LNSM method

Method	AUC	AUPR	Hamming loss	Ranking loss	One-error	Coverage	Average precision
LNSM method	0.8941	0.4491	0.0444	0.0713	0.1633	790.9471	0.5126
WGTS Kernel	0.9055	0.4216	0.0453	0.0710	0.1604	784.4220	0.5066

Table 7.8 Performances of WGTS Kernel SVM and LNSM method for independent test

Method	AUC	AUPR	Hamming loss	Ranking loss	One-error	Coverage	Average precision
LNSM method	0.8722	0.3109	0.0373	0.1038	0.1851	1535.9223	0.3649
WGTS Kernel	0.9150	0.2921	0.0125	0.0780	0.1845	3.6038e+03	0.3473

in AUC, meaning that better specificity and sensitivity are obtained in WGTS kernel. A smaller one-error in WGTS kernel means that the fraction of instances whose top-ranked label is not in the relevant label set is smaller. Besides, WGTS kernel is superior in Ranking Loss, Coverage as well. While LNSM shows superiority in AUPR, Average Precision and Hamming Loss.

Furthermore, we conducted the independent test to evaluate different methods where we evaluated their prediction capability for new drugs in the independent test. In the SIDER 4 dataset, 771 drugs were used as the training set, and 309 newly added drugs were used as the testing set. We still compare the results with the most recent proposed LNSM method. It can be seen that WGTS kernel is clearly superior in AUC measure, Hamming Loss and Ranking Loss. One-error measure in both methods are similar to each other. For LNSM method, Average Precision, AUPR and Coverage are clearly better recorded. Overall, WGTS kernel is comparable to LNSM method (Table 7.8).

7.4 Conclusions

In this chapter, we propose a simple and efficient Regularized Regression model (RR) for drug side-effects prediction. The regression-based model is efficient in model parameter estimation and the accuracy of the model is comparable to some of the existing approaches including Decision Tree algorithm, K-nearest Neighbors algorithm and Support Vector Machines. Taking into consideration on the practicability in not only improving accuracy but also AUC measures etc., a weighted generalized t-student kernel was proposed. The kernel has been compared with the most recent method for drug side-effect profiles predictions: Linear Neighbor Similarity Method (LNSM). On the one hand, the WGTS kernel is expected to straighten out brilliant future studies to understand the adverse or side-effects in the processing of drug design. For example, avoiding some chemical substructures might help avoid a set of drug side-effects. On the other hand, the predictive model is supposed to reduce the cost of side-effects elucidation for the pharmaceutical industry. Our work provides a promising perspective towards the drug development process.

References

Atias N, Sharan R (2011) An algorithmic framework for predicting side effects of drugs. J Comput Biol 18:207–218

Boughorbel S, Tarel J, Fleuret F (2004) Non-mercer kernels for SVM object recognition. In: British machine vision conference, BMVC 2004, Kingston, UK, September 7–9, 2004. Proceedings, pp 1–10 (2004). https://doi.org/10.5244/C.18.16. https://doi.org/10.5244/C.18.16

Bresso E, Grisoni R, Marchetti G, Karaboga AS, Souchet M, Devignes MD, Tabbone MS (2013) Integrative relational machine-learning for understanding drug side-effect profiles. BMC Bioinform 14:207

Butina D, Segall MD, Frankcombe K (2002) Predicting ADME properties in silico: methods and models. Drug Discov Today 7:S83–S88

Byvatov E (2003) Comparison of support vector machine and artificial neural network systems for drug/nondrug classification. J Chem Inf Comput Sci 43:1882–1889

Chen B, Wild D, Guh R (2009) Pubchem as a source of polypharmacology. J Chem Inf Model 49:2044–2055

Consortium, T.U (2010) The universal protein resource (UniProt) in 2010. Nucleic Acids Res 38:D142–D148

Cruz-Monteagudo M, Gonzles-Daz H, Uriarte E (2006) Simple stochastic fingerprints towards mathematical modeling in biology and medicine 2. unifying Markov model for drug side effects. Bull Math Biol 68:1527–155

Drug side effect prediction through linear neighborhoods and multiple data source integration (2016)

Edda K, Rebecca CW, Ursula K (2010) Biochemical network-based drug-target prediction. Curr Opin Biotechnol 21:511–516

Ekins S (2004) Docking and scoring in virtual screening for drug discovery: methods and applications. Drug Discov Today 9:276–285

Finn R, Tate J, Mistry J, Coggill P, Sammut JHH, Ceric G, Forslund K, Eddy S, Sonnhammer E, Bateman A (2008) The Pfam protein families database (2008) Nucleic Acids Res 36:D281–D288

Fukuzaki M, Seki M, Kashima H, Sese J (2009) Side effect prediction using cooperative pathways. In IEEE international conference on bioinformatics and biomedicine, pp 142–147

Golub GH, Loan CFV (1996) Matrix computations, 3rd edn. Johns Hopkins University Press, US

Iwata H, Mizutani S, Tabei Y, Kotera M, Goto S, Yamanishi Y (2013) Inferring protein domains associated with drug side effects based on drug-target interaction network. BMC Syst Biol 7(suppl 6):S18

Kuhn M, Campillos M, Letunic I, Jensen L, Bork P (2010) A side effect resource to capture phenotypic effects of drugs. Mol Syst Biol 6:643

Liu M, Wu Y, Chen Y, Sun J, Zhao Z, Chen X, Matheny ME, Xu H (2012) Large-scale prediction of adverse drug reactions using chemical, biological, and phenotypic properties of drugs. J Am Med Inform Assoc 19:e28–e35

Ma'ayan A, Jenkins SL, Goldfarb J, Lyengar R (2007) Network analysis of FDA approved drugs and their targets. Mt Sinai J Med 74:27–32

Nacher JC, Schwartz JM (2008) A global view of drug-therapy interations. BMC Pharmacol 8:5
Pauwels E, Stoven V, Yamanishi Y (2011) Predicting drug side-effect profiles: a chemical fragment-based approach. BMC Bioinform 12:169
Pearlstein RA, Vaz RJ, Kang JS, Chen XL, Preobrazhenskaya M, Shchekotikhin AE, Korolev AM, Lysenkova LN, Miroshnikova OV, Hendrix J, Ramppe D (2003) Characterization of HERG potassium channel inhibition using CoMSiA 3D QSAR and homology modeling approaches. Bioorg Med Chem Lett 13:1829–1835
Rarey M (1996) A fast flexible docking method using an incremental construction algorithm. J Mol Bol 261:470–489
Roche O, Trube G, Zuegge J, Pflimlin P, Alanine A, Schnelder G (2002) A virtual screening method for prediction of the HERG potassium channel liability of compound libraries. ChemBioChem 3:455–459
Scheiber J, Jenkins JL, Chetan S, Sukuru K, Bender A, Mikhailov D, Milik M, Azzaoui K, Whitebread S, Hamon J, Urban L, Glick M, Davies JW (2009) Mapping adverse drug reactions in chemical space. J Med Chem 52:3103–3107
Yamanishi Y, Kotera M, Kanehisa M, Goto S (2010) Drug-target interaction prediction from chemical, genomic and pharmacological data in an integrated framework. Bioinformatics 26:i246–i254
Yen PF, Mital DP, Srinivasan S (2011) Prediction of the serious adverse drug reactions using an artificial neural network model. Int J Med Eng Inform 3:53–59
Yildirim MA, Goh KI, Cusick ME, Barabasi AL, Vidal M (2007) Drug-target network. Nat Biotechnol 25:1119–1126
Zhang W, Liu F, Luo L, Zhang J (2015) Predicting drug side effects by multi-label learning and ensemble learning. BMC Bioinform 16:365
Zuegge J, Fechner U, Roche O, Parrott NJ, Engkvist O, Schneider G (2002) A virtual screening method for prediction of the HERG potassium channel liability of compound libraries. QSAR Comb Sci 21:156–249

Chapter 8
Single Cell RNA-Sequencing Data Analysis

8.1 Introduction

A transcriptome analysis utilizing single cell RNA sequencing (scRNA-Seq) has been one of the most attractive topics among recent research activities. The core technique of scRNA-Seq is to employ the advanced sequencing technologies to sequence cDNAs prepared from a single cell to obtain information about the cell's RNA content. scRNA-Seq thus offers gene expression measurements at single cell resolution. This unprecedented resolution into cell states allows the investigation of population heterogeneity as well as genetic and epigenetic variability in a cellular system (Eberwine et al. 2014; Stegle et al. 2015). For example, a popular study has conducted clustering analysis to identify cell subpopulations from a set of heterogeneous cells, hoping for a better understanding of cell function and dysfunction (Eberwine et al. 2013).

Despite the rapid advancement in scRNA-Seq technologies, multiple types of noise prevail in the single-cell experiments and cannot be overlooked. One source of noise is the biological fluctuation in both global and local perspectives (Shapiro et al. 2013), e.g., unwanted cell-to-cell variations. There are also noises from the scRNA-Seq protocols, e.g., the technical biases caused by pipetting errors, temperature difference, PCR amplifications, etc. These noises have led to many challenging issues in scRNA-Seq data analysis, including but not limited to high rates of dropout events, batch effects and unwanted cell-to-cell variations (Brennecke et al. 2013). The prevalence of dropout events would lead to zero-inflated data. Batch effects usually occur due to inconsistencies in library preparation of RNA samples (for sequencing) across different biological labs and thus confound true gene expression differences. Unwanted cell-to-cell variations are attributable to cell size, cell cycle state, and other factors that are irrelevant for cell type identification. If these issues are not managed properly, the results can be significantly affected. We refer to Yuan et al. (2017) for a comprehensive review and discussion on issues in single-cell analysis.

H. Jiang and W.-K. Ching, *Kernel Methods for Omics Data Mining*, Intelligent Control and Learning Systems 10, https://doi.org/10.1007/978-981-95-3129-5_8

scRNA-Seq data is noisy and of high dimensionality. Many clustering methods have been proposed to deal with data structure in high dimensionality and noise distributions. Among those, some efforts designed new (dis)similarity measures which were implemented in traditional clustering algorithms such as hierarchical or k-means clustering. Shared Nearest Neighbor (SNN), a commonly used secondary similarity measure (Guha et al. 1999; Ertöz et al. 2003), is expressed as a function of shared fixed-sized neighborhoods determined by the primary measure, e.g., Euclidean norm. It has been proved to be robust and produce relatively stable clustering results compared to those based on primary measures (Houle et al. 2010). Guha et al. (1999) proposed a robust hierarchical clustering algorithm for dealing with categorical attributes such as attributes described by different colors. The algorithm uses the number of neighborhood information to measure the similarity of samples instead of merely using the attribute values of sample pairs. However, the algorithm is not quite fit for single cell data sets where scRNA-Seq values are not categorical. On the other hand, in Ertoz et al., SNN clustering was proposed for handling high dimensional data which has been constructed based on the notion of DBSCAN by a new definition of density and the core points, and hence the number of optimal clusters was determined automatically. SNN-Cliq (Xu 2015), as an extension of SNN clustering algorithm, was further developed based on a quasi-cliq clustering method to identify tight groups, where similarity measure has been constructed based on neighborhood ranking. However, the drawback of the algorithm lies in large scale single cell clustering where many noisy clusters are detected.

Some researchers employed the well-known Pearson correlations or Euclidean distances as measures but implemented them in a newly designed clustering algorithm. The Rare Cell Type Identification algorithm identifies disease-specific cells through k-means clustering (Guha et al. 1999), where the first step involves cell similarity construction under Pearson correlation coefficient. One of the drawbacks lies in convergence to a local minimum which may produce counterintuitive results. The PhenonGraph algorithm (Levine et al. 2015) constructs k-nearest neighbor graph to study cell phenotypes, where the distance is measured under Euclidean distance. This algorithm is a supervised one based on the construction of Jaccard graph and the dissimilarity between cells is evaluated from a local perspective. The application to unsupervised cases is not clear. Wang et al. (2017) proposed a kernel based similarity learning algorithm for analysis of scRNA-Seq data, where RBF kernel is utilized with Euclidean norm as distance measurement. Teschendorff and Enver (2017) introduced Partitioning Around Medoids (PAM) algorithm with Pearson correlation metric to infer cell clusters. It works with a generalization of the Manhattan norm to define distance between data-points instead of L_2-norm. However, the algorithm needs to firstly know the number of cell populations, which restricts the generalization ability to unknown cell type cases. Vladimir et al. (2016) recently developed a consensus clustering framework for single cell clustering, where a number of distance measures were considered in cell dis(similarity) construction, and a final consensus similarity matrix was obtained for hierarchical clustering. However, all these methods evaluate the dissimilarity of cells locally without taking the cellular microenvironment into consideration.

As discussed above, a central problem in clustering analysis of single cells is quantifying the relationships between cells. However, in general, scRNA-seq data is of high dimensionality, noisy, sparse and heterogeneous (Xu 2015). These properties make conventional (dis)similarity measures less effective and reliable (Beyer et al. 1999). In this chapter, inspired by the previous methods of measuring cell-to-cell similarity using neighborhood information, we propose a new measure for any pair of cells called **Corr**, which defines a cell-to-cell "differentiability correlation" for scRNA-Seq data taking into consideration on the expression patterns of surrounding cells from a global perspective. In particular, this "differentiability correlation" assesses cell-to-cell relationships based on gene differential patterns. It has a form similar to Gamma correlation, which evaluates all pair-wise similarities between cells from a global viewpoint to ensure a robust association assessment on any two cells. To perform clustering analysis of cells, we borrowed the framework of hierarchical clustering, but using our '**Corr**' as the cell-cell similarity measure and a new rule based on variance analysis to decide where to cut the hierarchical dendrogram. The newly developed dendrogram-cutting rule can be used to determine the number of clusters (or cell subpopulations) automatically. This proposed algorithm is compared with SNN-Cliq and several other clustering methods for their performance in recovering biologically meaningful cell types when applied to a number of real scRNA-Seq datasets. The effectiveness of the algorithms was evaluated by internal criteria (clustering number and accuracy) and external criteria (purity, adjusted rand index (ARI), F1-measure). Moreover, when computing **Corr**, an intermediate step generates the "differentiability vectors" that reveal global expression pattern in the whole environment, thus potentially providing a new means to identify biomarkers of diseases from single cell data. Prognosis analyses on independent datasets of cancers validated the effectiveness of our method in identification of robust biomarkers for Kaplan-Meier test.

8.2 Methodology

It is known that cellular microenvironment or cell-cell interaction plays a critical role in many biological processes (Federico and Giordano 2010), and can be engineered to improve cell based drug testing (Bhadriraju and Chen 2002) or targeted therapies for diseases (Gong et al. 2005). It is hence desirable, at least to some extent, to account for the effects of microenvironment or cell-cell interaction when assessing the relationships between cells. In this chapter, under the belief that cells with similar expression patterns would likely have similar functions, we define a new pairwise similarity measure based on scRNA-Seq data to assess potential functional relationships between cells. This measure evaluates "differentiability correlation", i.e., the correlation between differential expression statuses of the genes in two cells (when each cell is compared against most other cells). It incorporates the microenvironment that evaluates the relationship of two considered cells by taking into consideration on all the other surrounding cells from a global perspective.

With this new "differentiability correlation" employed, we will identify clusters of cells (i.e., cell type identification) using a Hierarchical Clustering Analysis (HCA) procedure. As a popular clustering method, HCA not only groups together cells but also provides a natural way to graphically represent all the cells in a hierarchical structure, allowing a thorough inspection on the relationships between cells and clusters of cells. We also develop a new criterion for determining the number of clusters under HCA. The method is described in detail in the following section.

8.2.1 Pairwise Cell Similarity Measure—Differentiability Correlation

We assume that there are n cells, and denote the gene expression profile for cell i by

$$\mathbf{X}_i = (x_{i1}, x_{i2}, \ldots, x_{ip}),$$

where p is the number of genes and $i = 1, 2, \ldots, n$.

To define the "differentiability correlation" between cells i and j, we first identify two "feature" gene sets for each cell. In more details, for cell i, we will identify the gene sets $\mathbf{V}_{i_j}^+$ and $\mathbf{V}_{i_j}^-$, where $\mathbf{V}_{i_j}^+$ consists of genes that show a relatively higher expression level in cell i than the gene's average expression level across all other cells excluding cell j, and similarly $\mathbf{V}_{i_j}^-$ consists of genes with relatively lower expressions in cell i:

$$\mathbf{V}_{i_j}^+ = \left\{ k | x_{ik} > \frac{(\sum_{l=1}^n x_{lk}) - x_{ik} - x_{jk}}{n-2} \right\}, \tag{8.1}$$

$$\mathbf{V}_{i_j}^- = \left\{ k | x_{ik} < \frac{(\sum_{l=1}^n x_{lk}) - x_{ik} - x_{jk}}{n-2} \right\}. \tag{8.2}$$

Using $\mathbf{V}_{i_j}^+$ and $\mathbf{V}_{i_j}^-$, we further denote the differential status for gene k in cell i as:

$$U_{i_jk} = \begin{cases} 1, & k \in V_{i_j}^+ \\ -1, & k \in V_{i_j}^- \\ 0, & \text{otherwise} \end{cases} \tag{8.3}$$

Similarly, we can define $U_{j_ik}, k = 1, \ldots, p$, for cell j. Then we define the dissimilarity (or semi-distance) between cell i and cell j by 1 minus the "differentiability correlation" between U_{i_j} and U_{j_i}, expressed as follows:

$$S_{ij} = 1 - \frac{\sum_{k=1}^p (U_{i_jk} - \overline{U_{i_j}})(U_{j_ik} - \overline{U_{j_i}})}{\sqrt{\sum_{k=1}^p (U_{i_jk} - \overline{U_{i_j}})^2}\sqrt{\sum_{k=1}^p (U_{j_ik} - \overline{U_{j_i}})^2}} \tag{8.4}$$

where $\overline{U_{i_j}} = \sum_{k=1}^{p} U_{i_j k}/p$ and $\overline{U_{j_i}} = \sum_{k=1}^{p} U_{j_i k}/p$. Note that the differentiability correlation $(1 - S_{ij})$ relies on U_{i_j} and U_{j_i}, which were defined through comparing cells i and j against all other cells in the population, leading to an evaluation of the expression relationship between cells i and j through a global perspective. This measure shares many nice properties of the SIDEseq measure in Schiffman et al. (2017), as both methods are able to incorporate information from all cells when evaluating the similarity between any two cells. But compared to SIDEseq, this measure is expected to be even more robust against cell heterogeneity and data noise since it considers the relationship of cell-specific gene expression patterns over the cell populations. This measure is also related to Gamma coefficient (Goodman and Kruskal 1954), where expression patterns resemble the order vector. However, our measure calculates the correlation between two pattern vectors while the gamma coefficient considers the ratio of different order number.

8.2.2 *Determining the Number of Clusters Based on Variance Analysis*

If we determine the number of clusters by simply using a divisive (or top-down) hierarchical clustering algorithm (HCA), all cells start in one cluster, and splits are performed recursively as one moves down the hierarchy until every cell is separated. However, to effectively determine the number of clusters in HCA, we here propose an optimal cutting of the HCA dendrogram based on variance analysis.

8.2.2.1 Review of Variance Analysis

Let $\mathbf{Y}_{ij}$ denote the random response for the ith ($i = 1, 2, \ldots, n_j$) observation in the jth ($j = 1, 2, \ldots, s$) treatment group. Assume $\mathbf{Y}_{ij}$ follows the following linear model:

$$\mathbf{Y}_{ij} = \mu + \delta_j + \varepsilon_{ij},$$

where μ represents the average effect which is common to all treatments, δ_j denotes the jth treatment effect (with constraint $\sum_{j=1}^{s} n_j \delta_j = 0$), and ε_{ij}'s are the i.i.d. random error terms that are distributed as $N(0, \sigma^2)$.

Based on the above model, we can determine the differences among various treatment groups by the analysis of variance (ANOVA) followed by an F-test with $H_0 : \delta_1 = \delta_2 = \ldots = \delta_s = 0$. The ANOVA is based on the decomposition of total variance in data into within-group variance (considered error, denoted as SSW) and between-group variance (considered meaningful difference among group means, denoted as SSB):

$$\text{SST} = \text{SSW} + \text{SSB}$$

where

$$\begin{cases} \text{SST} = \sum_{j=1}^{s} \sum_{i=1}^{n_j} (\mathbf{Y}_{ij} - \overline{\mathbf{Y}})^2 \\ \text{SSW} = \sum_{j=1}^{s} \sum_{i=1}^{n_j} (\mathbf{Y}_{ij} - \overline{\mathbf{Y}}_{.j})^2 \\ \text{SSB} = \sum_{j=1}^{s} n_j (\overline{\mathbf{Y}}_{.j} - \overline{\mathbf{Y}})^2 \end{cases} \tag{8.5}$$

where $\overline{\mathbf{Y}} = \frac{1}{n} \sum_{j=1}^{s} \sum_{i=1}^{n_j} \mathbf{Y}_{ij}$ and $\overline{\mathbf{Y}}_{.j} = \frac{1}{n_j} \sum_{i=1}^{n_j} \mathbf{Y}_{ij}$. The F-test statistic is defined as follows:

$$\frac{\text{SSB}/(s-1)}{\text{SSW}/(n-s)},$$

the ratio of two measures of variability. When H_0 is true, or when there are no significant differences among the means of various treatment groups, the *average variability between groups* ($\frac{\text{SSB}}{s-1}$) will be expected to be comparable to the *average variability within groups* ($\frac{\text{SSW}}{n-s}$) and so the test statistic will likely be close to 1. Under the null model described above, the test statistic follows an F-distribution with degrees of freedom $(s-1, n-s)$. When H_0 is not true, the variability between groups will likely be large and so the test statistic will tend to be much larger than 1.

8.2.2.2 Optimal Cluster Number

Motivated by variance analysis, we here introduce a new measure for deciding an optimal number of clusters in HCA.

We denote the expression profile for gene j across n cells by $(x_{1j}, \ldots, x_{nj})$. Now assume there are s cell subpopulations and each cell belongs to one and only one subpopulation. We model the expected expression value of gene j in cell i by $E(X_{ij}) = \alpha_j + \sum_{k=1}^{s} z_{ik}\beta_k$, where z_{ik} is a binary membership indicator (i.e., $z_{ik} = 1$ if cell i belongs to subpopulation k, and $z_{j,k} = 0$ otherwise). Supposing we have s cell subpopulations, for each gene j, treating each cell subpopulation as a treatment group, we can define $\text{SST}_{j,s}$, $\text{SSB}_{j,s}$ and $\text{SSW}_{j,s}$ analogously as in Eq. (8.5). If the s cell subpopulations are well distributed, meaning that the cells of the same type are closely clustered while the cells of different types are distant, $r_{j,s} = \frac{\text{SSB}_{j,s}}{\text{SST}_{j,s}}$ is likely to be large.

Based on m pre-selected genes, we determine a potentially optimal number of clusters (denoted by C_m) under HCA by checking the changes of $R_s = \sum_{j=1}^{m} r_{j,s}$ as s increases (or equivalently, as the cutting threshold of the dendrogram decreases): C_m is the one when the first local maximum achieves. We compute R_s based on m top ranked differentially expressed genes across all the cells. To achieve a stable result, we repeatedly compute R_s and determine C_m across many different choices of m

and the set of pre-selected genes. We finally determine a stable optimal number of clusters C_{opt} as the most frequent among many C_m's we obtained.

8.2.2.3 Computational Complexity of the Algorithm

In this algorithm, one major computation lies in the differential gene set computation, which is of computational complexity $O(p)$. On the other hand, performing the algorithm for all possible pairs of cells, we can see that computational complexity of the algorithm is of $O(n^2 p)$ which depends on the number of attributes (e.g., genes) as well as the number of cells involved and thus is relatively time-consuming.

Note that differential sets $\mathbf{V}_{i_j}^{+}$ and $\mathbf{V}_{i_j}^{-}$ between cell i and cell j depend on both i and j, which take major computational cost, because we intend to isolate cell i and cell j and compare them with the remaining cells. However, if we relax such a condition by making them only depend on i, we can simply replace or approximate Eqs. (8.1)–(8.2) with

$$\mathbf{V}_i^{+} = \left\{ k | x_{ik} > \frac{\left(\sum_{l=1}^{n} x_{lk}\right) - x_{ik}}{n-1} \right\},$$

$$\mathbf{V}_i^{-} = \left\{ k | x_{ik} < \frac{\left(\sum_{l=1}^{n} x_{lk}\right) - x_{ik}}{n-1} \right\}$$

when n is relatively large. Clearly when n is large, $\frac{(\sum_{l=1}^{n} x_{lk})-x_{ik}-x_{jk}}{n-2}$ is very close to $\frac{(\sum_{l=1}^{n} x_{lk})-x_{ik}}{n-1}$. This kind of amendment in the algorithm would largely shorten the time complexity from $O(n^2 p)$ to $O(np)$ which makes large scale clustering feasible. For such a case, each differential set is not symmetric with respect to its indices i and j, i.e., generally $\mathbf{V}_i^{+} \neq \mathbf{V}_j^{+}$ and $\mathbf{V}_i^{-} \neq \mathbf{V}_j^{-}$ with respect to cell-pair (i, j).

The algorithm of the proposed method **Corr** is given in Algorithm 1.

Algorithm 1 Framework of our algorithm **Corr** based on differentiability correlation and variance.

Input: The set of single cells, $P_n \in R^{n \times p}$;
Output: Cell types for the set of single cells, $L_n \in R^{n \times 1}$;
  Evaluate cell-pair (i, j) differentiability correlation for $i, j \in \{1, 2, \ldots, n\}$;
  Construct dissimilarity measure based on cell-pair differentiability correlations by Eq. (8.4);
  Determine Cluster Number C_{opt} based on variance analysis;
  Hierarchical Clustering with the above dissimilarity measure and cluster number.
  Return: L_n;

8.3 Numerical Experiments

To evaluate our algorithm **Corr** with differentiability correlation and variance based on hierarchical clustering for single cell RNA-Seq data, we introduce the following algorithms for comparison:

- **SNN-Cliq**
  SNN-Cliq (Xu 2015) is a recently proposed graph theory based clustering method that utilizes the concept of Shared Nearest Neighbor (SNN) to define cell similarity. The clustering output on single cell RNA-seq data is highly in accordance with the cell type origins.
- **Partitioning Around Medoids (PAM)**
  PAM (Teschendorff 2017) is the most common realization in k-medoids clustering. In the algorithm, centers are chosen from the given data points and a generalization of the Manhattan norm is used to define distance between data points. The average silhouette width is introduced to determine the optimal number of clusters after 200 rounds of k-medoids clustering are done. The final best clustering result is then generated with the selected optimal number.
- ***K*-means Clustering**
  K-means clustering is the most commonly used algorithm in clustering. Supposing that there are n observations $(\mathbf{x}_1, \mathbf{x}_2, \ldots, \mathbf{x}_n)$, k-means clustering aims to cluster the data set into K clusters $S = \{S_1, S_2, \ldots, S_K\}$ to minimize within cluster variance which can be described as the following optimization problem:

$$\arg\min_S \sum_{i=1}^{K} \sum_{\mathbf{x} \in S_i} ||\mathbf{x} - \mu_{\mathbf{i}}||^2 = \sum_{i=1}^{K} |S_i| \mathrm{var} S_i$$

  where $\mu_{\mathbf{i}}$ is the mean of points in S_i. In this algorithm, the optimal number of clusters is determined using the same rule as PAM.
- **Hierarchical Clustering with Euclidean Distance**
  Hierarchical clustering with Euclidean distance is the most frequently used measure in data (dis)similarity evaluation. We incorporate it as a comparison partner and the optimal cluster number is determined using the same method as proposed in **Corr**.
- **Hierarchical Clustering with Spearman Distance**
  Hierarchical clustering with Spearman distance evaluates data (dis)similarity from a correlation perspective. We also incorporate it as a comparison partner and the optimal cluster number is determined using the same method as proposed in **Corr**.

We report the results of various methods for the considered data sets. The data sets used can be downloaded from NCBI (National Center for Biotechnology Information) GEO, and we will have the detailed descriptions on the data sets.

- **Islet Single Cells**
  Six known human islet cell types (alpha cells, beta cells, delta cells, pp cells, acinar cells and duct cells) were identified from this single-cell RNA-Seq data set based on the expression of known marker genes (Li et al. 2015). In total, there are 72 single cells involved, 12 of which are of unknown types, including 2 delta cells. Hence we exclude 12 undefined single cells, leaving 60 single cells for verification of the methods. In the data set, there are 18 alpha cells, 12 beta cells, 11 acinar cells, 8 duct cells , 2 delta cells and 9 pp cells. Following the filtering method of Xu (2015) and Ramsköld et al. (2012), we discarded genes with average RPKM less than 20 across all 60 cells, leaving over 4000 genes.
- **Human Cancer Cells**
  The data set from Ramsköld et al. (2012) used a single-cell RNA-Seq platform named Smart-Seq for data extraction. RPKM gene expressions are used to quantify the single cells. There are 8 human embryonic stem cells hESC (8 cells), 4 cells from prostate cancer cell lines LNCap (4 cells), 4 PC3 (4 cells), 6 putative melanoma CTCs (6 cells) from peripheral blood, 4 cells from melanoma cell lines SKMEL5 (4 cells), 3 UACC257 cells (3 cells), and 4 cells from bladder cancer cell line T24 (4 cells). Following the filtering method of Xu (2015) and Ramsköld et al. (2012), we discarded genes with average RPKM less than 20 across all 33 cells, leaving over 3000 genes.
- **Human Embryo Stem Cells**
  This data set is obtained from Yan et al. (2013) and uses 124 individual cells in various developmental stages from human pre-implantation embryos. The human embryonic stem cells are extracted using a highly sensitive sequencing technique. The data set covers 7 early developmental stages: metaphase II oocyte (3 cells), zygote (3 cells), 2-cell-stage (6 cells), 4-cell-stage (12 cells), 8-cell-stage (20 cells), morula (16 cells) and late blastocyst at hatching stage (30 cells). The data set also includes an eighth stage of development of primary outgrowth during human embryonic stem cell (hESC) derivation (34 cells). Different from Xu (2015) who only used cells from the first seven early developmental stages, we used all 124 cells for the clustering analysis.
- **Allodiploid Embryonic Stem Cells**
  This data set involves mRNA profiles of allodiploid embryonic stem cell lines from mice and rats, analyzed using the Illumina HiSeq 2000 platform (Li et al. 2016). Single-cell RNA-Seq was conducted to check the transcriptomes of single allodiploid embryonic and differentiated cells. The quality of sequencing reads was assessed using FastQC. Low quality bases were trimmed with a cutoff of Phred quality score 20 using Fastq Quality Trimmer program in FASTX-Toolkit. We focus on allodiploid embryonic stem cell line MR1-1 in this chapter where cell types contain G0/G1 stage embryonic stem cell and fibroblast single cells derived from MR1-1 mouse chimaera, labeled by ESC and mFibroblast.
- **Mouse Embryo Stem Cells**
  This data set refers to the existence of inter-blastomere differences in 2-cell and 4-cell mouse embryos (Biase et al. 2014). The hypothesis has been certified by the related experiments. Within the dataset, 1857 million SMART-Seq reads were

generated from 49 single cells composed of nine 1-cell (zygote), 10 midstage 2-cell, and five 4-cell embryos.

The clustering results are summarized in Fig. 8.1.

8.3.1 Results for Islet Data

In Islet data set, 6 types of cells are considered: alpha, beta, acinar, duct, delta and pp. From the results as shown in Fig. 8.1a, we found that our proposed algorithm **Corr** yields the best result. The k-medoids algorithm generated only 2 clusters: pp cells are regarded as significantly different from other types of cells, and the difference among other types of cells cannot be detected. The k-means algorithm results show only 2 clusters in the considered data set as well. Slightly different from the k-medoids algorithm, k-means algorithm cannot clearly distinguish pp cells from other type of cells, where 2 pp cells are clustered into the remaining cluster. SNN-Cliq finds 11 clusters where delta cells are clustered together with duct cells. Moreover, the algorithm grouped alpha cells into 3 clusters, beta cells into 2 clusters, and pp cells into 3 clusters. On the other hand, our method also has better performance than those hierarchical clustering based algorithms. In the Spearman algorithm, 3 clusters are found, whereas alpha, beta, delta, and most of the pp cells are merged into one single cluster. Duct cells and acinar cells are regarded to be explicitly different from other cells. There are only 2 clusters found in Euclidean algorithm. Similar to the k-means algorithm, the Euclidean algorithm regards almost all types of cells as one single type, with pp cells being divided into two clusters. Our **Corr** algorithm has been shown to accurately cluster alpha, acinar, beta, duct and pp cells into different clusters, with only one acinar cell having been wrongly clustered. 3 alpha cells with 1 pp cell are clustered into a single scattered cluster. Delta cells are clustered near pp cells. Looking further at the results of the **Corr** algorithm, we found that the wrongly clustered 'acinar' cell was also considered to be isolated from other 'acinar' cells in the SNN-Cliq algorithm, and it is clustered in the 'duct' cell cluster in both algorithms. Comparing all the considered algorithms, we can conclude that the **Corr** algorithm can correctly find the right cluster number and further cluster the single cells into the desired clusters. Other algorithms like Euclidean and K-means algorithms underestimate the cluster number, while the SNN-Cliq algorithm over-estimates the cluster number within the data set.

Regarding the optimal cluster number determination, we choose the optimal cluster number based on factorial analysis of variance for the three hierarchical clustering based algorithms: **Corr**, Euclidean and Spearman. The results are shown in Fig. 8.2, where the subfigures on the left hand side show the optimal cluster number distribution in **Corr**, Euclidean and Spearman. The final optimal cluster number is determined as the most frequently appeared one. The subfigures on the right-hand side report the changes in the suggested optimal cluster number when the number of differentially expressed attributes increases. Figure 8.2 shows the distribution

Fig. 8.1 Clustering results from different algorithms for considered datasets. The compared algorithms are **Corr**, Euclidean, Spearman, 'Kmedoids', 'Kmeans' and 'SNN-Cliq'. The first column under name **Corr** stands for our **Corr** algorithm, the second column named Euclidean refers to hierarchical clustering with Euclidean distance, the third column represents hierarchical clustering with Spearman distance, the last column stands for SNN-Cliq, and similarly the fourth and fifth columns represent k-medoids clustering and k-means clustering. The column on the leftmost lists the cell type, and the columns indicated with different colors refer to the clustering results of cell type. And the involved datasets are **a** islet data; **b** human cancer data; **c** human embryo data; **d** Allodiploid data; **e** mouse embryo data; **f** ovarian cancer data. In the heatmap, each row stands for an individual cell; each column corresponds to the clustering result produced by one of the six methods. Cells that are grouped in the same cluster by a method are displayed in the same color in the column

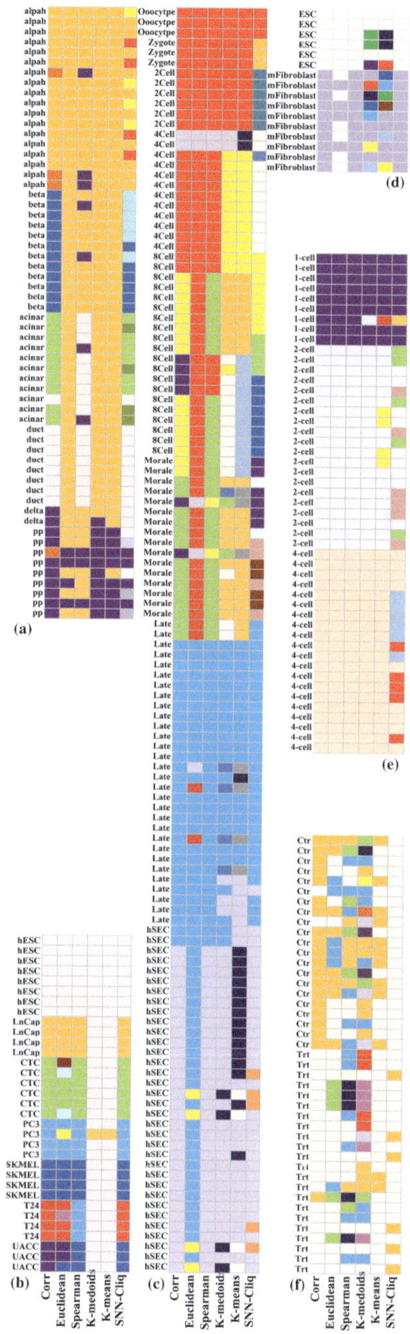

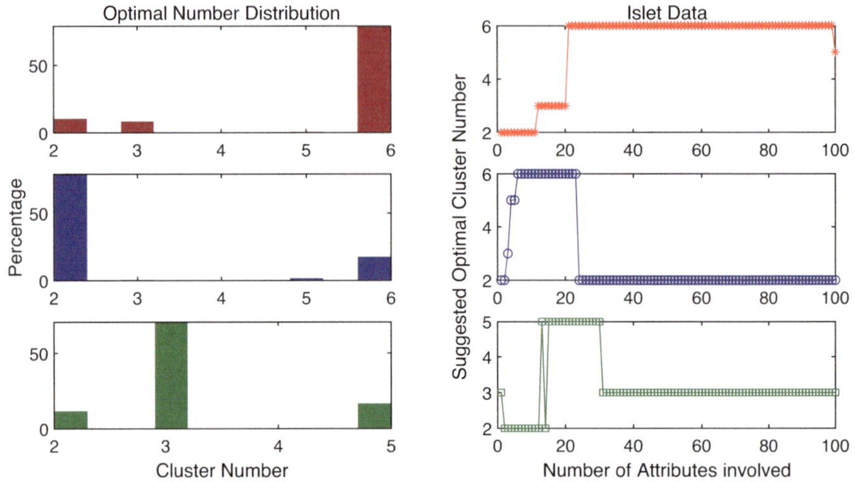

Fig. 8.2 Optimal cluster number determination with hierarchical clustering methods: islet data

of the suggested optimal cluster number when the number of involved differential attributes permutes from 1 to 100 ($m = 100$). In the **Corr** algorithm, the most frequently selected cluster number is 6, achieving almost 80% in all the suggested optimal cluster numbers. In the Euclidean algorithm, the most frequently selected cluster number is 2, achieving almost 80% in all the suggested optimal cluster numbers. In the Spearman algorithm, the most frequently selected cluster number is 3, achieving around 70% in all the suggested optimal cluster numbers. Figure 8.3 shows the optimal number determination for k-medoids and K-means algorithms. For k-medoids algorithm, 10 runs of k-medoids clustering were conducted on islet data to generate a relatively robust and stable result. The top left subfigure corresponds silhouette value distribution and the top right subfigure corresponds the corresponding average silhouette value distribution. The figure shows that the optimal cluster number is 2 for 'k-medoids' algorithm. Similarly we found that the optimal cluster number for 'k-means' algorithm is 2 as well.

Further analysis of the hierarchical clustering results for islet data are shown in Fig. 8.4. **Corr** and Spearman algorithms obviously outperform Euclidean algorithm as we could not find tightly clustered cells using Euclidean algorithm. In the **Corr** and Spearman algorithms, several tight clusters can be found. Employing variance analysis, we determined the optimal cluster number for each algorithm. We found that **Corr** algorithm is the most accurate with only 1 pp cell and 3 alpha cells clustered in the right hand side as noise clusters. When we further assessed the hierarchical relationships among the clusters, we found that acinar and duct cells are more closely clustered. Studies in mice have demonstrated that acinar cells can transdifferentiate to ductal cells (Mukhi 2011) because of inherited relationship between those types of cells. Alpha , beta , delta and pp cells are more closely clustered in **Corr** algorithm. We further found that alpha, beta and delta cells are actually T cells. This further

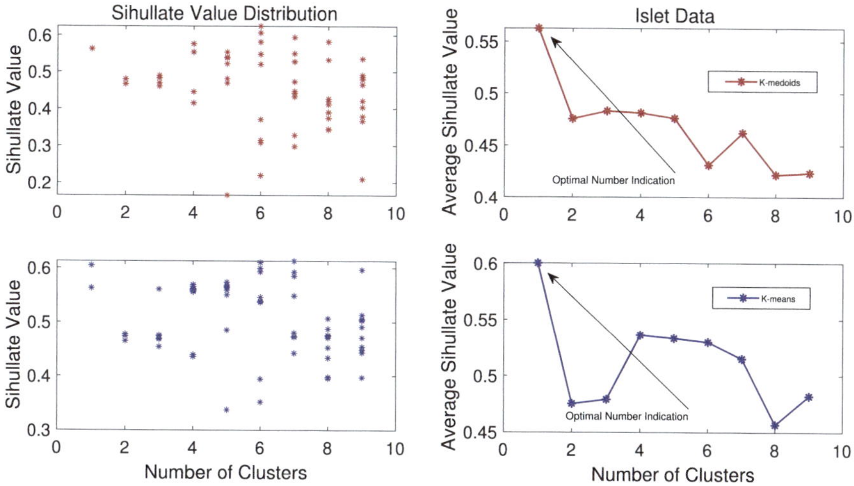

Fig. 8.3 Optimal cluster number determination with K-medoids and K-means methods: islet data

illustrates that **Corr** algorithm can help to determine the cell types and hierarchical relationship among the clusters.

8.3.2 Results for Human Cancer Data

There are 7 types of cells in human cancer data set. Following the data preprocessing (Xu 2015), we selected attributes with RPKM $\geq$ 20 in at least one cell for data analysis. Considering SNN-Cliq algorithm, log transformation ($\log_2(x + 1)$) was introduced to reduce the effect of highly expressed genes. However, we did not do any transformation on the data in our **Corr** algorithm.

Looking at the clustering results for different algorithms as shown in (Fig. 8.1b), we make some conclusions. Using **Corr** algorithm, the resulting cluster number is 7 with 7 clusters each corresponding to a unique cell type. Each cell type is clearly identified. For Euclidean algorithm, the number of clusters is defined to be 10 after calculation. There are a number of single data clusters. For 'CTC' cell line alone, 3 clusters are detected, whereas for 'PC3', 'UACC' and 'T24' cell lines respectively, 2 clusters are identified. For Spearman algorithm, the clustering results are better than Euclidean algorithm, with 5 clusters identified. Similar to 'Corr' algorithm, 'hESC', 'LnCap' and 'CTC' types are successfully clustered. But the algorithm groups 'PC3' and 'T24' in the same cluster, and groups 'SKMEL' and 'UACC' in the same cluster. Using SNN-Cliq algorithm, 6 clusters were yielded, with SKMEL5 and UACC257 cells grouped into one single cluster. Note that SKMEL5 and UACC257 are melanoma cell lines and the difference between them should be relatively small. Hence, SNN-Cliq could not detect the slight differences between the two related cell

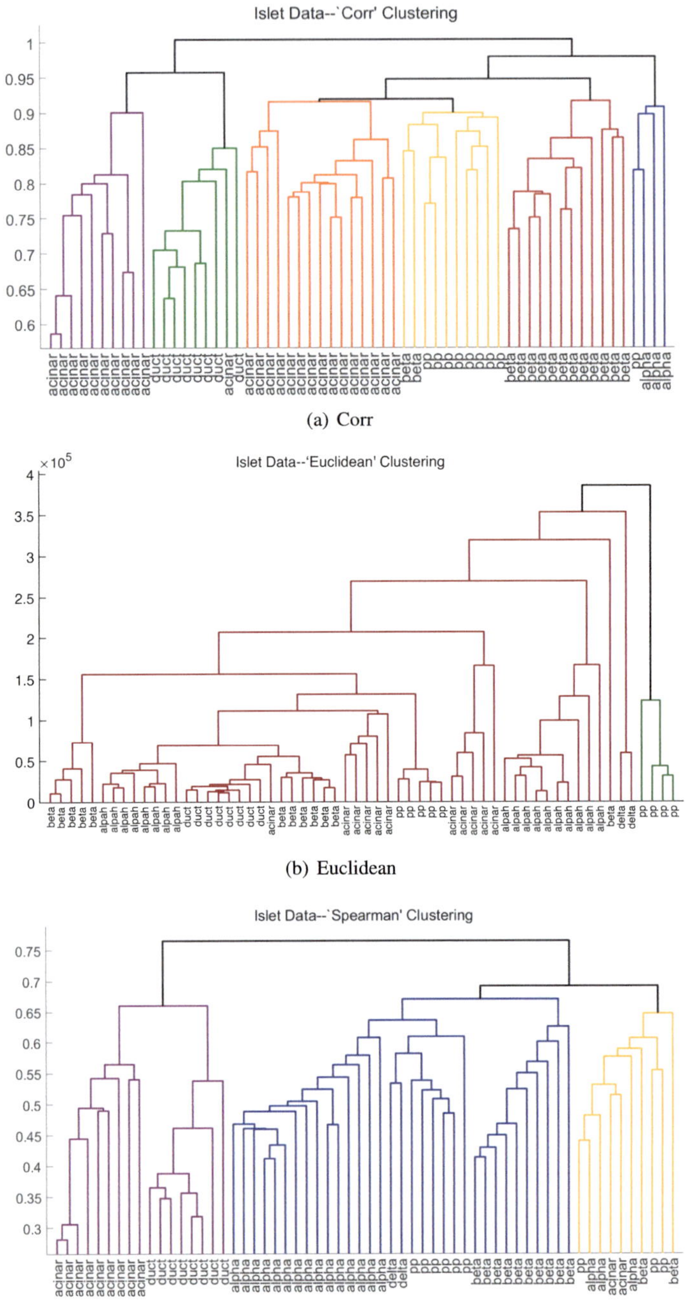

Fig. 8.4 Hierarchical clustering representations for islet data

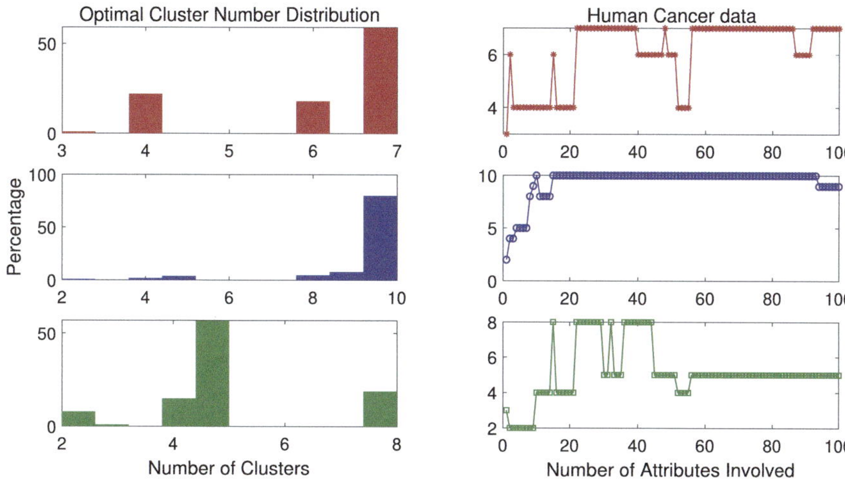

Fig. 8.5 Optimal cluster number determination with hierarchical clustering methods in human cancer data

lines. Notably, **Corr** algorithm could capture the slight difference between these two types, successfully splitting them into two different types. k-medoids algorithm and K-means algorithm showed only 2 clusters, with all but one cells grouped into a cluster, leaving one 'PC3' cell as a singleton cluster.

Figures 8.5 and 8.6 illustrate the determination of optimal cluster numbers for all algorithms except 'SNN-Cliq'. In Fig. 8.5, the subfigures on the left hand side show the optimal cluster number distribution using **Corr**, Euclidean and Spearman algorithms, and the final optimal cluster number is determined as the most frequently appeared one. Subfigures on the right hand side report the changes in the suggested optimal cluster number when the number of the involved differentially expressed attributes increases, where the number of involved differential attributes permutes from 1 to 100 ($m = 100$). Similarly, in Fig. 8.6, it can be seen that the optimal cluster numbers in **Corr**, Euclidean, Spearman, k-medoids and K-means algorithms are 7, 10, 5, 2, and 2, respectively.

We further analyzed the hierarchical clustering results for human cancer data as shown in Fig. 8.7. We found that **Corr** algorithm can clearly distinguish various cell status, besides 'hESC' cells cluster separately from other types of cells. On the contrary, Euclidean algorithm did not capture cell variability. Spearman algorithm has an advantage over Euclidean algorithm, but we found that 'hESC' cells are not isolated from other cells, rather clustered near T24 and PC3 cells. Further analysis of the hierarchical relationship by **Corr** algorithm indicates that hESC cells can be isolated from other types of cells, which is consistent with literature and our usual understanding. SKMEL and UACC are closely clustered as they are from melanoma cell line. PC3 and LNCaP are closely clustered because they are both prostate cancer cells. Notably, the PC3 prostate cancer cells are clustered nearer to

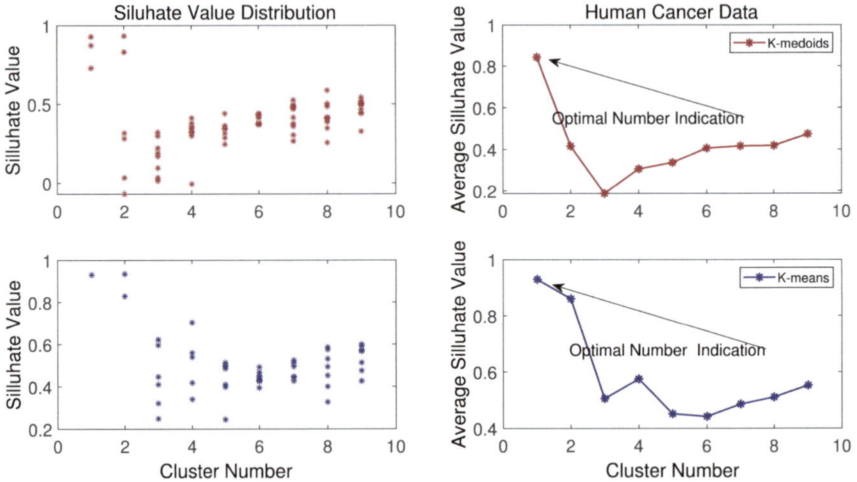

Fig. 8.6 Optimal cluster number determination with K-medoids and K-means methods in human cancer data

the T24 bladder cancer cells than to the other LNCap prostate cancer cells. This might contain significant biological meaning and should be further investigated using gene ontology or functional experimental analysis.

8.3.3 Results for Human Embryo Data

In scRNA-Seq clustering analysis for Human Embryo data, attributes with RPKM > 0.1 in at least one cell are selected. We can see the comparison results for different methods as shown in Fig. 8.1c. Using **Corr** algorithm, the 124 single cells are clustered into 6 major clusters. Oocyte, zygote, 2-cell and 4-cell at very early developmental stages are clustered into a single cluster. 8-cell and Morule are clustered into another single cluster. hESC cells are well separated from late blastocyst cells. However, 4 8-cell cells and 2 Morule cells are wrongly clustered. Results received using Spearman algorithm and **Corr** are similar where oocyte, zygote, 2 cell and 4-cell in very early developmental stages are clustered into a single cluster. The number of clusters is 5, 'Late' and 'hESC' cell types are well distinguished and most of the '8-cell', 'Morule' cells are merged into one single cluster, with 2 'hESC' cells and two 'Morule' cells separately designated as one cluster. Using Euclidean algorithm, we detected only 4 clusters, while the rest of the cells are pooled in by 2 clusters. Morule cells are clustered into a single cluster. Moreover, 4 'hESC' cells and 2 'Late' cells separately are designated as one cluster as well. For SNN-Cliq algorithm, the default parameters were introduced: $r = 0.7, m = 0.5$; that the final clustering yielded 13 clusters. The method could distinguish cells at the very early

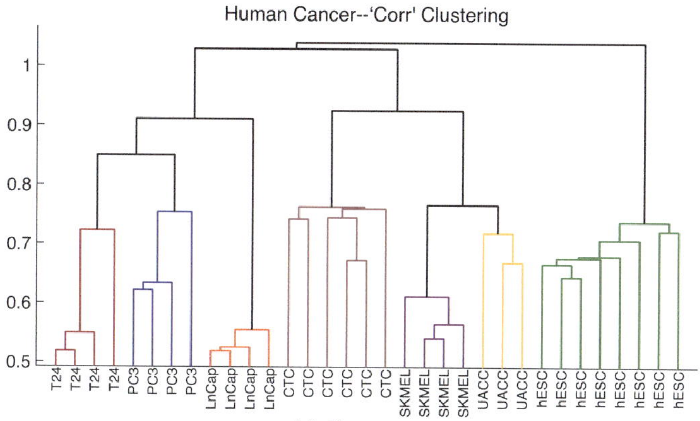

(a) Corr

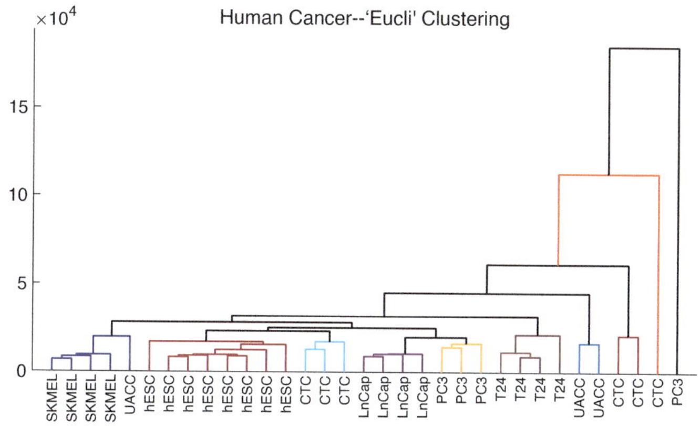

(b) Euclidean

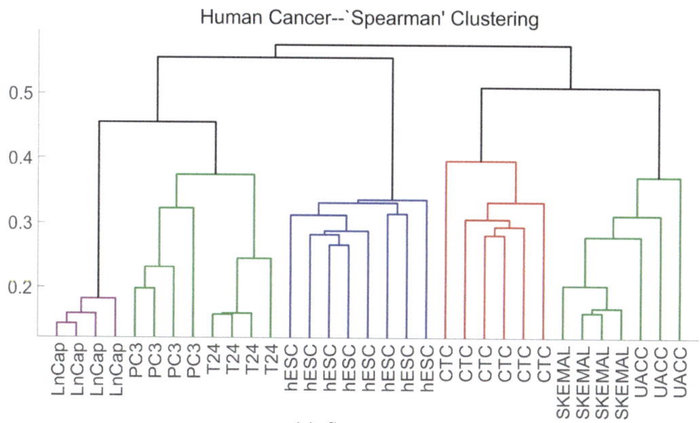

(c) Spearman

Fig. 8.7 Hierarchical clustering representations for human cancer data

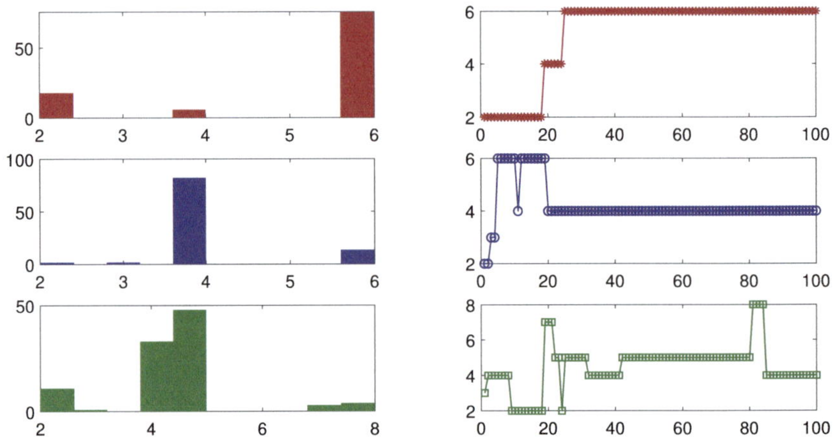

Fig. 8.8 Optimal cluster number determination with hierarchical clustering methods in human embryo data

stage of development: Oocyte, Zygote and 2-cell. However, a number of clusters were generated within 8-cell, Morule and hESC stage cells separately. Late cells are separately clustered. The algorithm could not clearly differentiate stem cells from other type of cells.

In k-medoids algorithm, 9 clusters were detected and 4-cell stage cells were well separated from other cells. The 'hESC' cells are partitioned into two clusters, very similar to SNN-Cliq algorithm. Similar to SNN-Cliq, k-medoids algorithm could not clearly identify Morule cells, generating a number of noise clusters. Using K-means algorithm, the cluster number is 9; oocyte, zygote and 2-cell cells are grouped into one cluster, and 4-cell stage cells are well separated. For cells in other stages, more than two clusters were detected even in a single stage, e.g., for hESC cells, more than 3 clusters are observed.

The cluster number determination and hierarchical clustering results are shown in Figs. 8.8, 8.9, and 8.10, respectively.

8.3.4 Results for Allodiploid Data

The results of Allodiploid data analysis are summarized in Fig. 8.1d. 16 cells were assessed, of which 6 are embryonic stem cells and 10 are mouse fibroblast cells. Using **Corr** algorithm, we could perfectly partition the cells into two separated groups. SNN-Cliq and Spearman algorithm generated the same results. Other methods brought unsatisfactory results. The cluster number is 2 for Euclidean Hierarchical Clustering, but the majority of mouse fibroblast cells were included into the 'ESC' cells cluster. The cluster number for k-medoids algorithm and K-means algorithm

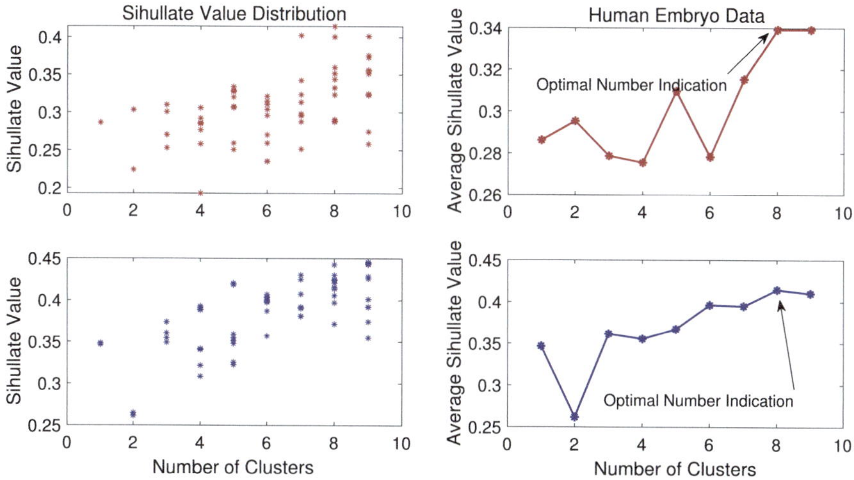

Fig. 8.9 Optimal cluster number determination with K-medoids and K-means methods in human embryo data

are both 10, generating a number of noise clusters. For mouse fibroblast cells cluster that includes only 10 cells, both algorithms detected 7 clusters.

The determination of optimal cluster number is shown in Figs. 8.11 and 8.12, where the number of involved differential attributes permutes from 1 to 100 ($m = 100$). Figure 8.11 shows that the optimal number is 2 for **Corr**, Euclidean, and Spearman algorithms . Figure 8.12 records the average silhouette width of k-medoids clustering and K-means clustering algorithm for MR11 cell line. The silhouette value is a measure of similarity for cell in its own cluster compared to cells in other clusters, ranging from -1 to 1. Hence, a large average silhouette value would indicate a better clustering result. For k-medoids clustering in MR11, optimal cluster number is 10 and for K-means clustering is 10.

Figure 8.13 reports the results on the hierarchical clustering algorithms including **Corr**, Euclidean, and Spearman. Looking at the hierarchical clustering result for each method, we found that for **Corr** algorithm helps to separate cell types clearly. Clusters are not so tightly grouped using Euclidean algorithm. Variance analysis finally indicates the number to be 2 and most of the fibroblast cells were clustered near hESC cells under Euclidean distance measure. Using Spearman algorithm, Embryo stem cells are clustered separately as shown in Fig. 8.13. Therefore, **Corr** and Spearman algorithms gave a correct description of the relationship between fibroblast cells and ESC cells, while Euclidean algorithm failed to do so. Looking at the hierarchical structure provided by **Corr** and Spearman algorithms, we observed that the structure of fibroblast cell cluster differs from each other, which may require further investigation.

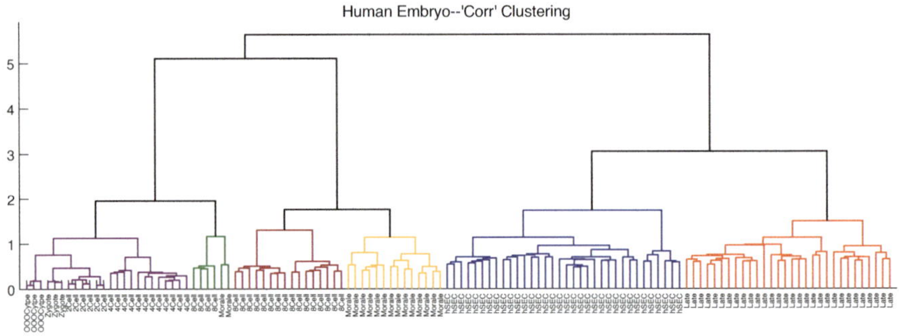

(a) Corr

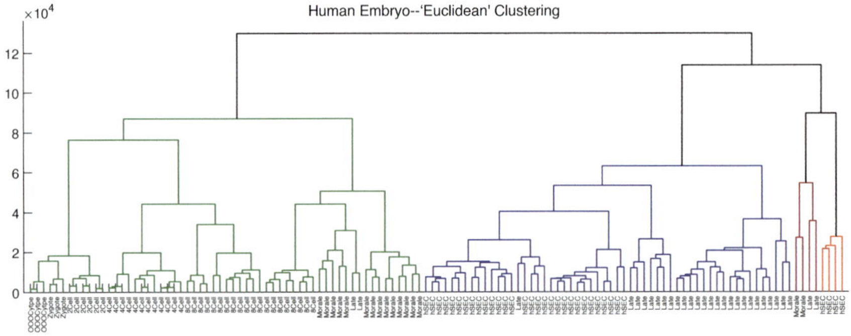

(b) Euclidean

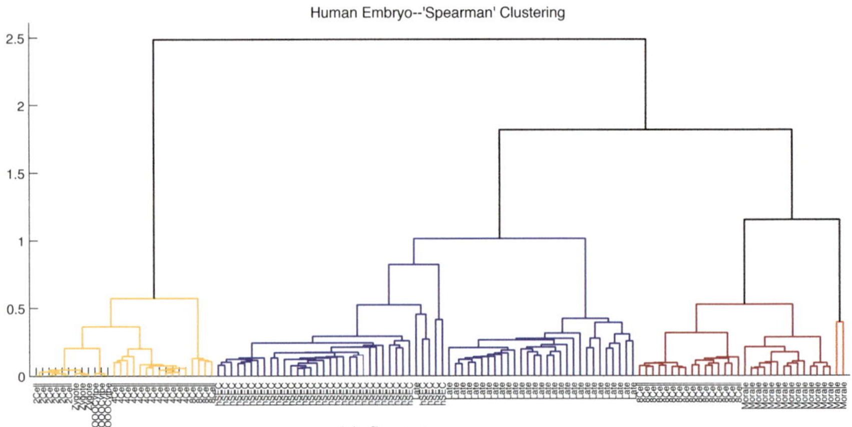

(c) Spearman

Fig. 8.10 Hierarchical clustering representations for human embryo data

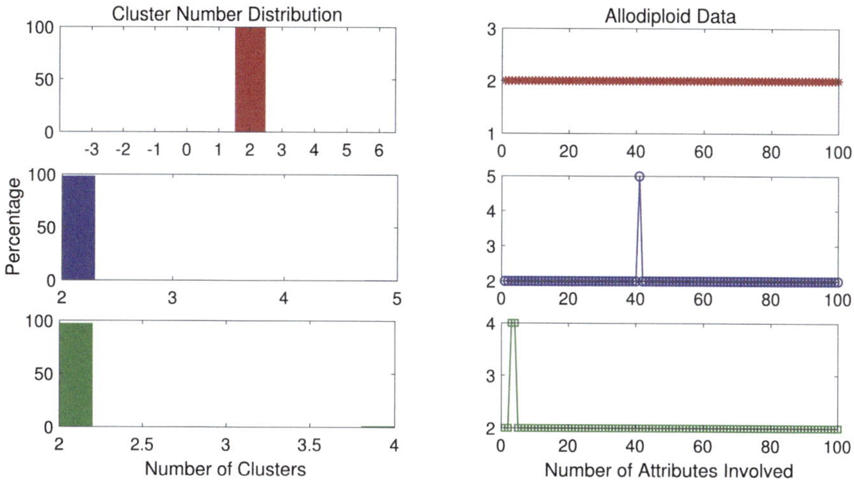

Fig. 8.11 Optimal cluster number determination with hierarchical clustering methods in Allodiploid stem cells

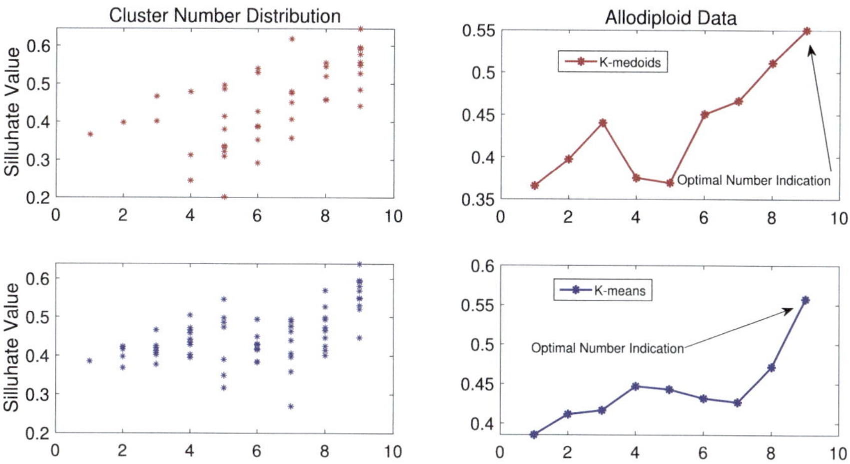

Fig. 8.12 Optimal cluster number determination with K-medoids and K-means methods in Allodiploid stem cells

8.3.5 *Results for Mouse Embryo Stem Cells*

For mouse embryo stem cells, hierarchical clustering based methods performed similarly and the optimal cluster number determined is uniformly 3, as shown in Fig. 8.1e. The number of involved differential attributes equals 100 ($m = 100$). In addition, **Corr**, Euclidean and Spearman correctly distinguished the 3 types of cells. In contrast, for K-means and k-medoids algorithms, the optimal cluster number are

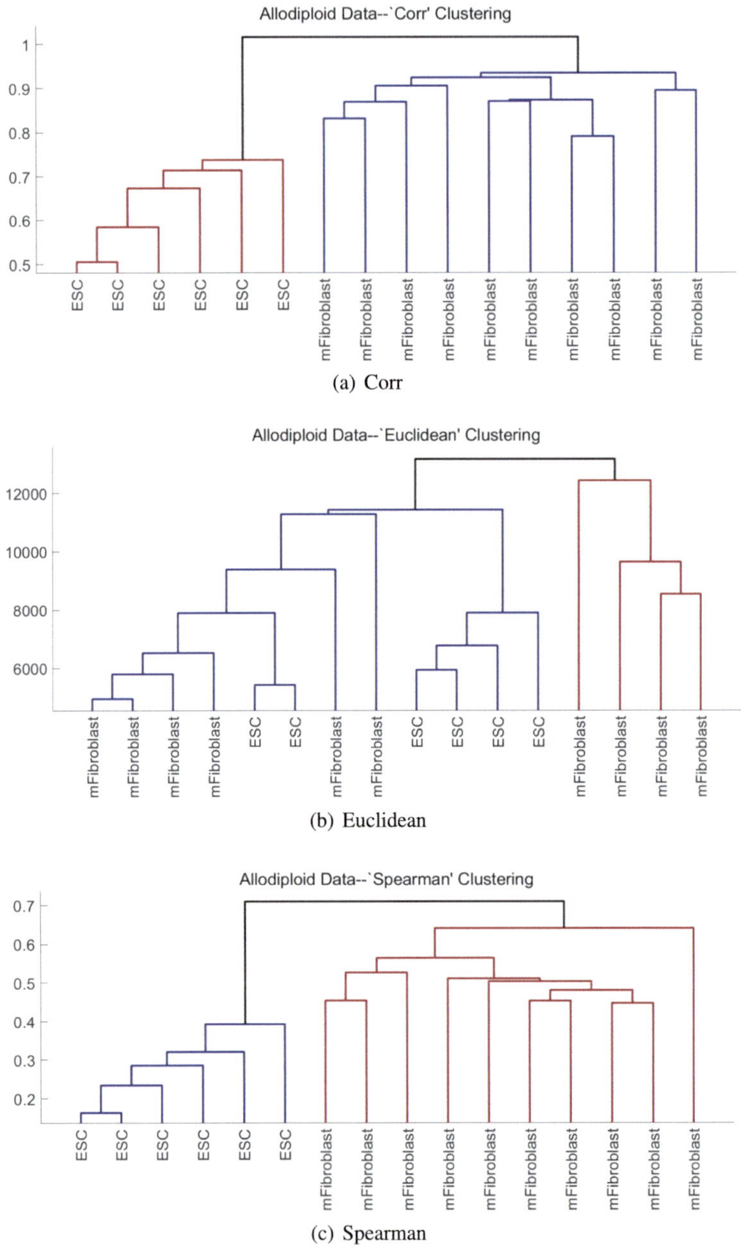

Fig. 8.13 Hierarchical clustering representations for Allodiploid stem cells

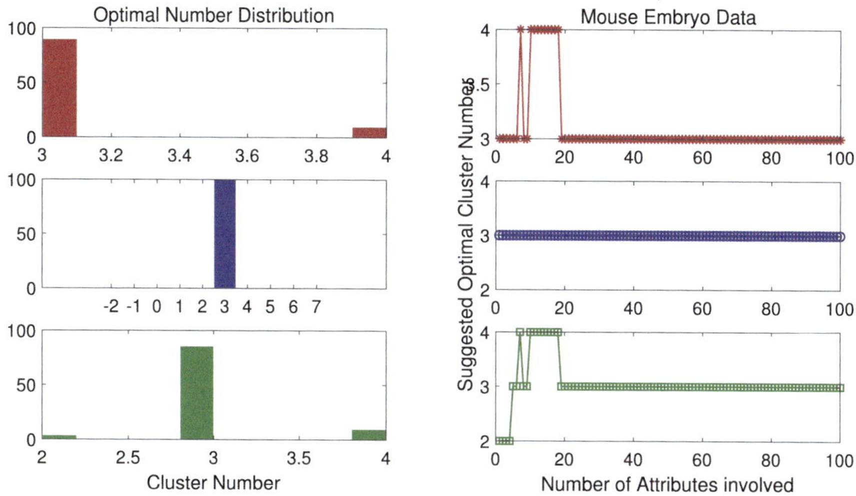

Fig. 8.14 Optimal cluster number determination with hierarchical clustering methods in mouse embryo data

4 and 3, respectively. k-medoids algorithm misclassified one 1-cell to 2-cell cluster. For K-means algorithm, 2-cell cluster was divided into two different groups. For SNN-Cliq algorithm, the clustering result is not satisfactory. The total number of clusters is 7, although there are only 3 truly different clusters. The corresponding graphical results are presented in Fig. 8.1e. And the number determination process is indicated on Figs. 8.14 and 8.15. Regarding the hierarchical clustering results, we could find differences from Fig. 8.16. **Corr** and Euclidean algorithms grouped 1-cell

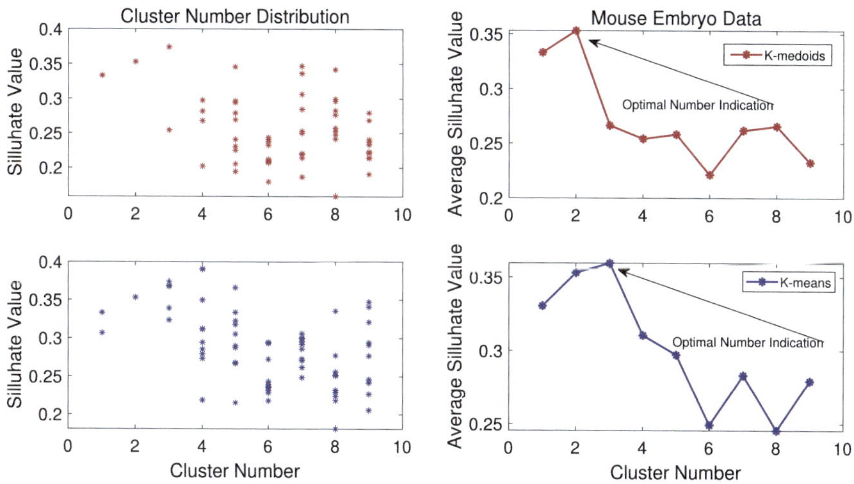

Fig. 8.15 Optimal cluster number determination with K-medoids and K-means methods in mouse embryo data

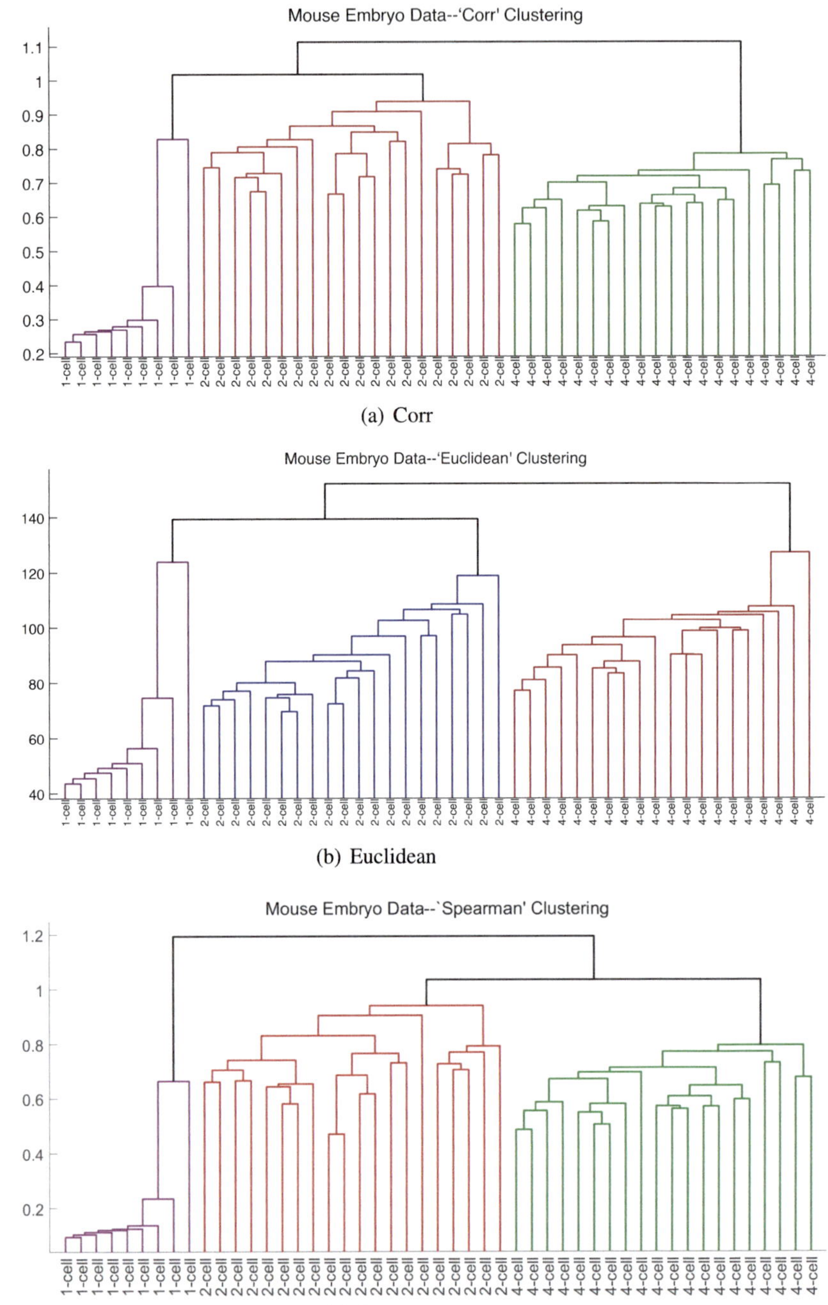

Fig. 8.16 Hierarchical clustering representations for mouse embryo data

and 2-cell more closely located, and Spearman algorithm considered 2-cell and 4-cell types more similar than others. It was shown previously in Yan et al. (2013) that inter-blastomere differences between 2- and 4-cell mouse embryos exist. Therefore, the hierarchical structures presented using **Corr** and Euclidean algorithms are more reasonable.

8.4 Discussions

8.4.1 Determination Methods of Optimal Cluster Number

We proposed variance analysis based algorithm for optimal cluster number determination in our 'Corr' method. Existing methods in optimal cluster number determination include Calinski-Harabasz index (Caliński and Harabasz 1974), where a method for identifying clusters of points in a multidimensional Euclidean space is described and a dendrite method for cluster analysis is proposed. Davies-Bouldin index (Davies and Bouldin 1979) proposed a measure indicating the similarity of clusters. The clusters were assumed to have a data density defined as a decreasing function of distance from a vector characteristic of the cluster. This measure can be used to infer the appropriateness of data partitions and can therefore be used to compare relative appropriateness of various divisions of the data. One of the frequently used measure, the average silhouette width (Rousseeuw 1987), provides an evaluation of clustering validity, and can be used to select an appropriate number of clusters. We compared our variance-analysis-based measure with the above 3 measures for determining an optimal number of clusters. The comparison results are included in Table 8.1 with detailed illustrations. It can be seen that in the presented examples, our new measure always works better than or at least equivalent to the other three measures. In particular, silhouette width and Davies-Bouldin index tend to get more clusters. Calinski-Harabasz (CH) index is more comparable to ours; this is expected since both measures are based on variance decomposition (or ANOVA). However, for its best performance, CH index requires a constant variance across the subpopulations (or individual clusters), for which scRNA-seq data usually do not have such a property. We consider this the main reason for the outperformance of our measure over CH index.

8.4.2 External Clustering Evaluation Measures

In addition to the clustering results with internal criteria such as clustering number and accuracy, we introduced external evaluation measures (i.e. purity, adjusted rand index (ARI), and F1-measure) on various scRNA-Seq methods as suggested in Xu (2015) for comparing the clustering ability.

Table 8.1 Optimal cluster number determination method

Datasets	Measures	Methods			
		'Variance analysis'	'Calinski-Harabasz'	'Silhouette'	'Davies-Bouldin'
Islet	Number	**6**	6	7	7
	Purity	**0.9333**	0.9333	0.9333	0.9333
	ARI	**0.8289**	0.8289	0.7703	0.7703
	F1-measure	**0.9102**	0.9102	0.8817	0.8817
Human cancer	Number	**7**	10	10	10
	Purity	**1**	1	1	1
	ARI	**1.0000**	0.8337	0.8337	0.8337
	F1-measure	**1.0000**	0.9307	0.9307	0.9307
Human embryo	Number	**6**	2	10	2
	Purity	**0.8871**	0.4355	0.8871	0.4355
	ARI	**0.7129**	0.3295	0.4865	0.3295
	F1-measure	**0.7964**	0.5097	0.6879	0.5097
Allipoloid	Number	**2**	2	10	10
	Purity	**1.0000**	1.0000	1.0000	1.0000
	ARI	**1.0000**	1.0000	0.2667	0.2667
	F1-measure	**1.0000**	1.0000	0.5833	0.5833
Mouse embryo	Number	**3**	2	10	3
	Purity	**1.0000**	0.81630	1.0000	1.0000
	ARI	**1.0000**	0.6951	0.6718	1.0000
	F1-measure	**1.0000**	0.8284	0.7927	1.0000
Ovarian TGFB	Number	**2**	2	10	2
	Purity	**0.9302**	0.9302	0.9302	0.9302
	ARI	**0.7341**	0.7341	0.1603	0.7341
	F1-measure	**0.9302**	0.9302	0.4887	0.9302

Table 8.2 lists the evaluation measures on representative scRNA-Seq methods in islet data, human cancer and human embryo data, Allodiploid data with cell line MR11 and mouse embryo data. The graphical results are shown in Fig. 8.17. The results for our **Corr** method are marked in bold font. Clearly, our **Corr** algorithm demonstrates the best overall performances when compared to other algorithms applying to all scRNA-seq datasets. For example, in Fig. 8.17a and Table 8.2 for Islet Data, we can see that **Corr** algorithm outperforms all the other algorithms including SNN-Cliq.

The row indicated with Islet (Table 8.2) demonstrates that ARI and F1-measure for **Corr** algorithm are clearly superior to other methods except for purity (Purity is slightly less than that of SNN-Cliq). Although SNN-Cliq is slightly better than **Corr** algorithm in purity, but from the other two robust measures 'ARI' and F1-measure, we can see that **Corr** algorithm is better. The reason why SNN-Cliq algorithm has a

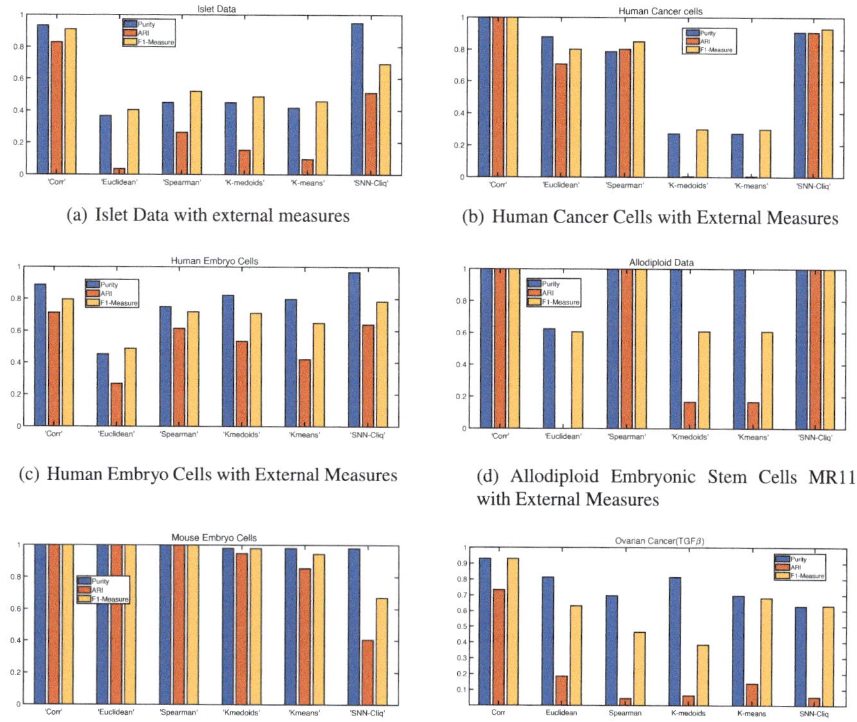

(a) Islet Data with external measures

(b) Human Cancer Cells with External Measures

(c) Human Embryo Cells with External Measures

(d) Allodiploid Embryonic Stem Cells MR11 with External Measures

Fig. 8.17 External measures

larger purity value is probably that SNN-Cliq algorithm generates more clusters (11 clusters) than the real number of analyzed cell types (6 types of cells).

In human cancer cells data as shown in Table 8.2 and Fig. 8.17b, we can see that **Corr** algorithm clearly identifies all the cell identities and hence the three considered measures in **Corr** algorithm are uniformly 1. The second best algorithm for this data set is SNN-Cliq algorithm, while k-medoids and K-means algorithms seem not suitable for handling this data set.

For human embryo cells, however, we note that Euclidean and Spearman algorithms could not capture the cell variability. k-medoids algorithm is better than K-means algorithm. Regarding the other four algorithms, we found that SNN-Cliq algorithm delivers the largest purity value , but **Corr** algorithm has the largest ARI value and F1-measure. Despite SNN-Cliq produces the highest purity value, we found that it has too many clusters, making each cluster having few samples, increasing the purity of the algorithm. Hence, large value of purity does not correspond to good performance of the method. If we combine the three measures together (either by arithmetic mean or by geometric mean), **Corr** outperforms other algorithms including SNN-Cliq. There is no dominant algorithm in discriminating the cell types within the data set. In conclusion, **Corr** and SNN-Cliq algorithms perform relatively better.

Table 8.2 External measures for the considered methods

Datasets	Measures	Methods					
		Corr	Euclidean	Spearman	'k-medoids'	'k-means'	'SNN-Cliq'
Islet	Purity	**0.9333**	0.3667	0.4500	0.4500	0.3667	0.9500
	ARI	**0.8289**	0.0354	0.2633	0.1532	0.0354	0.5109
	F1-measure	**0.9102**	0.4047	0.5197	0.4864	0.4047	0.6919
Human cancer	Purity	**1.0000**	0.8788	0.7879	0.2727	0.2727	0.9091
	ARI	**1.0000**	0.7065	0.8028	0.0057	0.0057	0.9079
	F1-measure	**1.0000**	0.8023	0.8498	0.2993	0.2993	0.9306
Human embryo	Purity	**0.8871**	0.4516	0.75	0.8225	0.7983	0.9677
	ARI	**0.7128**	0.2662	0.6149	0.5325	0.4193	0.6405
	F1-measure	**0.7964**	0.4863	0.7194	0.7112	0.6494	0.7841
Allipoloid	Purity	**1.0000**	0.6250	1.0000	1.0000	1.0000	1.0000
	ARI	**1.0000**	0	1.0000	0.1667	0.1667	1.0000
	F1-measure	**1.0000**	0.6071	1.0000	0.6071	0.6071	1.0000
Mouse embryo	Purity	**1.0000**	1.0000	1.0000	0.9796	0.9796	0.9796
	ARI	**1.0000**	1.0000	1.0000	0.9483	0.8532	0.4054
	F1-measure	**1.0000**	1.0000	1.0000	0.9792	0.9438	0.6711
Ovarian TGFB	Purity	**0.9302**	0.8140	0.6977	0.8140	0.6977	0.6279
	ARI	**0.7341**	0.1857	0.0462	0.0640	0.1397	0.0544
	F1-measure	**0.9302**	0.6333	0.4651	0.3848	0.6821	0.6311

Table 8.2 shows the external measure for the 6 algorithms in Allodiploid data with cell line MR11. It is found that **Corr**, Spearman and SNN-Cliq algorithms can correctly determine the cell types within the data set, yielding 100% accuracy for all considered measures. But for Euclidean, k-medoids and K-means algorithms, the results are not satisfactory.

Figure 8.17e shows the external measure for the 6 algorithms in mouse embryo data. It can be found that **Corr**, Spearman and Euclidean algorithms can correctly determine the cell types within the data set, yielding 100% accuracy in all considered measures, which implies that variance analysis based hierarchical clustering is a reliable option in cell type determination in this case. But for k-medoids and K-means algorithms, the results are relatively inferior although k-medoids is better than K-means. SNN-Cliq algorithm is not satisfactory, in particular for ARI and F1-Measure.

8.4.3 Application to Ovarian Cancer Single Cell Clustering

We utilize the new scRNA-Seq dataset consisting of 96 cells derived from the human epithelial ovarian cancer cells line, CAOV-3 (ATCC, Manassas, VA, USA (Schiffman et al. 2017). The ovarian cancer cells were sequenced in two batches of 48 cells each. One half of the cells in one batch were treated with TGFβ-1, and similarly half of the cells in the second batch were treated with thrombin. The remaining 48 cells in both batches were untreated, control cells. Since TGFβ-1 treatment is a well-studied inducer of EMT, the heterogeneity of the cellular phenotypes resulting from EMT in ovarian cancer cells would likely lead to an increased ability to escape early detection. We focused on TGFβ-1 batch trying to differentiate treatment cell from control cells. However, it is not an easy task for clearly distinguishing cells at two different conditions. The untreated control cells in both batches should not have significantly different expression profiles, but apparent differences were observed for control cells in the two batches. This is probably associated with technical noise or unwanted biological variability. Therefore, we tested the ability of our method to deal with such noise or biological variability.

Using the differentiability vector (the same as previous subsection) to represent the noisy data, we measured the cell dissimilarity with differentiability correlation and determined cluster number based on variance analysis. The clustering result is reported in Fig. 8.1f. The clustering numbers determined by the compared 6 methods were 2,4,5,10,2,2 for **Corr**, Euclidean, Spearman, k-medoids, K-means, and SNN-Cliq, respectively. We found that our **Corr**, K-means, and SNN-Cliq determines the correct cluster numbers. By further analysis on the clustering result, we found that **Corr** method yields the best result. It can cluster the cells into two separate types: control and treatment, and only 3 out of the 43 cells were wrongly clustered. For K-means and SNN-Cliq algorithms, the clustering results are different, but they share some similarity in that the majority of cells was grouped as one cluster. They can not clearly detect the differences between the two types of cells.

As the number determined by variance analysis is 2, we found that the wrongly clustered 3 cells are: two control cells and one treated cell. The purity, adjusted rand index and F1-measure are also reported in Table 8.2. We found that **Corr** algorithm shows the best performance, achieving purity and F1-measure 0.9304. The adjusted rand index is 0.7341. For the other algorithms, the best purity value is 0.8140, in Euclidean and k-medoids algorithms. The best F1-measure value is achieved in 'k-means' clustering algorithm, achieving 0.6821. The best adjusted rand index for other algorithms is achieved in Euclidean algorithm, and is only 0.1857. Figures 8.18 and 8.19 illustrate cluster number determination in the data set. The hierarchical representations for the **Corr**, Euclidean, and Spearman algorithms are given in Fig. 8.20.

From the results, we found that **Corr** algorithm is the best among the considered methods. In some of the cases, SNN-Cliq shows good performance similarly to **Corr** algorithm. However, there are occasions in which SNN-Cliq cannot compete with hierarchical based clustering methods including Euclidean and Spearman. Thus, **Corr** algorithm can provide an appropriate cell-similarity measure and also identify suitable cluster number.

When constructing our new cell-cell (dis)similarity measure employed in **Corr**, we used the sample mean expression (excluding cell i and cell j) to estimate/approximate the "expected" expression for the cell population. This approximation should be reasonable in general but likely works best for normally distributed data. The **Corr** algorithm provides an alternative cell-to-cell measure in differentiability vector based correlation construction. More importantly, we also introduced

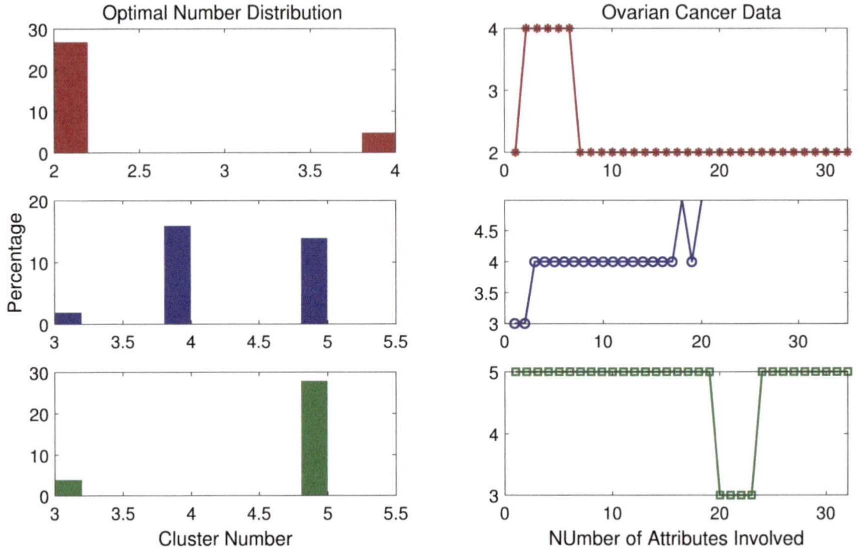

Fig. 8.18 Optimal cluster number determination with hierarchical clustering methods in ovarian cancer data

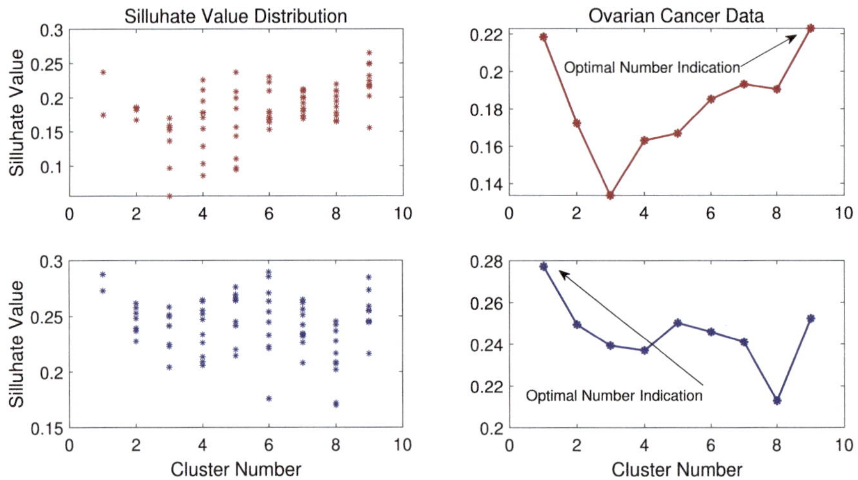

Fig. 8.19 Optimal cluster number determination with K-medoids and K-means methods in ovarian cancer data

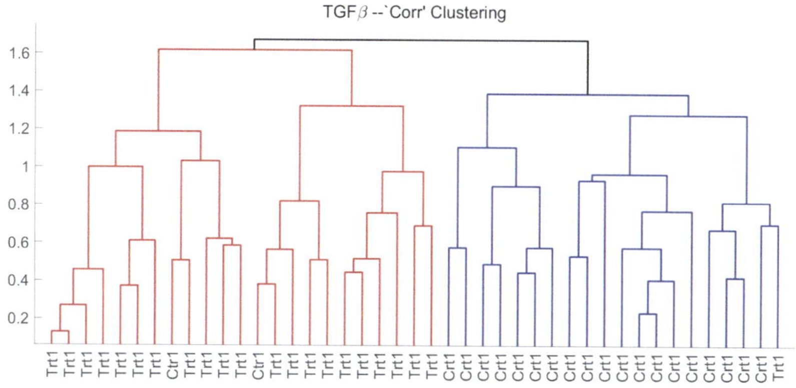

(a) Corr

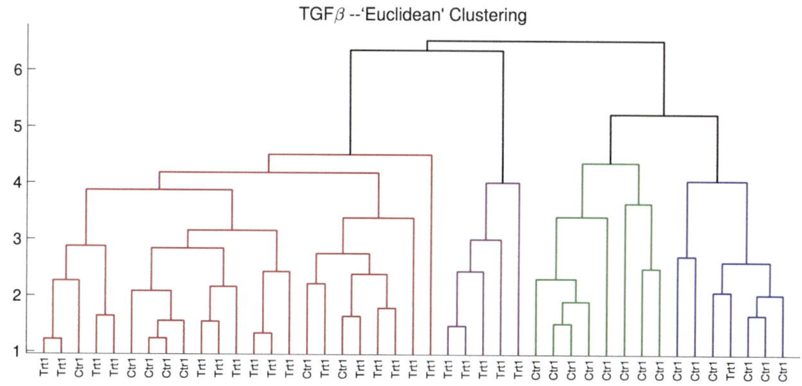

(b) Euclidean

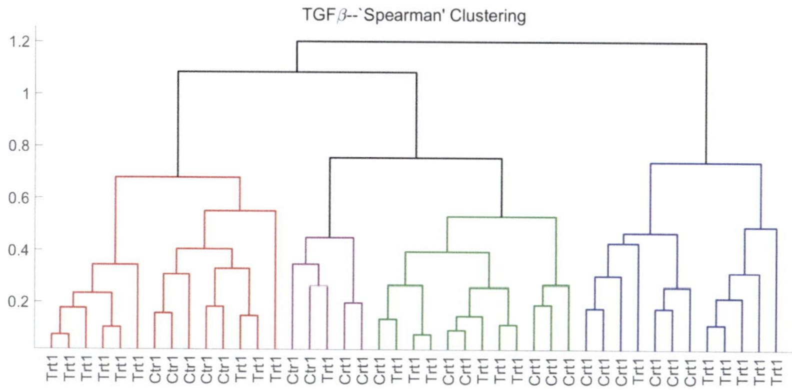

(c) Spearman

Fig. 8.20 Hierarchical clustering representations for TGFβ treated cells

a variance analysis that can systematically determine the number of clusters in the hierarchical clustering analysis.

8.5 Summary

scRNA-Seq analysis provides a new way of cell composition analysis at various developmental stages. As a fundamental problem in grouping individual cells based on their noisy gene expression values, scRNA-seq clustering is developed to understand pathology of developmental processes. We proposed a novel measure of differentiability correlation for evaluating cell dissimilarity that fits the framework of hierarchical clustering. Using variance analysis, we determined optimal cluster number. We therefore propose a new method **Corr** for understanding cell functions based on scRNA-seq data even with strong noise or fluctuations.

Our **Corr** algorithm is characterized by a list of notable features. Firstly, the algorithm takes into consideration the micro-environment of cell populations in dissimilarity construction, providing a more robust relationship assessment, i.e., cell-pair differentiability correlation. Furthermore, **Corr** algorithm incorporates factorial analysis of variance in optimal cluster number determination which is a new way in this field. The algorithm can automatically determine the optimal cluster number without a need for number specifications, and it can always suggest a correct cluster number for the respective data set. Notably, there is no requirement for setting extra parameters. **Corr** algorithm shows outstanding performance in benchmark or real experimental data sets, handling data with various cluster structures, against various exiting approaches in terms of internal criteria (clustering number and accuracy) and external criteria (purity, ARI, and F1-measure). **Corr** algorithm can clearly recognize embryo stem cells and other type of cells in various stages, capturing the cell-to-cell variability. The data normalization based on differentiability transformation (or differentiability vector) proves to be a reliable way to identify significant genes related to the biological processes or phenotypes while traditional differential gene expression fails to do so. And the application in ovarian cancer single cell clustering shows the ability of **Corr** algorithm in dealing with noise or unwanted biological variability, was also validated by the prognosis analysis of independent dataset.

References

Beyer KS, Goldstein J, Ramakrishnan R, Shaft U (1999) When is "nearest neighbor" meaningful? In: International conference on database theory

Bhadriraju K, Chen CS (2002) Engineering cellular microenvironments to improve cell-based drug testing. Drug Discov Today 7(11):612–20

Biase FH, Cao X, Zhong S (2014) Cell fate inclination within 2-cell and 4-cell mouse embryos revealed by single-cell rna sequencing. Genome Res 24:1787–1796

Brennecke P, Anders S, Kim JK, Kolodziejczyk AA, Zhang X, Proserpio V, Baying B, Benes V, Teichmann SA, Marioni JC, Heisler MG (2013) Accounting for technical noise in single-cell rna-seq experiments. Nat Methods 10(11):1093–1095

Caliński T, Harabasz J (1974) A dendrite method for cluster analysis. Commun Stat Theory Methods 3:1–27

Davies DL, Bouldin DW (1979) A cluster separation measure. IEEE Trans Pattern Anal Mach Intell PAMI-1(2):224–227

Eberwine JH, Sul JY, Bártfai T, Kim J (2013) The promise of single-cell sequencing. Nat Methods 11:25–27

Eberwine J, Sul J, Bartfai T et al (2014) The promise of single-cell sequencing. Nat Methods 11:25–27

Ertöz L, Steinbach MS, Kumar V (2003) Finding clusters of different sizes, shapes, and densities in noisy, high dimensional data. In: Proceedings of 2nd SIAM international conference on data mining

Federico M, Giordano A (2010) Cancer stem cells and microenvironment. Springer New York, New York, NY, pp 169–185

Gong Q, Ou Q, Ye S, Lee WP, Cornelius J, Diehl L, Lin WY, Hu Z, Lu Y, Chen Y, Wu Y, Meng YG, Gribling P, Lin Z, Nguyen K, Tran T, Zhang Y, Rosen H, Martin F, Chan AC (2005) Importance of cellular microenvironment and circulatory dynamics in b cell immunotherapy1. J Immunol 174:817–826

Goodman LA, Kruskal WH (1954) Measures of association for cross classifications, iv: simplification of asymptotic variances. J Am Stat Assoc 49:732–764

Guha S, Rastogi R, Shim K (1999) Rock: a robust clustering algorithm for categorical attributes. In: Proceedings 15th international conference on data engineering (Cat. No. 99CB36337), pp 512–521. https://doi.org/10.1109/ICDE.1999.754967

Houle ME, Kriegel HP, Kröger P, Schubert E, Zimek A (2010) Can shared-neighbor distances defeat the curse of dimensionality? In: International conference on statistical and scientific database management

Kiselev VY, Kirschner K, Schaub MT, Andrews TS, Yiu A, Chandra T, Natarajan KN, Reik W, Barahona M, Green AR, Hemberg M (2016) Sc3 - consensus clustering of single-cell rna-seq data. Nat Methods 14:483–486. https://api.semanticscholar.org/CorpusID:10927079

Levine JH, Simonds EF, Bendall SC, Davis KL, ad David Amir E, Tadmor MD, Litvin O, Fienberg HG, Jager A, Zunder ER, Finck R, Gedman AL, Radtke I, Downing JR, Pe'er D, Nolan GP (2015) Data-driven phenotypic dissection of aml reveals progenitor-like cells that correlate with prognosis. Cell 162:184–197. https://api.semanticscholar.org/CorpusID:11608684

Li J, Klughammer J, Farlik M, Penz T, Spittler A, Barbieux C, Berishvili E, Bock C, Kubicek S (2015) Single-cell transcriptomes reveal characteristic features of human pancreatic islet cell types. EMBO Rep 17:178–187

Li X, Cui XL, Giang Wang J, Wang Y, Li Y, Wang L, Wan H, Li T, Feng G, Shuai L, Li ZK, Gu Q, Hao J, Wang L, Zhao XY, Liu Z, Wang XJ, Li W, Zhou Q (2016) Generation and application of mouse-rat allodiploid embryonic stem cells. Cell 164:279–292

Mukhi S, Brown DD (2011) Transdifferentiation of tadpole pancreatic acinar cells to duct cells mediated by notch and stromelysin-3. Dev Biol 351:311–317

Ramsköld D, Luo SJ, Wang YC, Li R, Deng Q, Faridani OR, Daniels GA, Khrebtukova I, Loring JF, Laurent LC, Schroth GP, Sandberg R (2012) Full-length mrna-seq from single cell levels of rna and individual circulating tumor cells. Nat Biotechnol 30:777–782. https://api.semanticscholar.org/CorpusID:6705114

Rousseeuw PJ (1987) Silhouettes: a graphical aid to the interpretation and validation of cluster analysis. J Comput Appl Math 20:53–65

Schiffman C, Lin C, Shi F, Chen L, Sohn LL, Huang H (2017) Sideseq: a cell similarity measure defined by shared identified differentially expressed genes for single-cell rna sequencing data. Stat Biosci 9:200–216

Shapiro EY, Biezuner T, Linnarsson S (2013) Single-cell sequencing-based technologies will revolutionize whole-organism science. Nat Rev Genet 14:618–630
Stegle O, Teichmann SA, Marioni JC (2015) Computational and analytical challenges in single-cell transcriptomics. Nat Rev Genet 16:133–145
Teschendorff AE, Enver T (2017) Single-cell entropy for quantification of differentiation potency from a cell's transcriptome. Nat Commun 8:15599
Wang B, Zhu J, Pierson E, Ramazzotti D, Batzoglou S (2017) Visualization and analysis of single-cell rna-seq data by kernel-based similarity learning. Nat Methods 14:414–416 (2017)
Xu C, Su Z (2015) Identification of cell types from single-cell transcriptomes using a novel clustering method. Bioinformatics 31:1974–1980
Yan et al (2013) Single-cell rna-seq profiling of human preimplantation embryos and embryonic stem cells. Nat Struct Mol Biol 20(9):1131
Yuan G, Cai L, Elowitz MB, Enver T, Fan G, Guo G, Irizarry RA, Kharchenko PV, Kim J, Orkin SH, Quackenbush J, Saadatpour A, Schroeder T, Shivdasani RA, Tirosh I (2017) Challenges and emerging directions in single-cell analysis. Genome Biol 18:84

Chapter 9
Kernel Non-negative Matrix Factorization Framework for Single Cell Clustering

9.1 Introduction

RNA-sequence (RNA-Seq) measures the abundance of RNA transcripts, enabling the study of transcriptional structures, gene expression levels and so on (Wang et al. 2009). Bulk cell RNA-Seq technology has become one of the most popular technologies for transcriptome profiling. However, it cannot address cellular heterogeneity problem for its inability to isolate individual cells from complex organisms and to measure the corresponding transcriptional activity. Recent advances in single cell RNA-Seq technology allow for quantification of intra-population heterogeneity across a range of cellular states at the level of single cell (Wei and Li 2018). Consequently, scRNA-seq has gradually become the method of choice for understanding cellular heterogeneity in different complex biological conditions: such as cell type identification (Grün et al. 2015; Jiang et al. 2016; Tsoucas and Yuan 2018), cell development processes (Bendall et al. 2014; Yan et al. 2013; Chu et al. 2016; Farrell et al. 2018), cancer evolution (Gao and Ni 2017; Brady and McQuerry 2017; Kim and Gao 2018), and tumor heterogeneity (Mann et al. 2016; Hou et al. 2016; Giustacchini et al. 2017; Roerink et al. 2018).

scRNA-seq data is structurally identical to that obtained from a bulk expression experiment, often has high dimension and is highly noisy. In particular, scRNA-seq data is extremely sparse, having a lot of zeros. This is a typical phenomenon in scRNA-seq data where a gene is observed at a moderate expression level in some cell but undetected in other cells (Kharchenko et al. 2014), making further analysis more difficult and challenging.

One way to deal with scRNA-seq data is to find an accurate representation for the high dimensional, noisy and sparse data. Several imputation approaches have been designed in the recent years, all of which have various model assumptions. Bayesian approaches include BISCUIT, URSM and SAVER (Prabhakaran et al. 2016; Zhu et al. 2017; Huang et al. 2018) where the former two methods were reported to be computational comprehensive. DrImpute (Gong et al. 2018) imputes zero values in

H. Jiang and W.-K. Ching, *Kernel Methods for Omics Data Mining*, Intelligent Control and Learning Systems 10, https://doi.org/10.1007/978-981-95-3129-5_9

scRNA-seq data by averaging strategy within the same cluster, scImpute (Wei and Li 2018) recovers gene expression profiles through non-negative least square model, and MAGIC (Dijk et al. 2018) imputes zero values through Markov affinity graph. Taking into consideration on the high dimensionality in scRNA-seq data, researchers have also developed several dimension reduction methods. Identification of Highly Variable Genes (HVG) assumes that genes with high level of variance are caused by biological effects rather than mere technical noise (Bacher and Kendziorski 2016). Brennecke et al. (2013) used a gamma generalized linear model to estimate the highly variable genes. BiSiCS (Vallejos et al. 2015) introduces Poisson-Gamma hierarchical models to identify highly variable genes. In Kim et al. (2015), a simulation based framework was proposed to test the highly variable genes. M3Drop (Andrews and Hemberg 2018) implements two dropout-based feature selection methods with specific models for the null expectation. Another main approach for dealing with the curse of dimensionality is to project the high dimensional scRNA-seq data into a lower dimensional space. In Pierson and Yau (2015) zero-inflated factor analysis was applied to the scRNA-seq data. Note that t-SNE is the most frequently used method for visualizing high dimensional datasets (Macosko et al. 2015; Baron et al. 2016; Wei and Li 2018). However the drawback of which lies in the stochastic nature in producing different embeddings for the same dataset. As a nonlinear projection method, diffusion maps preserve local and distant relationships between data points and it is very suitable for large data sets (Haghverdi et al. 2016).

Much effort has been devoted to find accurate representation of scRNA-seq data either in terms of imputation or dimension reduction. However, most of the methods rely on different kinds of model assumptions thereby restricting the applications. Some related work tried to seek an appropriate description on the relationship within the high dimensional, sparse and noisy scRNA-seq data. SNN-Cliq (Chen and Zhengchang 2015) defines the similarity between two data points using connectivity in the neighborhood, proposing a shared nearest neighborhood (SNN) similarity measure. However, the nearest neighbor identification in high dimensional data needs careful specification and the inherent graph structure in scRNA-seq data cannot always be properly described. SIMLR (Wang et al. 2017) presents a multi-kernel learning framework to obtain the similarity between data points using a linear combination of Gaussian kernel functions under different variance settings. It needs the predefinition of cluster number within the data set to start the learning process, and the usage of Gaussian kernels in measuring data similarity may not always be suitable for it sometimes can make the learning process stuck into overfitting. SC3 (Kiselev et al. 2017) combines PCA and K-means clustering algorithm to construct a consensus similarity measure for the scRNA-seq data, proves to be a very robust method in identifying cellular heterogeneity. One of the main highlights in the method lies in the Cluster-based Similarity Partitioning Algorithm (CSPA) for consensus matrix construction, contributing to the stable and powerful performance. But in the preprocessing, PCA as a linear dimension reduction method may not be appropriate for all the scRNA-seq data. Jiang et al. (2018) proposed a new similarity construction method using cell-pair correlation, and the method shows robust power in cell type identification for small scRNA-seq data sets. The constructed similarity measure can be rewritten as a dot product and therefore can be regarded as a data transformation method. Results show that the transformation method gives a better representation on the original data and can help discover potential biomarkers.

In this chapter, we focus on cell type identification problem and we will develop a kernel non-negative matrix factorization framework for learning similarity in the scRNA-seq data. The constructed kernel models the nonlinear relationship within the scRNA-seq data, and after non-negative matrix factorization we obtain a low dimensional representation for the original data. Through the usage of CSPA, we finally construct a consensus matrix for measuring the relationships among the data points.

9.2 Methodology

Assume we have an expression matrix from scRNA-seq data denoted as $V = [v_1, v_2, \ldots, v_n] \in R^{p\times n}$, where n is the number of cells and p is the number of attributes used to represent a cell. In the following, we will first give a brief introduction to non-negative matrix factorization and then we will propose our kernel non-negative matrix factorization framework.

9.2.1 *Preliminaries: Non-negative Matrix Factorization (NMF)*

NMF (Lee and Seung 1999) realizes non-negative factorization on V by finding two non-negative matrices:

$$W = [w_1, w_2, \ldots, w_k] \in R^{p\times k}$$

and

$$H = [h_1, h_2, \ldots, h_n] \in R^{k\times n}$$

such that

$$V \approx WH$$

where k is a specified parameter of reduced dimensionality, the columns of W represent the base vectors for transforming the original data V, and columns of H correspond to the coefficients describing each cell.

The solutions of W, H can be found through solving the following optimization problem

$$\min_{W \geq 0, H \geq 0} \sum_{i \in \{1,\ldots,p\}, j \in \{1,\ldots,n\}} \left(V_{ij} \log \frac{V_{ij}}{(WH)_{ij}} - V_{ij} + (WH)_{ij} \right),$$

where the objective function is actually the KL-divergence between V and WH.

However, NMF is essentially linear hence can not fully capture the nonlinear structures embedded in the scRNA-seq data. Kernel non-negative matrix factorization (KNMF) (Zhang et al. 2006; Pan et al. 2011) as an nonlinear extension can be incorporated into scRNA-seq data analysis.

Assume we have a nonlinear mapping ϕ from R^p to a vector feature space F of higher dimension or infinity dimension

$$\phi : v \in R^p \rightarrow \phi(v) \in F.$$

Therefore, we have $\phi(V) = [\phi(v_1), \phi(v_2), \ldots, \phi(v_n)]$. In a similar fashion to NMF, KNMF also tries to find two non-negative matrix W_ϕ, H_ϕ such that

$$\phi(V) \approx W_\phi H_\phi.$$

When the nonlinear mapping ϕ is of infinity dimension, it is impractical to factorize $\phi(V)$ in a direct manner. But from $\phi(V) \approx W_\phi H_\phi$, we can derive the formula in the following:

$$\phi(V)^T \phi(V) \approx \phi(V)^T W_\phi H_\phi.$$

The formula indicates that $K = \phi(V)^T \phi(V) \in R^{n \times n}$ is a valid kernel matrix and $\phi(V)$ is exactly the kernel induced nonlinear mapping. Therefore, $K = W_\phi^K H_\phi$, $W_\phi^K = \phi(V)^T W_\phi$ shares the same formalism with that of NMF, where W_ϕ^K are the bases for kernel matrix K and H_ϕ represents the coefficients matrix as dimension reduced representation for V. KNMF (Zhang et al. 2006; Pan et al. 2011) naturally extends the NMF framework where it needs a careful description on the nonlinear mapping on the original data V, or alternatively constructing a delicate kernel for describing the relationship between different data points in scRNA-seq data set.

9.2.2 KDCorr: Kernel on Differentiability Correlation

There are a number of popular kernels:

- Linear Kernel

$$K(\mathbf{x}, \mathbf{x}') = \mathbf{x}^T \mathbf{x}',$$

  which is an inner product of $\mathbf{x}$ and $\mathbf{x}'$ in $\mathbf{R}^\mathbf{p}$.
- Polynomial kernel

$$K(\mathbf{x}, \mathbf{x}') = (\mathbf{x}^T \mathbf{x}' + 1)^d.$$

- Gaussian Radial Basis Function (RBF) kernel

$$K(\mathbf{x}, \mathbf{x}') = \exp(-d||\mathbf{x} - \mathbf{x}'||^2)$$

where d is parameter.

While scRNA-seq data is of high dimensionality, highly sparse and noisy, the above kernels may not be appropriate. In Wang et al. (2017), authors proposed using a linear combination of RBF kernel functions under different variance settings, but the selection of variance is also a problem need to be addressed. Jiang et al. (2018) proposed to use cell-pair correlation for modeling cellular relationships,

$$Dis_{ij} = 1 - \frac{\sum_{k=1}^{p}(U_{i_jk} - \overline{U_{i_j}})(U_{j_ik} - \overline{U_{j_i}})}{\sqrt{\sum_{k=1}^{p}(U_{i_jk} - \overline{U_{i_j}})^2}\sqrt{\sum_{k=1}^{p}(U_{j_ik} - \overline{U_{j_i}})^2}} \tag{9.1}$$

where U_{i_jk} is discrete version of gene expression representing differential status for gene k in cell i when coupled with cell j for measuring similarity between cell i and cell j. The method is applicable for small data sets, taking into nonlinear relationship within cells, but it is not efficient when the involved number of cells become relatively large. We here propose a kernel incorporating the advantages shown in Jiang et al. (2018), and is efficient for dealing with large scale data sets.

In the first step, we define a continuous version of differentiability for each cell i in gene k.

$$V_{i_k} = x_{ik} - \frac{\left(\sum_{l=1}^{n} x_{lk}\right) - x_{ik}}{n-1}.$$

In the later step, we calculate the differentiability correlation among the given n cells in the data set

$$\text{DCorr}(i, j) = \frac{\sum_{k=1}^{p}\left(V_{i_k} - \overline{V_k}\right)\left(V_{j_k} - \overline{V_k}\right)}{\sqrt{\sum_{k=1}^{p}\left(V_{i_k} - \overline{V_k}\right)^2}\sqrt{\sum_{k=1}^{p}\left(V_{j_k} - \overline{V_k}\right)^2}}$$

where $\overline{V_k} = \sum_{l=1}^{n} V_{l_k}/n$.

The KDCorr kernel is then constructed as

$$\text{KDCorr}(i, j) = \exp^{\left(\frac{1}{2}(\text{Dcorr}(i,j)-1)\right)}, i, j \in \{1, 2, \ldots, n\}. \tag{9.2}$$

It can be easily proved that KDCorr is a valid kernel as by kernel trick (Shawetaylor and Cristianini 2004).

9.2.3 KDCorr for Kernel Non-negative Matrix Factorization Framework in Cellular Heterogeneity Analysis

KDCorr kernel evaluates the nonlinear relationship among cells in scRNA-seq data. Suppose we have a factorization $K = W_\phi^K H_\phi$,where $W_\phi^K \in R^{n\times k}$ and $H_\phi \in R^{k\times n}$, we can then use H_ϕ as the low-dimension representation for the original data and perform clustering to discover different cell types.

The algorithm of the proposed method KDCorr is illustrated in the following.

Algorithm 2 Framework of our algorithm KDCorr based on kernel non-negative matrix factorization.

Input: The set of single cells, $P_n \in R^{n\times p}$;
Output: Cell types for the set of single cells, $L_n \in Z_+^{n\times 1}$;
Evaluate continuous version of differentiability correlation for $i, j \in \{1, 2, \ldots, n\}$;
Construct KDCorr kernel by Eq. (9.2);
Determine Cluster Number C_{opt} based on Diffusion Maps and variance analysis;
Consensus$^+$ Clustering with the above similarity measure and cluster number.

- for certain k, perform KNMF on KDCorr : $K = W_{\phi_k}^K H_{\phi_k}$.
- Consensus clustering on H_{ϕ_k} to obtain $L_{n_k} \in Z_+^{n\times 1}$.
- Consensus clustering on $L_{n_k} \in Z^{n\times 1}$ based on CSPA.

Return: L_n.

9.2.4 Optimal Cluster Number: Diffusion Maps with Variance Analysis

When the number of involved cells becomes large, the variance analysis based optimal cluster number is no longer efficient (Jiang et al. 2018). Here we propose to use diffusion maps to construct a method for determining optimal cluster number C_{opt} as it is very suitable for large data sets. We first evaluate the intrinsic dimension n_t embedded in the data set P_n with maximum likelihood estimation, and then perform diffusion maps with the denoted dimension n_t to obtain the transform data P_{n_t}. In the later stage, we introduce the same framework of variance analysis in Jiang et al. (2018) to obtain the final C_{opt}. We perform hierarchical clustering on P_{n_t} for different number of given clusters s, and check the changes of $R = \sum_{j=1}^m r_j$ as s increases, and compute the most frequent number determined among many C_m's we obtained, where m denotes the number of pre-selected genes.

9.3 Results

It is widely accepted that distinct cell types express different sets of genes, but in scRNA-seq data, notable technical noise in single-cell transcriptomes makes cell type identification non-trivial. We tested KDCorr for capability of cell type identification using a number of scRNA-seq datasets in a variety of cell types (Dmitry et al. 2015; Kolodziejczyk et al. 2015; Ii 2017). The cell clustering results will be presented in comparison with three widely used single cell clustering algorithms: SNN-Cliq (Chen and Zhengchang 2015) that can reflect cell types of origins in a highly accurate manner, SIMLR (Wang et al. 2017): a stable multi-kernel learning framework for cell type identification and SC3 (Kiselev et al. 2017): a robust and accurate consensus clustering method. The clustering results are evaluated with two broadly used measures: Adjusted Rand Index (ARI) and Normalized Mutual Information (NMI). ARI is used to describe the agreement between two partitions, and NMI is often used in clustering to measure the similarity between two clustering results. They are important measurement indicator that can objectively evaluate the accuracy of comparing a community division with a standard division.

9.3.1 Performance on Neuronal Cells

This neuronal cell data set (Dmitry et al. 2015) contains 622 neuronal cells with sensory subtypes: peptidergic nociceptors, nonpeptidergic nociceptors, neurofilament containing and tyrosine hydroxylase containing. It was obtained from mouse dorsal root ganglion, generated by using Illumina Genome Analyzer IIx. The KNMF parameter k is set to be 16. For the hierarchical clustering with low dimensional representation generated by KNMF, the consensus parameter is set to be 30. The consensus$^+$ parameter is set to be 10. As shown in Fig. 9.1, the ARI value by KDCorr is 0.9373, NMI value is 0.9113. In comparison, the robust and accurate SC3 method achieves ARI value 0.8849, NMI value 0.8736, ranking the second best. SIMLR by similarity learning shows 0.6820 in ARI value, and 0.7476 in NMI value. SNN-Cliq finds 110 quasi-cliques, merged into 29 clusters, and the final ARI value is 0.2677, with NMI value 0.4819.

It should be noted that we need to specify the number of clusters in advance in both SC3 and SIMLR, we all use the correct cluster number 4 as input for the two methods. While in KDCorr, we estimated the number of clusters using diffusion maps and variance analysis. We calculated the intrinsic dimension for neuronal cell data set to be 98, and conducted further variance analysis. Figure 9.2 illustrates the determination of the optimal cluster numbers for KDCorr, the final optimal cluster number is determined as the most frequently appeared one. We can see that diffusion maps with variance analysis helps determine the right cluster number, however, in SNN-Cliq, the cluster number estimated as 29 tends to be much larger than the real one.

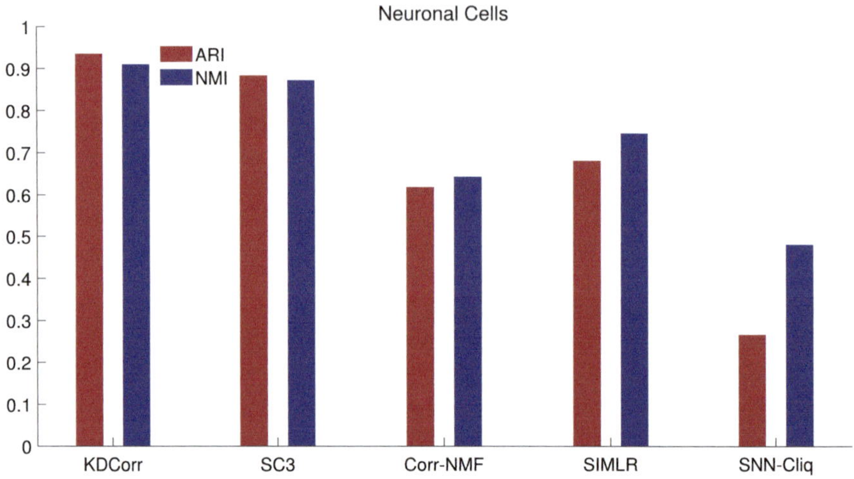

Fig. 9.1 Evaluation of clustering accuracy by ARI and NMI in neuronal cells

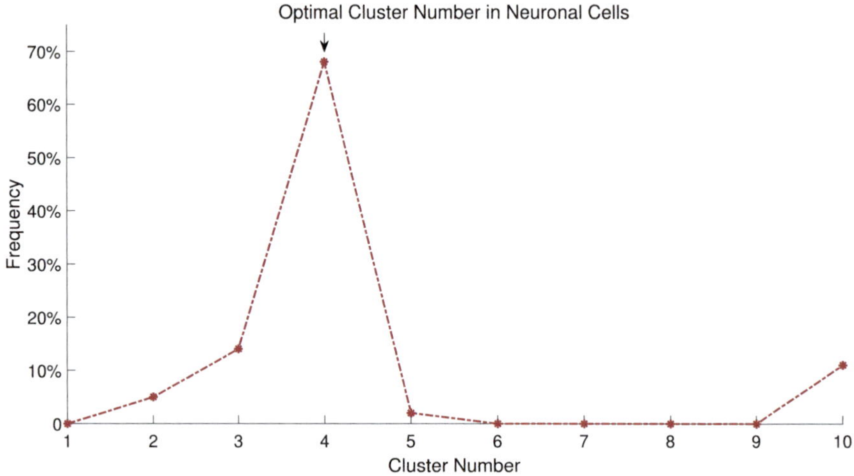

Fig. 9.2 Cluster number determination in neuronal cells by KDCorr

9.3.2 Performance on Pluripotent Cells

The pluripotent cell data set contains 704 mESCs (mouse embryonic stem cells) involving 3 different culture conditions. It was obtained from a stem cell study considering the influence of culture conditions on pluripotent states of mESCs. The data set is available at ArrayExpress database (http://www.ebi.ac.uk/arrayexpress) under accession number E-MTAB-2600. The KNMF parameter k is set to be 9. For the hierarchical clustering with low dimensional representation generated by

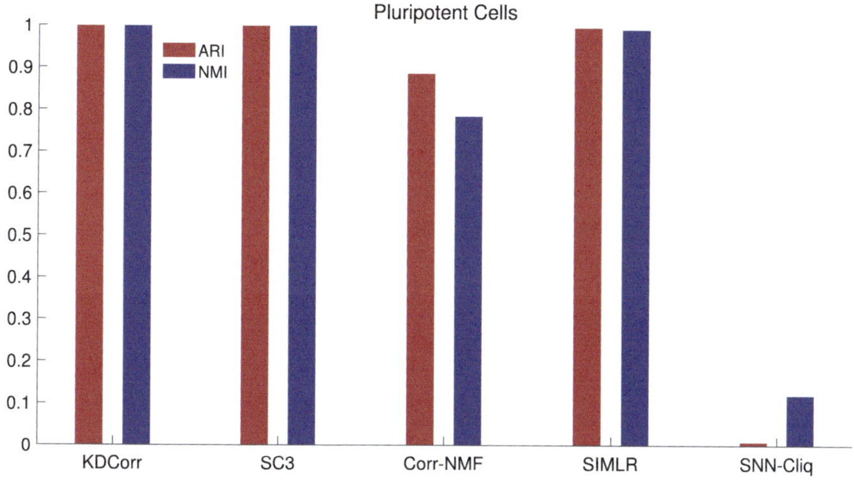

Fig. 9.3 Evaluation of clustering accuracy by ARI and NMI in pluripotent cells

KNMF, the consensus parameter is set to be 30. The consensus$^+$ parameter is set to be 10. The ARI value by KDCorr is 1, NMI value is 1, showing in Fig. 9.3. In comparison, the robust and accurate SC3 method achieves ARI value 1, NMI value 1. Both KDCorr and SC3 show 100% in accuracy, showing that they can accurately distinguish mESCs in different culture conditions. SIMLR by similarity learning shows 0.9960 in ARI value, and 0.9915 in NMI value, which is almost 100% correct. SNN-Cliq finds 29 quasi-cliques, merged into 3 clusters, and the final ARI value is 0.0096, with NMI value 0.1205. From the results we know that SNN-Cliq as a graph clustering algorithm may not be quite appropriate for this data set.

We calculated the intrinsic dimension estimated by maximum likelihood estimation for pluripotent cell data set as 64, and conducted variance analysis in a further step to estimate the optimal cluster number. Figure 9.4 illustrates the determination of optimal cluster numbers for KDCorr, the final optimal cluster number is determined as the most frequently appeared one. It is very clear that the optimal cluster number is 3, occupying over 80% in the suggested optimal numbers. We can see that diffusion maps with variance analysis helps determine the right cluster number. It is interesting to see that in SNN-Cliq, the cluster number estimated as 3 is also correct. However, the clustering performance in SNN-Cliq is quite unsatisfactory.

9.3.3 Performance on PBMCs

We adopted an immune cell data set (https://www.nature.com/articles/nmeth.4179) (Ii 2017) using Seq-Well technology, that is more prone to drop out and noise errors. In the dataset, there are 4296 cells with 602 cells likely representing single-cell

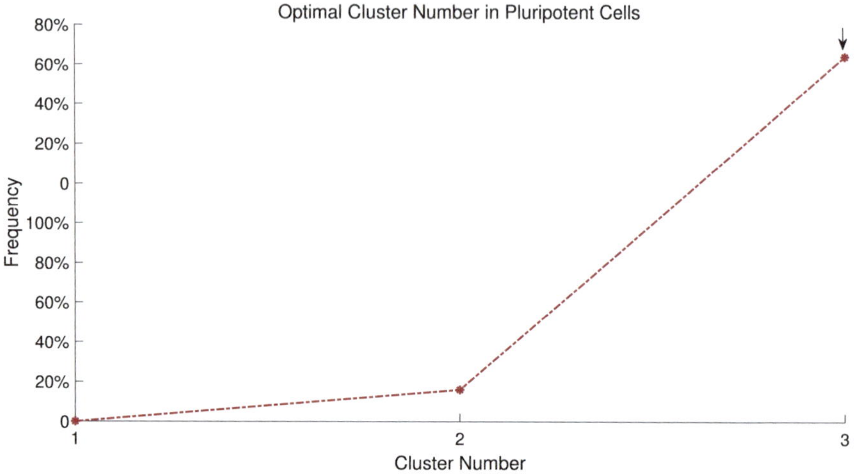

Fig. 9.4 Cluster number determination in pluripotent cells by KDCorr

libraries of low complexity removed. In total, there are 3694 cells, containing 6 different cell types: B cell, NK cell, monocyte cell, CD4+ cell, CD8+ cell, Dendritic cell. The KNMF parameter k is set to be 36. For the hierarchical clustering with low dimensional representation generated by KNMF, the consensus parameter is set to be 30. The consensus$^+$ parameter is set to be 10. The ARI value by KDCorr is 0.8725, NMI value is 0.7587, showing in Fig. 9.5. In comparison, the robust and accurate SC3 method achieves ARI value 0.7927, NMI value 0.7061, inferior to KDCorr. SIMLR by similarity learning shows 0.6454 in ARI value, and 0.6200 in NMI value. SNN-Cliq finds 502 quasi-cliques, merged into 56 clusters, and the final ARI value is 0.3987, with NMI value 0.4959. From the results we know that SNN-Cliq as a graph clustering algorithm may not be quite appropriate for this data set.

We calculated the intrinsic dimension estimated by maximum likelihood estimation for PBMC data set as 86, and conducted variance analysis in a further step to estimate the optimal cluster number. Figure 9.6 illustrates the determination of optimal cluster numbers for KDCorr, and the final optimal cluster number is determined as the most frequently appeared one. It is very clear that the optimal cluster number is 6, which dominates the whole suggested cluster numbers. We can see that diffusion maps with variance analysis helps determine the right cluster number. In comparison with SNN-Cliq, the cluster number estimated as 56, providing an unreliable estimation on the cluster number. The clustering performance in SNN-Cliq is unsatisfactory as well.

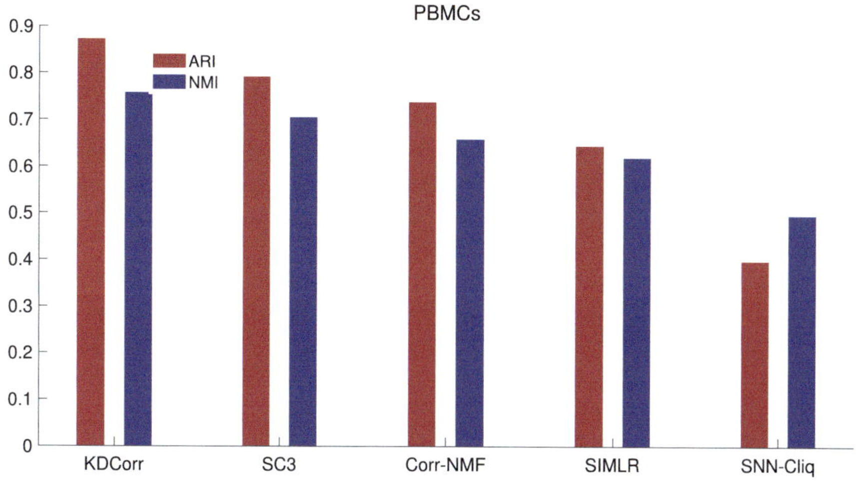

Fig. 9.5 Evaluation of clustering accuracy by ARI and NMI in PBMCs

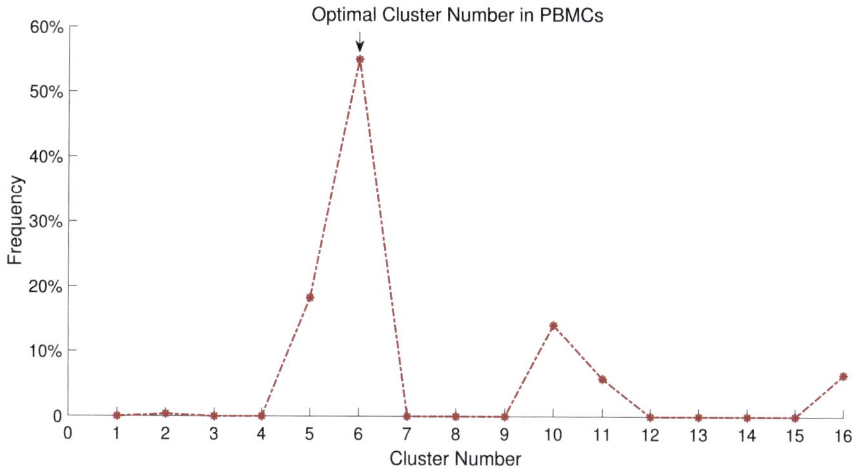

Fig. 9.6 Cluster number determination in PBMCs by KDCorr

9.4 Discussions

In the results part, we have included a comparison partner Corr-NMF apart from SC3, SIMLR and SNN-Cliq. 'Corr-NMF' is different from KDCorr in the kernel construction part. Since we know that KDCorr as a kernel is induced by DCorr where DCorr itself is a valid kernel as well, therefore we also want to test if Corr-NMF can be suitable for dealing with scRNA-seq data. Based on the computational results, we can have the following discoveries.

- KDCorr is the best among all the comparison partners, achieving the best in both ARI and NMI values in all the considered data sets. In pluripotent cell data set, the data is relatively clean, KDCorr and SC3 show 100% in both ARI and NMI values, perfectly distinguish cells in different culture conditions, SIMLR also achieves 0.9980 in ARI value, 'Corr-NMF' yields 0.8861 in ARI value. SNN-Cliq only achieves 0.0096 in ARI value, near 0. In neuronal cell data set with mediate noise, KDCorr can still show its power in cell type identification. SC3 ranked the second best and SIMLR is the third, achieving 0.6820 in ARI value. SNN-Cliq only shows 0.2677 in ARI value. In PBMCs data set with strong noise, KDCorr can show 0.8741 in ARI value, SC3 obtains 0.7927 accordingly. Corr-NMF is the third for this data set, superior to SIMLR who obtains 0.6454 in ARI value. SNN-Cliq only shows 0.3987 in ARI value.
- SNN-Cliq seems inappropriate for dealing with large scale scRNA-seq data sets. In neuronal cell data set and PBMCs data set, SNN-Cliq cannot give a relatively reasonable estimation on the cluster number, much larger than the truth. The evaluation measures are also not satisfactory. In particular for pluripotent cell data set, although SNN-Cliq provides accurate estimate on the cluster number within the data set, the ARI value and NMI value is almost 0.
- SC3 can demonstrate its ability in cell type identification. Although it cannot compete with KDCorr, it is the most robust and efficient method among the other competitors. There is no dominant method in SIMLR and Corr-NMF. In neuronal cell data set and pluripotent cell data set, SIMLR is better than Corr-NMF and in PMBCs data set Corr-NMF is better than SIMLR.

KDCorr as a kernel may provide a relatively clear representation on the cellular relationships. Hence, we checked if t-SNE with the similarity matrix KDCorr may provide a proper low dimensional visualization on the highly noisy and sparse scRNA-seq data. Figure 9.7 shows that t-SNE with KDCorr can help preserve local structures better than t-SNE with SIMLR. There are 6 types of cells involved, and cells with type 0, 3, 4, 5 are clearly distinguished, leaving cells in type 1 and 2 blended in KDCorr. In SIMLR, we can see that cells in type 3 and 5 are perfectly isolated from other cells. But cells in type 0 are divided into two subclusters, and cells with type 1, 3, 4 are blended together. Similarly in the other two datasets, we can also see that KDCorr can provide clear representation on the cellular relationships.

Regarding the selection of k, we predetermined a feasible range of k values related to the number of determined optimal cluster number, k_{opt}^2. We tested over a range of k values around k_{opt}^2 to check if consensus$^+$ KDCorr is robust or not. We found that the consensus$^+$ framework helps to guarantee a robust and stable performance in clustering. As shown in Fig. 9.8, in neuronal cells data, the performance of consensus$^+$ KDCorr is very stable when $k \in (16, 20)$. When k is chosen in a relatively small number, the performance is relatively less stable, but stable in a overall manner. And for pluripotent cells data, the performance is also very stable for $k \in (5, 13)$. For PMBC data, when $k \in (31, 40)$, the performance of consensus$^+$ KDCorr over multiple runs tends to be stable.

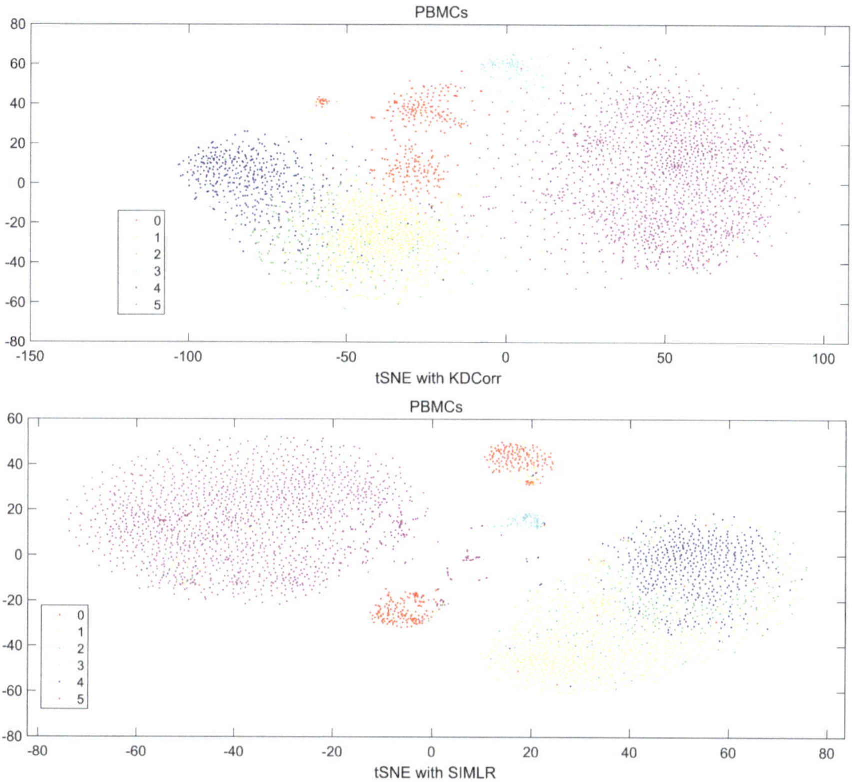

Fig. 9.7 t-SNE in PBMCs by KDCorr and SIMLR

Even when consensus$^+$ KDCorr is less stable for some certain k, we still can help identifying a near optimal clustering result through developing a measure to detect the block structure embedded in the new kernels. It is reasonable to assume that cells in the same cluster tend to be more similar to each other. We first reformulate the constructed kernel KDCorr after clustering result is obtained, where the new matrix is reordered so that entries for cells in the same cluster are put together. Therefore, ignoring the similarities within the clusters, the similarities between clusters should be relatively small. Hence the block structure measure F_{BLS} is defined as the norm of reordered KDCorr matrix accounting for the cell similarities between clusters.

We determine the final clustering output when F_{BLS} achieves the lowest value over multiple runs. It provides a new way to evaluate the non-negative matrix factorization result as well as the clustering result. And we found that the determined clustering result is quite stable for different values of k.

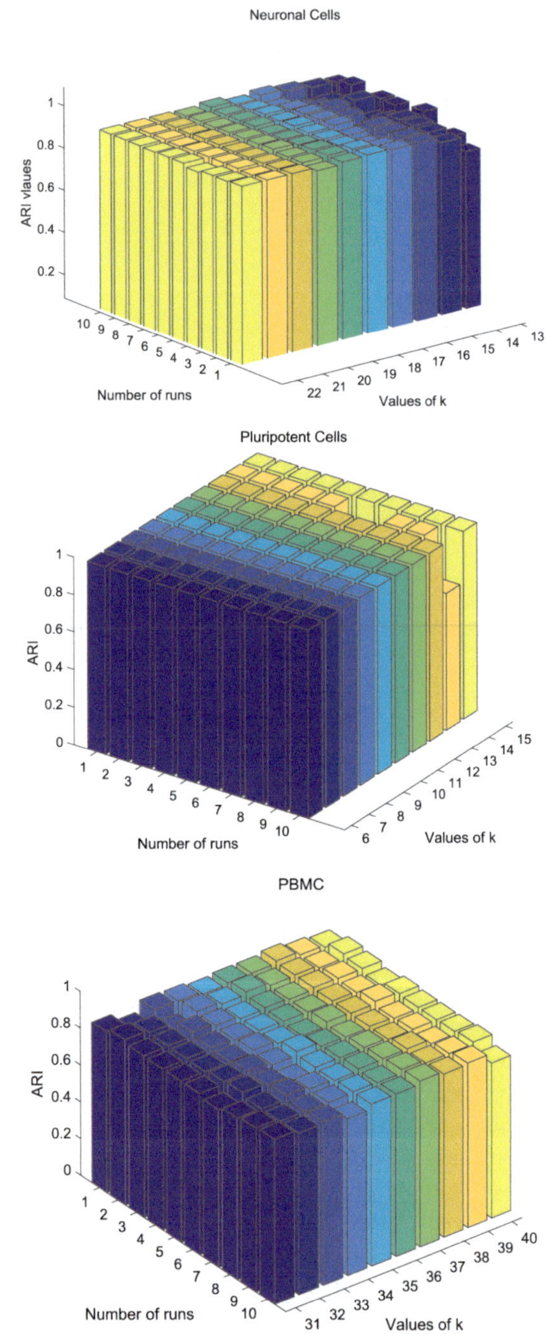

Fig. 9.8 Stability of consensus^{+} KDCorr

9.5 Conclusions

In this chapter, we proposed kernel non-negative matrix factorization framework for single cell clustering. The KDCorr kernel provides a proper evaluation on cell similarity based on cell-pair differentiability correlation for nonlinear and noisy scRNA-seq data. And the consensus$^+$ framework provides a stable way for scRNA-seq data analysis. Experiments under different evaluation metrics support the effectiveness and feasibility of our proposed method. Besides, the cluster number determination method based on diffusion maps and variance analysis is a robust approach for estimating the intrinsic clusters embedded in the high-dimensional and noisy data.

References

Andrews TS, Hemberg M (2018) Dropout-based feature selection for scrnaseq. Bioinformatics

Bacher R, Kendziorski C (2016) Design and computational analysis of single-cell rna-sequencing experiments. Genome Biol 17(1):63

Baron M, Veres A, Wolock S, Faust A, Gaujoux R, Vetere A, Ryu JH, Wagner B, Shen-Orr S, Klein A (2016) A single-cell transcriptomic map of the human and mouse pancreas reveals inter- and intra-cell population structure. Cell Syst 3(4):346–360.e4

Bendall SC, Davis KL, ad David Amir E, Tadmor MD, Simonds EF, Chen TJ, Shenfeld DK, Nolan GP, Pe'er D (2014) Single-cell trajectory detection uncovers progression and regulatory coordination in human B cell development. Cell 157(3):714–725

Brady SW, McQuerry JA, Qiao Y et al (2017) Combating subclonal evolution of resistant cancer phenotypes. Nat Commun 8:1231

Brennecke P, Anders S, Kim JK, Kołodziejczyk AA, Zhang X, Proserpio V, Baying B, Benes V, Teichmann SA, Marioni JC (2013) Accounting for technical noise in single-cell rna-seq experiments. Nat Methods 10(11):1093–1095

Chen X, Zhengchang S (2015) Identification of cell types from single-cell transcriptomes using a novel clustering method. Bioinformatics 31(12):1974–80

Chu LF, Leng N, Zhang J, Hou Z, Mamott D, Vereide DT, Choi J, Kendziorski C, Stewart R, Thomson JA (2016) Single-cell rna-seq reveals novel regulators of human embryonic stem cell differentiation to definitive endoderm. Genome Biol 17(1):173

Dijk DV, Sharma R, Nainys J, Yim K, Kathail P, Carr AJ, Burdziak C, Moon KR, Chaffer CL, Pattabiraman D (2018) Recovering gene interactions from single-cell data using data diffusion. Cell 174(3):S0092867418307,244

Dmitry U, Alessandro F, Saiful I, Hind A, Peter L, Daohua L, Jens HL, Jesper H, Olga K, Kharchenko PV (2015) Unbiased classification of sensory neuron types by large-scale single-cell rna sequencing. Nat Neurosci 18(1):145–153

Farrell JA, Wang Y, Riesenfeld SJ, Shekhar K, Regev A, Schier AF (2018) Single-cell reconstruction of developmental trajectories during zebrafish embryogenesis. Science 360:eaar3131

Gao Y, Ni X, Guo H et al (2017) Single-cell sequencing deciphers a convergent evolution of copy number alterations from primary to circulating tumor cells. Genome Res 27:1312–1322

Giustacchini A, Thongjuea S, Barkas N, Woll PS, Povinelli BJ, Booth CAG, Sopp P, Norfo R, Rodriguez-Meira A, Ashley N (2017) Single-cell transcriptomics uncovers distinct molecular signatures of stem cells in chronic myeloid leukemia. Nat Med 23(6):692

Gong W, Kwak IY, Pota P, Koyano-Nakagawa N, Garry DJ (2018) Drimpute: imputing dropout events in single cell rna sequencing data. BMC Bioinform 19(1):220

Grün D, Lyubimova A, Kester L, Wiebrands K, Basak O, Sasaki N, Clevers H, van Oudenaarden A (2015) Single-cell messenger RNA sequencing reveals rare intestinal cell types. Nature 525:251–255

Haghverdi L, Büttner M, Wolf FA, Buettner F, Theis FJ (2016) Diffusion pseudotime robustly reconstructs lineage branching. Nat Methods 13(10):845

Hou Y, Guo H, Cao C, Li X, Hu B, Zhu P, Wu X, Wen L, Tang F, Huang Y (2016) Single-cell triple omics sequencing reveals genetic, epigenetic, and transcriptomic heterogeneity in hepatocellular carcinomas. Cell Res 26(3):304–319

Huang M, Jingshu W, Eduardo T, Hannah D, Sydney S, Roberto B, Murray JI, Arjun R, Mingyao L, Zhang NR (2018) Saver: gene expression recovery for single-cell rna sequencing. Nat Methods

Ii MHW (2017) Seq-well: portable, low-cost rna sequencing of single cells at high throughput. Nat Methods 14(4):395–398

Jiang L, Chen H, Pinello L, Chen Y (2016) GiniClust: detecting rare cell types from single-cell gene expression data with Gini index. Genome Biol 17:144

Jiang H, Sohn LL, Huang H, Chen L (2018) Single cell clustering based on cell-pair differentiability correlation and variance analysis. Bioinformatics 34(21):3684

Kharchenko PV, Silberstein L, Scadden DT (2014) Bayesian approach to single-cell differential expression analysis. Nat Methods 11(7):740

Kim JK, Kolodziejczyk AA, Ilicic T, Teichmann SA, Marioni JC (2015) Characterizing noise structure in single-cell rna-seq distinguishes genuine from technical stochastic allelic expression. Nat Commun 6:8687–8687

Kim C, Gao R, Sei E et al (2018) Chemoresistance evolution in triple-negative breast cancer delineated by single-cell sequencing. Cell 173:879–893

Kiselev VY, Kirschner K, Schaub MT, Andrews T, Yiu A, Chandra T, Natarajan KN, Reik W, Barahona M, Green AR (2017) Sc3: consensus clustering of single-cell rna-seq data. Nat Methods 14(5):483–486

Kolodziejczyk A, Kim JK, Tsang JH, Ilicic T, Henriksson J, Natarajan K, Tuck A, Gao X, Bühler M, Liu P (2015) Single cell rna-sequencing of pluripotent states unlocks modular transcriptional variation. Cell Stem Cell 17(4):471–485

Lee DD, Seung HS (1999) Learning the parts of objects by non-negative matrix factorization. Nature 401(6755):788–791

Macosko E, Basu A, Satija R, Nemesh J, Shekhar K, Goldman M, Tirosh I, Bialas A, Kamitaki N, Martersteck E (2015) Highly parallel genome-wide expression profiling of individual cells using nanoliter droplets. Cell 161(5):1202–1214

Mann KM, Newberg JY, Black MA, Jones DJ, Amaya-Manzanares F, Guzman-Rojas L, Kodama T, Ward JM, Rust AG, van der Weyden L (2016) Analyzing tumor heterogeneity and driver genes in single myeloid leukemia cells with sbcapseq. Nat Biotechnol 34(9):962–972

Pan B, Lai J, Chen WS (2011) Nonlinear nonnegative matrix factorization based on mercer kernel construction. Pattern Recogn 44(10):2800–2810

Pierson E, Yau C (2015) Zifa: Dimensionality reduction for zero-inflated single-cell gene expression analysis. Genome Biol 16(1):241

Prabhakaran S, Azizi E, Carr A, Pe'Er D (2016) Dirichlet process mixture model for correcting technical variation in single-cell gene expression data. In: International conference on machine learning

Roerink SF, Sasaki N, Lee-Six H, Young MD, Alexandrov LB, Behjati S, Mitchell TJ, Grossmann S, Lightfoot H, Egan DA (2018) Intra-tumour diversification in colorectal cancer at the single-cell level. Nature 556(7702):102–102

Shawetaylor J, Cristianini N (2004) Kernel methods for pattern analysis: pattern analysis

Tsoucas D, Yuan G (2018) Giniclust2: a cluster-aware, weighted ensemble clustering method for cell-type detection. Genome Biol 19:58

Vallejos CA, Marioni JC, Richardson S (2015) Basics: Bayesian analysis of single-cell sequencing data. Plos Comput Biol 11(6):e1004,333

Wang Z, Gerstein M, Snyder M (2009) Rna-seq: a revolutionary tool for transcriptomics. Nat Rev Genet 10:57–63

Wang B, Zhu J, Pierson E, Ramazzotti D, Batzoglou S (2017) Visualization and analysis of single-cell rna-seq data by kernel-based similarity learning. Nat Methods 14(4):414

Wei VL, Li JJ (2018) An accurate and robust imputation method scimpute for single-cell rna-seq data. Nat Commun 9(1):997

Yan L, Yang M, Guo H, Yang Y, Wu J, Li R, Liu P, Lian Y, Zheng X, Yan J, Huang J, Li M, Wu X, Wen L, Lao K, Li R, Qiao J, Tang F (2013) Single-cell RNA-Seq profiling of human preimplantation 115 embryos and embryonic stem cells. Nat Struct Mol Biol 20:1131–1139

Zhang D, Zhou ZH, Chen S (2006) Non-negative matrix factorization on kernels

Zhu L, Jing L, Devlin B, Roeder K (2017) A unified statistical framework for single cell and bulk rna sequencing data. Ann Appl Stat 12(1):609–632

Chapter 10
Deep Neural Network with Kernel Nonnegative Matrix Factorization for Single Cell Clustering

10.1 Introduction

Single cell RNA sequencing (scRNA-seq) technology provides the unprecedented possibility for analyzing the heterogeneity between cells by profiling gene expression in single cells. In the recent years, a number of scRNA-seq methods have been developed, most of which have similar characteristics of cell isolation, reverse transcription, etc., (Svensson 2017; Ziegenhain 2017). It is worth mentioning that current methods generate large and complex scRNA-seq data that require specialized analysis techniques to facilitate accurate data interpretation. Besides, technical noise and random transcription bring considerable challenges to the downstream analysis.

scRNA-seq data has three main characteristics: high dimensionality, sparsity and nonlinearity. These properties are non-negligible as they pose obstacles for downstream analysis such as differential gene expression and heterogeneity analysis etc. Various techniques have been proposed to deal with the above-mentioned issues. Dimensionality reduction methods such as unified manifold approximation and projection (UMAP) (Becht et al. 2019) and t-SNE are popular for high-dimensional data visualization, imputation methods such as magic (David et al. 2018) and SAVER (Huang et al. 2018) are used for dealing with sparsity problems and nonlinear relationship evaluation for modeling the scRNA-seq data.

To fully understand the complexity of cellular heterogeneity, appropriate design of clustering methods would play a critical role. Conventional approaches realize heterogeneity by reducing the dimensionality of scRNA-seq data via projecting it into a low dimensional space; and use the traditional machine learning clustering algorithm for heterogeneity analysis, such as k-means, hierarchical clustering, density clustering, graph based clustering and so on.

Taking into consideration on the special property that scRNA-seq data possessed, clustering methods designed for scRNA sequence data, such as SC3 (Kiselev et al. 2017), Seurat (Satija et al. 2015), SIMLR (Wang et al. 2017), Scanpy (Wolf et al. 2018), Jiang et al. (2021) have been proposed. SC3 performs consistent clustering on

H. Jiang and W.-K. Ching, *Kernel Methods for Omics Data Mining*, Intelligent Control and Learning Systems 10, https://doi.org/10.1007/978-981-95-3129-5_10

single cell data by parallelization methods. Seurat and Scanpy are single-cell analysis frameworks with similar performance. By default, they use Louvain algorithm and k-nearest neighbor method to segment cells with similar gene expression and realize cell recognition. SIMLR is based on kernel similarity learning to cluster single-cell data. When the number of cells is small, the performance of SC3 is better than other methods on average. The result of Scanpy is similar to that of Seruat. For large-scale single-cell data clustering, the computational complexity of SC3 is quite high. SC3 is not suitable for the analysis of a large number of single cell data.

In the analysis of large-scale scRNA-seq data, some methods use integrated or parallel computing to complete such a high amount of computation. Sharp (Wan et al. 2022) is to cluster millions of cells by integrating random projection method. bigSCale (Iacono et al. 2018) uses a large sample size to estimate high-precision and comprehensive noise numerical models. Sharp (Wan et al. 2022) improves the dimensionality reduction method. bigSCale's model can quantify the distance between cells. Both of them use hierarchical clustering to cluster the data, but their accuracy is still low. The SSCC (Ren et al. 2019) framework proposed by Ren uses feature engineering and projection technology to improve the clustering framework with sub sampling and classification. However, it uses traditional clustering and classification algorithms. The influence of the deviation introduced by subsampling is also not considered. In this chapter, we combine kernel non-negative matrix factorization clustering with deep neural network classification. Instead of clustering the whole data directly, we first determine the optimal representative data for clustering, followed by classifying the remaining data. We use the idea of stratified sampling to select the representative samples, and determine the optimal partition of clustering samples and classification samples based on KL divergence. A deep neural network based classification method is introduced for further classification problem to ensure the discrimination power on the whole data.

The rest of this chapter is organized as follows. We propose the method including framework design, partition optimization, clustering and classification in Sect. 10.2. In Sect. 10.3, experimental results are shown, followed by discussions on the advantages and disadvantages of the method. Finally, conclusions will be made in Sect. 10.4.

10.2 Materials and Methods

Two major motivations drive our way in designing the framework for large-scale single cell heterogeneity analysis. Large-scale scRNA-seq data for its high dimensionality, sparsity and complexity brings high computational complexity as well as low discrimination power for traditional heterogeneity analysis methods. In order to cope with the above challenges, we propose an optimal partition based framework where we initially select representative subset V_s from the whole single cell gene expression matrix $V \in R^{N \times p}$, and conduct clustering to achieve a robust and clear discrimination on the cells involved in the representative data. The rest of the data

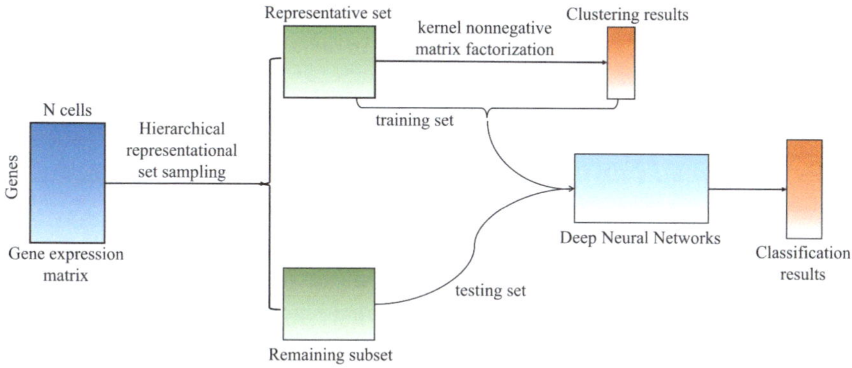

Fig. 10.1 Framework design

is used as a testing set, where the deep neural network classification algorithm is used to entangle the heterogeneity embedded. The graphical framework is shown in Fig. 10.1.

10.2.1 The Hierarchical Representative Set Selection

In the selection of representative set, we use the idea of hierarchical sampling as shown in Fig. 10.2. First, we use the farthest point sampling (FPS) method to locate K center points $c_1, c_2, \ldots, c_K$, and assign the other samples to the K blocks centered at the K center points. The assignment guarantees that the sample has the shortest distance with the assigned center. We use apricot (Schreiber et al. 2019), a python package that has been developed, to filter M/K representative data from each block according to the module optimization algorithm, and then merge the data filtered

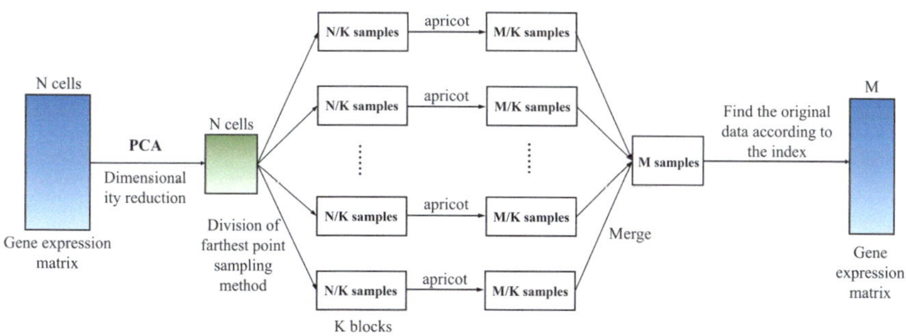

Fig. 10.2 Flow chart of hierarchical representative set selection

from each block together. The selected data set V_s follows similar distribution with the original data V.

10.2.2 Optimal Partition Criterion

From the above subsection we know that the hierarchical representative set selection method can ensure the representativeness of the selected data set, (Tung and Kingsford 2021) but how to determine the optimal representative set D_s^* is a problem need to be addressed. We develop an optimal partition criterion by calculating the KL divergence between the sample distribution of the representative set and the remaining data distribution.

We assume that the probability distribution of representative set V_s and remaining set V_r follows multivariate Gaussian distribution, where the probability density functions are $p_1(x \mid \mu_1, \Sigma_1)$ and $p_2(x \mid \mu_2, \Sigma_2)$, respectively. Here

$$p_1(x \mid \mu_1, \Sigma_1) = \frac{1}{(2\pi)^{\frac{p}{2}}} e^{-\frac{1}{2}(x-\mu_1)^T \Sigma_1^{-1}(x-\mu_1)}$$

and

$$p_2(x \mid \mu_2, \Sigma_2) = \frac{1}{(2\pi)^{\frac{p}{2}}} e^{-\frac{1}{2}(x-\mu_2)^T \Sigma_2^{-1}(x-\mu_2)}.$$

The KL divergence of the two multivariate Gaussian distributions can be represented as follows:

$$\begin{aligned} D(p_1 \,||\, p_2) = 1/2\Big[&\log\tfrac{\det(\Sigma_2)}{\det(\Sigma_1)} - p + \operatorname{tr}(\Sigma_2^{-1}\Sigma_1) \\ &+(\mu_2-\mu_1)^T \Sigma_2^{-1}(\mu_2-\mu_1)\Big]. \end{aligned} \tag{10.1}$$

In the case of high-dimensional single cell data, the KL divergence computation in Eq. (10.1) will be time consuming. Here, we use the top 20 principal components to represent the original data, and calculate KL divergence accordingly. The best partition is determined when the KL divergence between distributions $p_1(x \mid \mu_1, \Sigma_1)$ and $p_2(x \mid \mu_2, \Sigma_2)$ generated by V_s and V_r achieves the optimal.

10.2.3 KNMF Based Clustering

Given the high-dimensionality and nonlinearity embedded in the gene expression matrix $V = [v_1, v_2, \ldots, v_N]^T$, we construct a nonlinear mapping

$$\phi : v_i \in R^p \rightarrow \phi(v_i) \in F \quad \phi(V) = [\phi(v_1), \phi(v_2), \ldots, \phi(v_N)]^T$$

to model the original data matrix V, where F is a vector feature space of high dimension. The mapping induced kernel matrix K ($K(i, j) = \phi(v_i)^T \phi(v_j), i, j = 1, 2, \ldots N$) is expressed as follows:

$$K(i, j) = \frac{\sum_{k=1}^{p}(v_{i_k} - \bar{v_i})(v_{j_k} - \bar{v_j})}{\sqrt{\sum_{k=1}^{p}(v_{i_k} - \bar{v_i})^2}\sqrt{\sum_{k=1}^{p}(v_{j_k} - \bar{v_j})^2}}, \qquad i, j = 1, 2, \ldots, N$$

where $\bar{v_i} = \sum_{k=1}^{p} v_{ik}/p$.

We propose kernel non-negative matrix factorization (KNMF) to extract the representation H_ϕ of V in reduced dimensions:

$$K_{n\times n} \approx (W_\phi)_{n\times k}(H_\phi)_{k\times n} \tag{10.2}$$

and W_ϕ is the coefficient matrix and H_ϕ is the base matrix.

Therefore, by performing NMF on the kernel matrix K, (Zhang et al. 2006) we can obtain the dimension reduced representation of V, denoted as W. Compared with traditional NMF, KNMF can extract nonlinear and complex features hidden in the original data using kernel induced nonlinear mapping.

In order to guarantee a robust and accurate differentiation on the involved cells described by W, we perform consensus clustering strategy on the embedding matrix W. The factorization of K into $W \times H$ may vary from time to time, (Lee and Seung 1999) hence the consensus strategy is applied by conducting a number of clustering on the generated matrix W to generate a consensus clustering result.

Algorithm 3 Consensus Strategy on KNMF based Clustering

For $i = 1$ to m
Perform KNMF $K = W_i \times H_i$;
Hierarchical clustering on W_i to get output labels L_i;
Generate Similarity matrix S_i from L_i;
End;
Consensus Similarity matrix $S = \frac{1}{m}\sum_{i=1}^{m} S_i$;
Hierarchical clustering on $1 - S$
Output the final clustering L.

10.2.4 DNN for Classification

The clustering result on the representative set V_s will serve as the gold standard for further heterogeneity analysis on the remaining V_r. We introduce feed-forward neural network with unidirectional multi-layer structure, with deep hidden layers for classification of the remaining data V_r.

The network training function is chosen as scaling convergent gradient algorithm (Moller 1993). It adjusts the step size by Levenberg-Marquardt method, by avoiding the line search of each iterative learning. Assume that step size a_k is adjusted each time according to the sign of λ_k, which are given below. The second-order term is calculated as follows:

$$\overline{s_k} = \frac{E'\left(v_k + \sigma_k \overline{\omega_k}\right) - E'\left(v_k\right)}{\sigma_k} + a_k \overline{\omega_k}.$$

The step size is defined as

$$\alpha_k = \frac{\mu_k}{\lambda_k} = \frac{-\overline{\omega_k}^T E'_{qw}\left(\bar{y}_1\right)}{\overline{\omega_k}^T E''(v)\bar{\omega}_k}$$

where $\bar{\omega}_1, \bar{\omega}_2 \ldots \bar{\omega}_n$ are the set of non-zero weight vectors. We have v is the weight vector in space R^n. $E(v)$ is the global error function, which could be the standard least square function or any other appropriate error function. $E'(v)$ is the gradient of error and $E'_{qw}\left(\overline{y_1}\right)$ is the quadratic approximation of error function. Here a_k is updated by

$$\overline{a_k} = 2\left(a_k - \frac{\lambda_k}{|\omega_k|^2}\right).$$

For more details, please refer to Moller (1993).

Cross entropy is chosen as loss function and we use Softmax regression to turn the result of forward propagation of neural network into a probability distribution. Softmax normalizes the outputs of multiple neurons to the (0, 1) interval. The output of Softmax can be regarded as probability distribution, which is often used for multi-label classification. In addition, cross entropy also uses sigmoid function, which can avoid the problem of reducing the learning rate of mean square error loss function when the gradient decreases. In this way, the learning rate can be controlled by the output error. When the error is large, the learning speed is fast. On the contrary, if the error is small, the learning speed becomes slow.

10.3 Results

10.3.1 Datasets

In this chapter, we adopt two real-world single-cell sequencing data sets to test our framework. They are COVID-19 dataset and Zeisel dataset (Zeisel et al. 2015). The COVID-19 dataset contained 8004 cells with 26,924 genes, containing 8 different types of cells. The Zeisel dataset contains 3005 cells from the mouse brain with 19,972 expressed genes, having 9 different types of cells (Table 10.1).

Table 10.1 Basic information of scRNA-seq dataset

Dataset	Size (cells, genes)	Clusters
COVID-19	(8004, 26,924)	8
Zeisel	(3005, 19,972)	9

10.3.2 Methods and Comparisons

In order to fully explore the capability of the framework in single cell heterogeneity analysis, we make method comparisons in three perspectives: clustering on representative data V_s, classification on remaining data V_r and overall clustering on V. Normalized mutual information (NMI) and adjusted Rand index (ARI) are used to evaluate the clustering results.

- NMI (Normalized Mutual Information)
  Suppose the label obtained by clustering algorithm is $A = \{A_1, A_2, A_3, \ldots, A_S\}$. The real label is $B = \{B_1, B_2, B_3, \ldots, B_T\}$. The overlapping part between A and B can be represented by a confusion matrix C with the size of $S \times T$.

$$\mathrm{NMI} = \frac{-2\sum_{i=1}^{S}\sum_{j=1}^{T} C_{i,j}\log\left(\frac{C_{ij}\times N}{C_{i-}\times C_{-j}}\right)}{\sum_{i=1}^{S} C_{i-}\log\left(\frac{C_{i-}}{N}\right) + \sum_{j=1}^{T} C_{-j}\log\left(\frac{C_{-j}}{N}\right)}$$

  where C_{ij} represents the number of cells belonging to cluster i of A and cluster j of B at the same time, N represents the total number of cells, C_{i-} is the number of cells in cluster i in A, C_{j-} is the number of cells in cluster j in B. The value range of NMI is [0, 1]. The better the performance of clustering method, the closer the value of NMI is to 1.
- ARI (Adjusted Rand Index)
  Suppose K represents the result of clustering prediction, and L is the real label of the data. Define rand index as

$$RI = \frac{A + B}{C_n^2}$$

  where n represents the total number of samples, C_n^2 is the number of unordered pairs from n samples, A is the number of unordered sample pairs which are assigned to the same cluster in both K and L, and B is the number of unordered sample pairs which are assigned to different clusters in both K and L. Because for two random partitions, the RI value is not a constant close to 0. Therefore, adjusted Rand index is proposed.

$$ARI = \frac{RI - E(RI)}{\max(RI) - E(RI)}$$

where $E(RI)$ is the expected rand index. The value range of ARI is $[-1, 1]$. The larger the value of ARI means that the clustering results are approximately consistent with the real situation. Moreover, the ARI of random clustering is very close to 0.

10.3.2.1 Comparison of Clustering Methods

Five representative clustering algorithms are introduced for clustering performance comparison, where details about the 5 methods are described below.

- SC3 (Kiselev et al. 2017) is essentially a consistent clustering algorithm. SC3 algorithm uses Euclidean, Pearson and Spearman to calculate the distance matrix of cells after filtering the original data. Then it reduces the dimension through PCA and Laplacian transformation to reduce the impact of noise on clustering. Finally, it calculates the consistency of multiple clustering results and obtains the optimal clustering results.
- bigSCale is a large single-cell data analysis framework. It uses a large sample size to estimate the numerical model of gene expression. This framework includes modules such as differential expression analysis and cell clustering. bigSCale constructed a probabilistic model to group cells with highly similar transcriptome. It standardizes the expression profile and uses hierarchical clustering to divide similar cells into groups. bigSCale defines a p-value to represent the possibility of changes between cells. The p-value was further corrected in the difference analysis. During clustering, bigSCale removes the genes with large changes and high similarity, and then calculates the distance between cells to generate a distance matrix. Finally, it uses hierarchical clustering method to cluster.
- K-means is the most popular and classic clustering algorithm. Its principle is to randomly select k points as the centroid of cluster. Then calculate the distance between the remaining samples and the centroid of each cluster, and assign each remaining sample to the nearest cluster. Finally, we calculate the new centroid of each cluster after classification. Repeat the process of selecting the centroid—calculating the distance and then classifying—selecting the new centroid again until each cluster is no longer changed.
- SIMLR (Wang et al. 2017) can be used for clustering and visualization by combining multiple kernels to learn similarity measures from single cell sequencing data. SIMLR learns the appropriate weights of multiple kernels, which are different measures of distance between cells, and constructs a symmetric similarity matrix according to the following optimization framework.

$$\begin{aligned}
& \min_{S,L,\omega} \sum_{i,j} K(v_i, v_j)S_{ij} + \beta \parallel S \parallel_F^2 \\
& \quad +\gamma tr(L^T(I_N - S)L) + \rho \sum_l \omega_l \log \omega_l \\
\text{s.t.} \quad & K(v_i, v_j) = \sum_l \omega_l K_l(v_i, v_j), \quad \sum_l \omega_l = 1, \quad \omega_l \geq 0 \\
& L^T L = I_C, \quad \sum_j S_{i,j} = 1, \quad S_{i,j} \geq 0, \quad i, j \in 1, 2, \ldots, n
\end{aligned}$$

where S represents the multi-kernel similarity matrix between cells, $K(v_i, v_j)$ is the distance between cell i and cell j. ω_l is the weight of each kernel K_l. The default implementation of SIMLR uses Gaussian kernels with various hyper-parameters. The similarity matrix S is obtained by using the framework, and then the clustering results of sequencing data can be obtained by clustering S.

- Hierarchical clustering is to create a hierarchical nested tree by calculating the similarity of different categories. First, each object is regarded as a cluster. Calculate the minimum distance between each two objects. Then merge the two clusters with the smallest distance into a new cluster. Recalculate the minimum distance between new clusters. Then we merge the two clusters with the minimum distance and calculate the new distance. When all the data are classified into one class or the number of iterations meets the termination conditions, the clustering process is stopped.

The compared clustering results on representative set are shown in Tables 10.2 and 10.3. For COVID-19 data set, 3200 cells are selected by stratified sampling to constitute representative set and used for KNMF-based clustering. The parameter rank r is set when the sum of squares of the first r singular values accounts for 98% of the sum of squares of all singular values, which is 23. The consistency parameters for consensus strategy and kernel non-negative matrix factorization are set to 20 and 10, respectively. The NMI score of KNMF-clustering is 0.87, and the ARI value is 0.82, which is higher than the other four clustering algorithms. SC3 ranks second with NMI value of 0.76 and ARI value of 0.77. The results of these two algorithms are significantly higher than the other three algorithms.

Table 10.2 NMI of clustering representative subsets under different algorithms

	KNMF	SC3	bigSCale	k-means	SIMLR	HC
COVID-19	0.87	0.76	0.49	0.30	0.47	0.68
Zeisel	0.80	0.74	0.69	0.31	0.43	0.6

Table 10.3 ARI of clustering representative subsets under different algorithms

	KNMF	SC3	bigSCale	k-means	SIMLR	HC
COVID-19	0.82	0.77	0.39	0.29	0.46	0.63
Zeisel	0.84	0.79	0.74	0.31	0.43	0.51

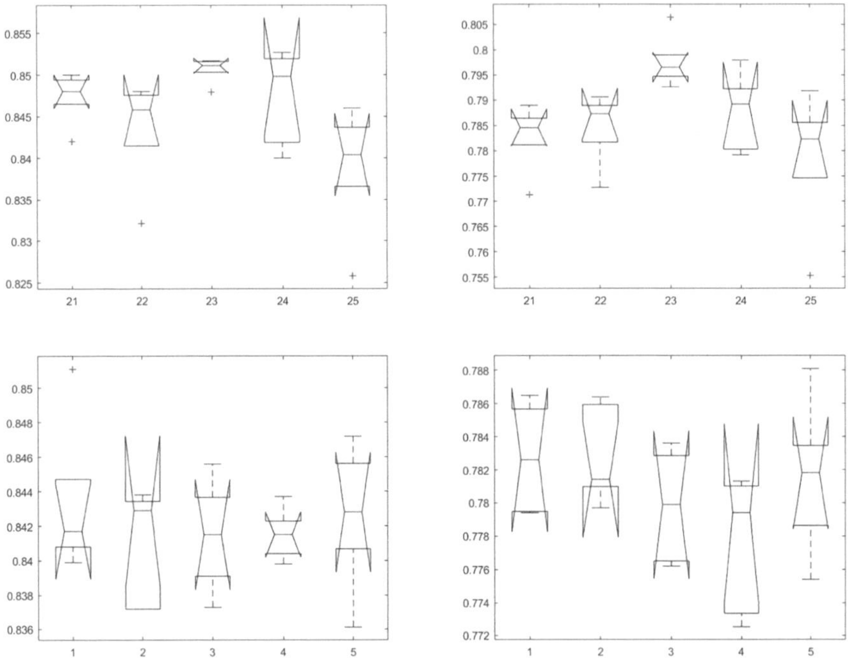

Fig. 10.3 Analysis of variance for r and samples

For the Zeisel dataset, the representative subset consists of 1500 selected cells. The parameter r is set in the same way as stated above, which is 50. The consistency parameter and consensus parameter are set to 20 and 10 as well. The NMI score of KNMF-clustering is 0.80 and the ARI value is 0.84, which is higher than the other four clustering algorithms. SC3 clustering results ranked second, whose NMI value and ARI value are 0.74 and 0.79, respectively. It is obvious that our KNMF-clustering algorithm is superior to other clustering algorithms, which will guarantee a relatively satisfactory training data for further classification purpose.

We consider whether the value of r will affect the clustering results, hence we analyze the performance on the same representative set when r value perturbs. Taking COVID-19 data set as an example, the results are shown in Fig. 10.3. When $\alpha = 0.05$, the p-value of NMI value is 0.0305, and the p-value of ARI is 0.0315, indicating that the choice of r has a statistically significant impact on the results.

In addition, we also consider whether screening different samples has an impact on the results under the optimal proportion. Similarly, taking COVID-19 data set as an example, we selected five representative set samples. Set the parameter r to 23 and analyze the variance of the results. Take $\alpha = 0.05$, the p-value of NMI is 0.0305, and the p-value of ARI is 0.0315. Both are greater than 0.05. We can think that under the optimal proportion, different samples have no significant statistical impact on the results.

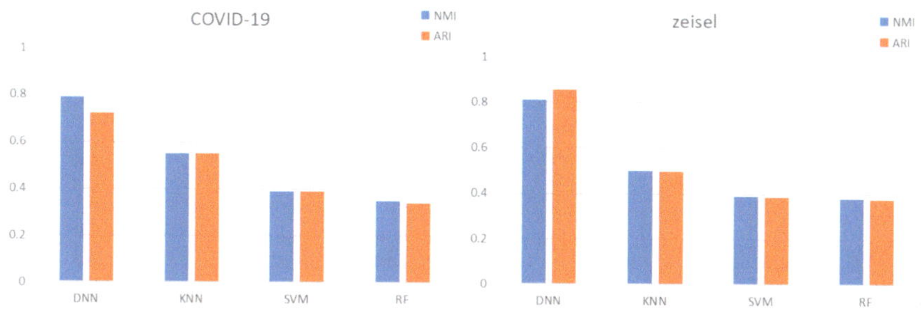

Fig. 10.4 Evaluation of clustering accuracy by ARI and NMI under different classification methods

10.3.2.2 A Comparison of Classification Methods

After clustering on the representative subset, we take the representative subset with clustering result as the training set. The remaining data V_r is used as the test set. The Deep Neural Network (DNN) classification algorithm is trained on V_s and applied on V_r to predict the labels accordingly. Three classification algorithms: k-nearest neighbor classification, support vector machine and random forest are incorporated for comparison.

For different classification methods, the clustering results of our framework are shown in Fig. 10.4. In the COVID-19 dataset, for the four classification methods, we used 3200 cells to predict the labels of the remaining 4804 cells. In deep neural network classification, the number of hidden layer neurons is set to 23. Finally, the NMI and ARI values of the whole framework cluster are 0.79 and 0.72, respectively. For Zeisel dataset, we employed 1500 cells to predict the labels of the remaining 1505 cells. In deep neural network classification, the number of hidden layer neurons is set to 12. The NMI value of the overall clustering result is 0.807 and the ARI value is 0.855. One can clearly see from Fig. 10.3 that the classification results of DNN are more accurate than the compared algorithms. Therefore, it is a very good decision to choose deep neural network to classify the remaining data.

10.3.3 Overall Comparison

Finally, we make full comparison of KNMF-DNN and other representative clustering methods on the whole data set, where SC3 (Kiselev et al. 2017), bigSCale (Iacono et al. 2018), SIMLR (Wang et al. 2017) and hierarchical clustering as the comparison partners. The results are shown in Tables 10.4 and 10.5, and KNMF-DNN shows clear superiority over the compared methods. Both KNMF clustering and SC3 suffer from high computational issue and run out of memory when dealing with COVID-19 dataset. For Zeisel dataset, the NMI and ARI of KNMF clustering and SC3 are

Table 10.4 NMI of clustering results under different clustering algorithms

NMI	KNMF-DNN	KNMF	SC3	bigSCale	SIMLR	HC
COVID-19	0.792	–	–	0.437	0.433	0.346
Zeisel	0.814	0.775	0.761	0.643	0.436	0.482

Table 10.5 ARI of clustering results under different clustering algorithms

ARI	KNMF-DNN	KNMF	SC3	bigSCale	SIMLR	HC
COVID-19	0.724	–	–	0.295	0.432	0.156
Zeisel	0.853	0.820	0.816	0.702	0.433	0.365

similar, ranking the second and third in the considered methods. The performance of bigSCale, SIMLR and hierarchical clustering is not satisfactory.

10.3.4 Comparison of Different Divisions

The number of representative subsets will affect the final result of our framework. We previously speculated that the KL divergence between the filtered sample data distribution and the remaining data distribution can determine the optimal sampling rate. We calculated the KL divergence corresponding to different sampling rates and fit it into a curve. The results are shown in Fig. 10.5.

For COVID-19 dataset, we can find that KL divergence is the smallest when the sampling rate is about 40%. The representative data we selected accounted for 40% of the total data. This means that the final result is better when about 3200 representative subsets are selected. For Zeisel dataset, KL divergence is small when the sampling rate is about 50%. We should select 1500 representative subsets for clustering.

The effectiveness of the above methods needs to be proved by experiments. We ensure that the steps and parameters of the framework remain unchanged, only the division proportion is different. For different representative subsets, the data are clustered by KNMF-DNN method. Finally, the corresponding KNMF-DNN clustering results under different sampling rates are shown in Fig. 10.5. From the figure, we can see that the final clustering is more accurate corresponding to the sampling rate with high KL divergence. This shows that it is feasible for us to use KL divergence to determine the optimal division.

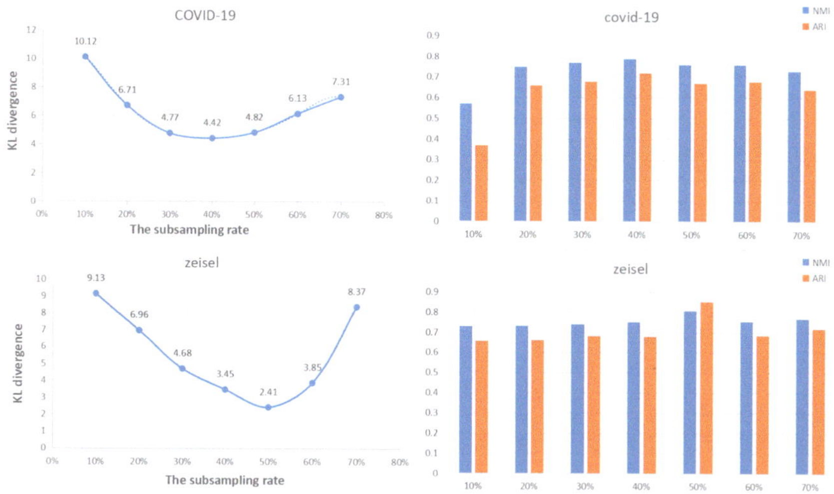

Fig. 10.5 KL divergence value, NMI value and ARI value corresponding to different sampling rates

10.4 Conclusions

In this chapter, we propose a novel framework for single cell sequencing data heterogeneity analysis. We integrate kernel non-negative matrix factorization (KNMF) with deep neural network aiming to ensure accurate heterogeneity analysis as well as computational feasibility. The framework consists of KNMF-clustering on representative set and classification with deep neural network on remaining subset. Optimal representative set selection is realized through KL divergence minimization based on stratifying sampling, and KNMF helps provide a proper evaluation on the nonlinear cellular relationships. Deep neural network for its discrimination ability contributes positively in heterogeneity analysis for the remaining cells. Results show that KNMF-DNN framework demonstrates excellent performance, and has potential in applications for large-scale single cell heterogeneity analysis.

References

Becht E, McInnes L, Healy J et al (2019) Dimensionality reduction for visualizing single-cell data using UMAP. Nat Biotechnol 37:38–44 January

David VD, Roshan S, Juozas N et al (2018) Recovering gene interactions from single-cell data using data diffusion. Cell 174:716–729

Huang M, Wang J, Torre E et al (2018) SAVER: gene expression recovery for single-cell RNA sequencing. Nat Methods 15:539–C542

Iacono G, Mereu E, Guillaumet-Adkins A, Corominas R et al (2018) bigSCale: an analytical framework for big-scale single-cell data. Genome Res 28:878–890

Jiang H, Yi M, Zhang S (2021) A kernel non-negative matrix factorization framework for single cell clustering. Appl Math Model 90:875–888 February

Kiselev V, Kirschner K, Schaub M et al (2017) SC3: consensus clustering of single-cell RNA-seq data. Nat Methods 14:483–486

Lee DD, Seung HS (1999) Learning the parts of objects by non-negative matrix factorization. Nature 401:788–791 October

Moller MF (1993) A scaled conjugate gradient algorithm for fast supervised learning. Neural Netw 6:525–533 January

Ren X, Zheng L, Zhang Z (2019) SSCC: a novel computational framework for rapid and accurate clustering large-scale single cell RNA-seq data. Genom Proteom Bioinform 17:201–210 April

Satija R, Farrell J, Gennert D, Schier A, Regev A (2015) Spatial reconstruction of single-cell gene expression data. Nat Biotechnol 33:495–502

Schreiber J, Bilmes J, Noble WS (2019) apricot: Submodular selection for data summarization in Python. J Mach Learn Res 21

Svensson B et al (2017) Power analysis of single-cell RNA-sequencing experiments. Nat Methods 14:381–387

Tung LH, Kingsford C (2021) Practical selection of representative sets of RNA-seq samples using a hierarchical approach. Bioinformatics 37(Supplement1):I334–I341

Wan S, Kim J, Won KJ (2022) SHARP: hyperfast and accurate processing of single-cell RNA-seq data via ensemble random projection. Genome Res 30:205–213 February

Wang B, Zhu J, Pierson E, Ramazzotti D, Batzoglou S (2017) Visualization and analysis of single-cell RNA-seq data by kernel-based similarity learning. Nat Methods 14:414-C416 April

Wolf FA, Angerer P, Theis FJ (2018) SCANPY: large-scale single-cell gene expression data analysis. Genome Biol 19(1):1–5 February

Zeisel A, Munoz-Manchado AB, Codeluppi S et al (2015) Cell types in the mouse cortex and hippocampus revealed by single-cell RNA-seq. Science 347:1138–1142 March

Zhang D, Zhou Z, Chen S (2006) Non-negative matrix factorization on kernels. In: Pricai 2006: trends in artificial intelligence, vol 4099, pp 404–412

Ziegenhain C et al (2017) Comparative analysis of single-cell RNA sequencing methods. Mol Cell 65:631–643

Chapter 11
Multi-omics Single-Cell Data Integration via High-Order Kernel Spectral Clustering

11.1 Introduction

The first advent of single cell RNA Sequencing (scRNA-seq) technology in 2009 (Tang et al. 2009) has triggered an explosion of research in generating high-resolution views of single-cell RNA-seq data, like Smart-seq (Daniel 2012) and Smart-seq2 (Picelli et al. 2014); efficient and effective Cel-Seq (Hashimshony and Wagner 2012), Cel-Seq2 (Hashimshony 2017); and quasilinear whole genome amplification method MALBAC (Zong and Lu 2012), etc. The exploration of cellular heterogeneity becomes feasible with scRNA-seq where traditional bulk sequencing data cannot reveal. Intratumoral heterogeneity of pancreatic ductal adenocarcinoma was highlighted in Peng (2019). Research in Bautista et al. (2021) provides significant insight on how cellular heterogeneity contributes to the induction of immune tolerance. In Zeng et al. (2022), single cell data was introduced to understand how disease heterogeneity links with therapy response in acute myeloid leukemia. In Sorek et al. (2021), transcriptional heterogeneity was discovered in disease-state neurons. A pan-cancer scRNA-seq dataset was introduced to conduct a systematic characterization of intratumour heterogeneity (Gavish et al. 2023). A comprehensive scRNA-seq analysis of over 895,000 peripheral blood mononuclear cells (PBMCs) was conducted to understand the role of innate immune cells in COVID-19 severity (Edahiro et al. 2023).

Apart from biological investigation in cellular heterogeneity using scRNA-seq techniques, effective and efficient computational methods have been extensively developed for addressing cellular heterogeneity problems. For instance, cell-pair differentiability correlation was proposed in evaluating cellular relationships (Jiang et al. 2018), and further incorporated for cellular heterogeneity analysis. CellVGAE (Buterez et al. 2021), an unsupervised framework with graph attention networks was proposed for scRNA-seq analysis. Semi-supervised clustering method (Chen et al. 2020) was also developed for analyzing scRNA-seq data. When scRNA-seq data is in relatively large scale, efficient hierarchical clustering algorithms (Zou et al. 2021;

H. Jiang and W.-K. Ching, *Kernel Methods for Omics Data Mining*, Intelligent Control and Learning Systems 10, https://doi.org/10.1007/978-981-95-3129-5_11

Jiang et al. 2021) were developed, such as kernel non-negative matrix factorization (Jiang et al. 2021); Also, method focused on similarity learning was proposed in Mei et al. (2021) for cell type identification. Recent progress has shed light on deep learning methods for scRNA-seq data representation and clustering (Yuan et al. 2021; Cheng and Ma 2022; Xiong et al. 2023).

Cell states are useful to understand the organization of tissues and organisms, which are determined by the interplay between transcriptome, proteome and epigenome etc. Multi-omics single-cell sequencing technologies, by parallel profiling multiple types of 'omics' expression in the same individual cells, enable the exploration of cellular heterogeneity in a systematic way. CITE-seq can simultaneously measure RNA expression and surface protein abundance via antibody-derived tags, and robust protein profiling contribute for better understanding of cell states (Stoeckius et al. 2017). scM&T-Seq allows for quantification of transcriptomic and epigenomic expression in the same individual cells (Angermueller 2016). Different 'omics' layers will together present more accurate and complete view of 'single cell state' and enable dissecting regulatory heterogeneity from complex cell populations.

A growing number of methods are in need and they have been proposed for integrating multi-omics data, with the rapid development of single cell multi-omics technologies. A major type of methods were designed for multi-omics data measured in different cells. Representatives include Zhana et al. (2018), a coupled non-negative matrix factorization method for scRNA-seq and scATAC-seq data integration. In Seurat (Stuart and Butler 2019), a statistical dictionary learning method was proposed to integrate scRNA-seq and scATAC-seq data. LIGER (Welch et al. 2019) was developed to align scRNA-seq data and single cell epigenomic data in a low-dimensional embedding space. MATCHER (Welch and Hartemink 2017) utilized latent variable model to evaluate the correlations between scRNA-seq data and single cell epigenomic measurements from different cells.

Data generated by simultaneous profiling of different modalities in the same cell require other types of methods to analyze. scAI (Jin et al. 2020) iteratively learns a low-dimensional representation for the multi-modal single cell data with a regularized matrix factorization framework. In BREM-SC (Wang et al. 2020), a Bayesian random effects mixture model was developed for joint clustering single cell transcriptomic and proteomic data generated by CITE-Seq. In Hao et al. (2021), modal weights in generating the weighted combination of modality affinities are designed to measure the final weighted similarity integrating multiple modalities of single cell data. How to adaptively and automatically determine the weighted combination of modal-specific 'similarities' or 'affinities' thus becomes an interesting topic. Taking into consideration on the inherent relationship between chromatin accessibility and gene expression, Duren et al. (2022) proposed a new concept: cis-regulatory potential to formulate a matrix factorization framework to integrate scRNA-seq data and scATAC-seq data. scAB (Zhang et al. 2022) integrates scRNA-seq data or scATAC-seq data with annotated bulk sequencing data incorporating knowledge and guided graph information. Deep learning frameworks such as GLUE (Cao and Gao 2022), scMCs (Ren et al. 2023) are also developed. The incorporation of knowledge would positively contribute to a better understanding of the cell states and characteristics described by single cell omics data.

However, the generalization ability in other multi-omics integration may be constrained. The development of integration techniques for single cell multi-omics data without knowledge information is in a growing need as well. In this chapter, we focus on integrative analysis of parallel multi-omics single-cell data. Most of the current methods mainly aim to model a common low dimensional embedding or unified relationship between cells. Taking into consideration of the sparsity and nonlinearity nature of single-cell data, also inspired by the above findings, we propose a multi-modal second-order neighborhood Laplacian matrix optimization framework for integrating multi-omics single cell data. The method is very flexible and robust and can be applied for efficiently integrating multi-omics data both in simulation and real-world data sets generated by scM&T-seq, CITE-Seq technologies, etc.

The chapter is structured as follows. In Sect. 11.2, we present preliminary information on the framework for multi-omics data integration. Section 11.3 presents the method scHoML for integrating multi-omics data. Experimental results are presented in Sect. 11.4. Section 11.5 discusses the application capability of scHoML. Finally, Sect. 11.6 concludes the chapter.

11.2 Preliminaries

In this section, we provide preliminary information on the framework for multi-omics data integration.

- **High-Order Networks**
  Assume single modal data set $X = [x_1, x_2, \dots, x_n]^T \in R^{n \times d}$, where n is the number of samples, d is the dimensionality of the attributes. We first present the high-order networks for the data set X modeling the connectivity of the data through definitions of adjacent matrices in different orders $W_i, i = 1, 2 \dots, U$.
  In the construction of the first-order adjacent matrix W_1,

$$w_{1,jk} = \begin{cases} A_{jk}, & \text{if a pair of vertices } (j,k) \text{ is connected} \\ 0, & \text{otherwise} \end{cases} \tag{11.1}$$

  where $A_{jk} = \exp(-\frac{\|x_j - x_k\|^2}{2\sigma^2}), 1 \le j, k \le n$. Here a pair of vertices (j, k) is connected if and only if vertex j is in the nearest neighbours of the vertex k.
  In the construction of high-order adjacent matrix W_i, we follow the similar concept in obtaining W_{i-1}. If $w_{i-1,j}$ is similar to $w_{i-1,k}$, vertex j is also similar to vertex k in a $i-1$th-order connectivity. Let $w_{i,j} = (w_{i,j1}, w_{i,j2}, \dots, w_{i,jn})$ represent the jth row of W_i, high-order adjacent matrix W_i, $i \ge 2$ can be derived in the following formulation.

$$
w_{i,jk} = \begin{cases} \exp\left(-\frac{\|w_{i-1,j}-w_{i-1,k}\|^2}{2\sigma^2}\right), & j \neq k, \text{if } \exists t, \text{ s.t.} \\ & w_{i-1,jt} > 0,\, w_{i-1,kt} > 0 \\ 0, & \text{otherwise} \end{cases} \tag{11.2}
$$

where $w_{i,jj} = 0$, $j = 1, 2, ...n$, making W_i satisfy the form of adjacent matrix.

- **High-Order Laplacian Matrix**
  The corresponding normalized Laplacian matrices in different orders can be derived based on W_i, $i = 1, 2, 3, \ldots$.
  Let $D_i \in \mathbb{R}^{n\times n}$ represent its ith-order degree matrix, a diagonal matrix and $D_{i,jj} = \sum_{k=1}^{n} w_{i,jk}$ The ith-order normalized Laplacian matrix can be defined as

$$
L^{(i)} = I_n - (D_i)^{-\frac{1}{2}} W_i (D_i)^{-\frac{1}{2}}, i = 1, 2, \ldots
$$

- **Multi-modal Laplacian Matrix**
  Suppose we have parallelled profiled single cell multi-omics data in V modals $X^{(1)}, X^{(2)}, \ldots, X^{(V)}$, where $X^{(i)} \in \mathbb{R}^{n\times d^{(i)}}$, $i = 1, 2, \ldots, V$ is the dataset of i-th modal and $d^{(i)}$ represents the attribute dimensionality of i-th modal.
  According to the steps in construction of high-order networks and high-order Laplacian matrix, we define $L_p^{(i)}$, $i = 1, 2, \ldots, U$ to represent the ith order normalized Laplacian matrix for the p-th modal, i.e., $L_p^{(i)} = I_n - (D_p^{(i)})^{-\frac{1}{2}} W_p^{(i)} (D_p^{(i)})^{-\frac{1}{2}}$, $p = 1, 2, \ldots, V$ where $W_p^{(i)} \in \mathbb{R}^{n\times n}$ represent ith-order adjacent matrix for p-th modal single cell data, $D_p^{(i)} \in \mathbb{R}^{n\times n}$ represent ith-order degree matrix for the p-th modal single cell data.
  Hence, in single cell data composed of V modals, we have in total $U \times V$ laplacian matrices for different modals and different orders.
- **Multi-modal Multi-order Laplacian Matrix Fusion**
  In multi-modal single cell data integration, how to integrate the modal-specific laplacian matrices to formulate a fused, appropriate laplacian matrix is a central and critical problem.
  Taking into consideration on the modal-specific laplacian matrices, we first integrate laplacian matrices for specific order i, $i = 1, 2, \ldots, U$ where

$$
\mathscr{L}_\mu^{(i)} = \sum_{p=1}^{V} \mu_p L_p^{(i)}, \sum_{p=1}^{V} \mu_p = 1, \mu_p \geq 0, p = 1, 2, \ldots, V,
$$

  to integrate modal-specific proximity information from multi-modal data.
  Secondly, incorporating high-order connectivity information embedded in the high-order laplacian matrix, we propose the linear combination of $\mathscr{L}_\mu^{(i)}$, $i = 1, 2, \ldots, U$ to formulate the fused Laplacian Matrix for multi-omics single cell data

$$
\mathscr{L}^* = \sum_{i=1}^{U} \lambda_i \mathscr{L}_\mu^{(i)}, \sum_{i=1}^{U} \lambda_i = 1, \lambda_i \geq 0, i = 1, 2, \ldots, U. \tag{11.3}
$$

Intuitively, we aim to approximate the fused Laplacian matrix $\mathscr{L}^*$ as the linear combination of different order Laplacian matrix $\mathscr{L}_\mu^{(i)}, i = 1, 2, \ldots, U$ respectively, to incorporate comprehensive structure information and seek better representation capability of the relationship described by multi-modal data.

11.3 Methods

The graph Laplacian serves as a powerful tool for learning embeddings that preserve the intrinsic geometric structure of the data. These embeddings effectively function as kernels that promote smoothness with respect to the underlying graph connectivity. In this section, we present the method for integrating multi-omics data, to optimize the fused Laplacian matrix (kernel), as well as obtaining the low-dimensional representation for the multi-omics data.

For single modal data, spectral clustering can be realized through solving optimization problem with given laplacian matrix L. In terms of multi-omics single cell data, the proposed Laplacian matrix $\mathscr{L}^*$ approximated by linear combination of different order modal-specific laplacian matrices in the form $\sum_{i=1}^{U} \lambda_i \mathscr{L}_\mu^{(i)}$ has several parameters yet to be determined.

How to automatically determine the parameters embedded in Laplacian matrix $\mathscr{L}^*$ and seek better representation capability of the common embedding for multi-modal data thus constitutes a critical challenge. Motivated by the framework of spectral clustering, we propose the optimization objective as minimization of $\mathrm{tr}(H^T \mathscr{L}^* H)$, while simultaneously seek optimized H as the low-dimensional embedding for the multi-modal data, and the optimization problem can be expressed as follows:

$$
\begin{aligned}
&\min_{\boldsymbol{\lambda}, H, \boldsymbol{\mu}} \mathrm{tr}(H^T \mathscr{L}^* H) + \|\mathscr{L}^* - \sum_{i=1}^{U} \lambda_i \mathscr{L}_\mu^{(i)}\|_F^2 \\
&s.t.\ \mathscr{L}_\mu^{(i)} = \sum_{p=1}^{V} \mu_p L_p^{(i)} (i = 1, 2, \ldots, U), \\
&\mathscr{L}^* \text{ is PSD}, \mathscr{L}_{jk}^* \leq 0, j \neq k \\
&H \in \mathbb{R}^{n \times c}, H^T H = I_c \\
&\boldsymbol{\mu} = [\mu_1, \mu_2, \ldots, \mu_V]^T, \|\boldsymbol{\mu}\|_1 = 1, \boldsymbol{\mu} \geq 0 \\
&\boldsymbol{\lambda} = [\lambda_1, \lambda_2, \ldots, \lambda_U]^T, \|\boldsymbol{\lambda}\|_1 = 1, \boldsymbol{\lambda} \geq 0.
\end{aligned}
\tag{11.4}
$$

11.3.1 Multi-modal Laplacian Matrix Optimization

High-order Laplacian matrix can model the hidden high-order connection information among data, but the value of order needs properly selected as too high order may distort the original relationship embedded in the data set. Hence, we focus on integration of Laplacian matrix in first-order and second-order, to preserve global data structure in a better manner, as well as improving learning performance. However, the positive-semi-definite property of $\mathscr{L}^*$ added in the constraints of the optimization problem makes the optimization problem hard and inefficient to solve. Taking into consideration on the original definition of Laplacian matrix $I_n - D^{-1/2}W_1D^{-1/2}$, and the symmetric property of W_1 that can be decomposed into eigen-matrix form $W_1 = \tilde{U}\Lambda\tilde{U}^T$, the optimization term $\mathscr{L}^*$ can be reformulated with $I_n - W\Lambda W^T$, hence we alternatively propose the final optimization problem in the following

$$\begin{aligned} \min_{\lambda, W, \Lambda, H, \boldsymbol{\mu}} \quad & \mathrm{tr}(H^T(I_n - W\Lambda W^T)H) \\ & + \|I_n - W\Lambda W^T - (\lambda\mathscr{L}_\mu^{(1)} + (1-\lambda)\mathscr{L}_\mu^{(2)})\|_F^2 \\ & s.t.\ \mathscr{L}_\mu^{(i)} = \sum_{p=1}^{V} \mu_p L_p^{(i)} (i = 1, 2), \\ & W, H \in \mathbb{R}^{n\times c}, W^TW = I_c, H^TH = I_c \\ & \boldsymbol{\mu} = [\mu_1, \mu_2, \ldots, \mu_V]^T, \|\boldsymbol{\mu}\|_1 = 1, \boldsymbol{\mu} \geq 0 \\ & 0 \leq \Lambda_{kk} \leq 1, k = 1, 2, \ldots, c, 0 \leq \lambda \leq 1. \end{aligned} \tag{11.5}$$

Here Λ is a diagonal matrix, and $0 \leq \Lambda_{kk} \leq 1$ makes sure the optimization stable.

Optimization Framework: Taking into consideration on the non-convexity of the above problem, we propose alternative optimization framework to solve the problem by updating each variable iteratively. For the convenience of optimization, we rewrite $\|I_n - W\Lambda W^T - (\lambda\mathscr{L}_\mu^{(1)} + (1-\lambda)\mathscr{L}_\mu^{(2)})\|_F^2$ into the following form:

$$\begin{aligned} \mathrm{tr}\Big[& I_n - 2W\Lambda W^T - 2(\lambda\mathscr{L}_\mu^{(1)} + (1-\lambda)\mathscr{L}_\mu^{(2)}) \\ & + 2W\Lambda W^T(\lambda\mathscr{L}_\mu^{(1)} + (1-\lambda)\mathscr{L}_\mu^{(2)}) \\ & + W\Lambda^2W^T + (\lambda\mathscr{L}_\mu^{(1)} + (1-\lambda)\mathscr{L}_\mu^{(2)})^2\Big]. \end{aligned}$$

The optimization process consists of the following five steps.

- **Updating** λ: Fixing W, Λ, H, $\boldsymbol{\mu}$, the update of λ can be realized through solving the optimization problem:

$$\min_{0\le\lambda\le1} \operatorname{tr}\left[(\lambda\mathscr{L}_\mu^{(1)} + (1-\lambda)\mathscr{L}_\mu^{(2)})^2\right] \\ - 2\operatorname{tr}\left[(I_n - W\Lambda W^T)(\lambda\mathscr{L}_\mu^{(1)} + (1-\lambda)\mathscr{L}_\mu^{(2)})\right] \tag{11.6}$$

Define

$$a = \operatorname{tr}\left[(\mathscr{L}_\mu^{(1)})^2 - 2\mathscr{L}_\mu^{(1)}\mathscr{L}_\mu^{(2)} + (\mathscr{L}_\mu^{(2)})^2\right] = \|\mathscr{L}_\mu^{(1)} - \mathscr{L}_\mu^{(2)}\|_F^2 \ge 0.$$
$$b = 2\operatorname{tr}\left[(\mathscr{L}_\mu^{(2)} - I_n + W\Lambda W^T)(\mathscr{L}_\mu^{(1)} - \mathscr{L}_\mu^{(2)})\right].$$

(1) If $a > 0$, we can obtain

$$\lambda = \begin{cases} 0, & \text{if } -\frac{b}{2a} < 0 \\ 1, & \text{if } -\frac{b}{2a} > 1 \\ -\frac{b}{2a}, & \text{otherwise} \end{cases}$$

(2) If $a = 0$, then we can deduce $b = 0$. In this case, We keep λ unchanged. That means if λ_k represent the value of λ in kth iteration, we will let $\lambda_k = \lambda_{k-1}$.

- **Updating $\boldsymbol{W}$**: Given fixed λ, Λ, H, $\boldsymbol{\mu}$, the update of $\boldsymbol{W}$ can be generated through the optimization problem below

$$\min_{W^T W = I_c} \operatorname{tr}(\Lambda W^T B W) \tag{11.7}$$

where $B = \lambda\mathscr{L}_\mu^{(1)} + (1-\lambda)\mathscr{L}_\mu^{(2)} - \frac{1}{2}HH^T$. The solution W of Eq. (11.7) can be calculated as the first c eigenvectors of B (Zhou et al. 2020).

- **Updating $\boldsymbol{\Lambda}$**: Given fixed λ, W, H, $\boldsymbol{\mu}$, we optimize the following problem to update $\boldsymbol{\Lambda}$:

$$\min_{0\le\Lambda_{ii}\le1,\, \Lambda_{ij}=0 (i\ne j)} \operatorname{tr}(\Lambda^2 + 2\Lambda C), \tag{11.8}$$

where

$$C = W^T\left[(\lambda\mathscr{L}_\mu^{(1)} + (1-\lambda)\mathscr{L}_\mu^{(2)}) - \frac{1}{2}HH^T\right]W - I_c$$

We can get:

$$\Lambda_{ii} = \begin{cases} 0, & C_{ii} \ge 0 \\ 1, & C_{ii} \le -1 \\ -C_{ii}, & \text{otherwise} \end{cases}$$

- **Updating $\boldsymbol{H}$**: Fixing λ, W, Λ, $\boldsymbol{\mu}$, the optimization problem with respect to H can be reduced into the following formula

$$\min_{H^T H = I_c} \operatorname{tr}(H^T(I_n - W\Lambda W^T)H) \tag{11.9}$$

Then we can obtain the solution H of Eq. (11.9) by calculating the first c eigenvectors of $I_n - W\Lambda W^T$.

- **Updating $\boldsymbol{\mu}$**: Given fixed λ, W, Λ, H, then we can optimize the problem in the following form:

$$\begin{aligned}\min_{\|\boldsymbol{\mu}\|_1=1,\boldsymbol{\mu}\geq 0} \operatorname{tr}\Big[& -2(\lambda\mathscr{L}_\mu^{(1)} + (1-\lambda)\mathscr{L}_\mu^{(2)}) \\ & + 2W\Lambda W^T(\lambda\mathscr{L}_\mu^{(1)} + (1-\lambda)\mathscr{L}_\mu^{(2)}) \\ & + (\lambda\mathscr{L}_\mu^{(1)} + (1-\lambda)\mathscr{L}_\mu^{(2)})^2\Big]\end{aligned} \tag{11.10}$$

The optimization problem can be rewritten as a standard quadratic programming formulation, which can be effectively solved with MATLAB *quadprog*.

The algorithm below presents the process of optimization for better understanding of scHoML.

Algorithm 4 High-order Laplacian Matrix Optimization for single cell multi-omics data: scHoML

Input: Datasets:$\{X_1, X_2, \ldots, X_V\}$, dimensionality of common embedding c, number of nearest neighbors k.
Output: Low dimensional Embedding $\boldsymbol{H}$
Compute $L_p^{(i)}$ of each modal X_p, $p = 1, 2, \ldots, V; i = 1, 2$.
Initialize λ, $\boldsymbol{W}$, $\boldsymbol{\Lambda}$, $\boldsymbol{\mu}$.
repeat
Update λ by solving optimization problem in Eq. (11.6).
Update $\boldsymbol{W}$ by solving Eq. (11.7).
Update $\boldsymbol{\Lambda}$ by solving Eq. (11.8).
Update $\boldsymbol{H}$ by solving Eq. (11.9).
Update $\boldsymbol{\mu}$ by solving Eq. (11.10).
until converge.

We now discuss the convergence and complexity of the proposed method.

- **Convergence Analysis**
Since Laplacian matrix is a positive semi-definite matrix, we can conclude that the objective function of scHoML takes zero as lower bound. Obtaining its global optimal solution is difficult, because the objective function is non convex. If alternative optimization framework is applied, the objective function value decreases while updating variables. Therefore, the algorithm will eventually converge to a local solution.
- **Complexity**
The computational complexity of scHoML is mainly caused by SVD decomposition when updating W and H, and its corresponding complexity is $O(n^3)$. Meanwhile, the complexity of updating λ and Λ is $O(1)$ and $O(n)$, respectively. Furthermore, to update μ, we need to solve a standard quadratic programming

problem. Let ε be the precision of the result and V be the number of modals, the complexity of solving the quadratic programming problem is $O(\varepsilon^{-1}V)$. If the algorithm has been run for t iterations, the total complexity of our method is $O(t(n^3 + n + \varepsilon^{-1}V))$. If $\varepsilon^{-1} \ll n^2$, the complexity of scHoML can be considered as $O(tn^3)$.

11.3.2 Clustering with Inferred Low-Dimensional Representation

In the optimization of high-order neighborhood Laplace matrix, we simultaneously obtain a common low dimensional embedding $H \in R^{n\times c}$ for the single cell multi-modal data. The cell sub-populations can be identified from the matrix H through appropriate evaluation on the cellular relationships between cells.

Assume $H = [h_1, h_2, \ldots, h_n]^T \in R^{n\times c}$, we model the distance between cell s and cell t $(s, t = 1, 2, \ldots, n)$ as

$$\mathrm{Dis}(s,t) = 1 - \frac{(h_s - \bar{h}_s)(h_t - \bar{h}_t)^T}{\sqrt{(h_s - \bar{h}_s)(h_s - \bar{h}_s)^T}\sqrt{(h_t - \bar{h}_t)(h_t - \bar{h}_t)^T}}$$

where $\bar{h}_s = \frac{1}{c}\sum_{j=1}^{c} x_{sj}$, $s = 1, 2, \ldots n$, and alternatively,

$$\mathrm{Dis}(s,t) = \sum_{k=1}^{c} |h_s(k) - h_t(k)|.$$

Agglomerative hierarchical clustering was performed on the constructed distance matrix to entangle the heterogeneity embedded in the cells.

An appropriate evaluation of the cluster number is critical. We here provide a grain to coarse design of the optimal cluster number. The cluster number is determined through solving the following optimization problems.

If the involved number of samples is small, we strive to evaluate the sample specific silhouette coefficient to measure the clustering matching degree and optimize the mean silhouette coefficient of all samples to determine the best cluster number $c^{\star}_{no}$:

$$c^{\star}_{no} = \mathrm{argmax}_{k\in\mathscr{K}} \sum_{i=1}^{n} (b_k(i) - a_k(i))/\max(a_k(i), b_k(i))$$

where $a_k(i) = \frac{1}{|C_I|-1}\sum_{j\in C_I, i\neq j} d(i,j)$ is the average distance from the i-th point to the other points in the same cluster I as i, and $b_k(i) = \min_{J\neq I}\frac{1}{|C_J|}\sum_{j\in C_J} d(i,j)$ is the minimum average distance from the i-th point to points in a different cluster J, minimized over clusters. For different cluster number $k \in \mathscr{K}$, we run agglomerative hierarchical clustering to generate different clustering results. If most samples have a high silhouette value, the clustering solution is believed appropriate.

If the involved number of samples is relatively large, we propose statistical measures in terms of variance for evaluation of cluster number appropriateness.

$$c_{no}^{\star} = \text{argmax}_{k \in \mathcal{K}} \frac{\text{tr}(\sum_{q=1}^{k} n_q (c_q - c_E)(c_q - c_E)^T)/(k-1)}{\text{tr}(\sum_{q=1}^{k} \sum_{x \in C_q} (x - c_q)(x - c_q)^T))/(n-k)},$$

where C_q is the set of all data in class q, c_q is the central point of class q, c_E is the central point of all data involved, and n_q is the total number of data points in class q. It is reasonable that we evaluate inter class variance and intra class variance to determine the optimal cluster number $c_{no}^{\star}$ when $\frac{\text{tr}(\sum_{q=1}^{k} n_q (c_q - c_E)(c_q - c_E)^T)/(k-1)}{\text{tr}(\sum_{q=1}^{k} \sum_{x \in C_q} (x - c_q)(x - c_q)^T))/(n-k)}$ achieves maximum.

11.4 Experiments

11.4.1 Datasets

We introduce a number of multi-modal single-cell data to test the performance of our proposed method.

- Simulation dataset 1.
  The data set is obtained from Jin et al. (2020), which consists of two simulated modals (paired scRNA-seq and scATAC-seq) at different noise levels. The ground truth data matrices were $X_1 = W_1 H$, $X_2 = W_2 H$, where $W_1 = W_1 + \rho E$, $W_2 = W_2 + \rho E$, E is the Gaussian noise with $\rho = 0.5$.

$$W_1(i, j) = \begin{cases} 1, & 1 \leq i \leq 100, j = 1; \\ 1, & 151 \leq i \leq 300, j = 2; \\ 1, & 501 \leq i \leq 800, j = 3; \\ 0, & \text{otherwise}; \end{cases} \tag{11.11}$$

$$W_2(i, j) = \begin{cases} 1, & 1 \leq i \leq 500, j = 1; \\ 1, & 1001 \leq i \leq 1500, j = 2; \\ 1, & 3001 \leq i \leq 3800, j = 3; \\ 0, & \text{otherwise}; \end{cases} \tag{11.12}$$

$$H(i,j)=\begin{cases}1, & i=1, 1\le j\le 70;\\ 1, & i=2, 71\le j\le 130;\\ 1, & i=3, 131\le j\le 200;\\ 0, & \text{otherwise};\end{cases} \tag{11.13}$$

Dropouts were generated by a Bernoulli distribution on X_1 and X_2 with the probabilities p_{1i}, p_{2j}, which were defined as $p_{1i}=e^{-\lambda_1 x_i^2}$, $p_{2j}=e^{-\lambda_2 y_j^2}$, where x_i is the mean expression level of the i-th cluster of X_1, y_j is the mean expression level of the j-th cluster of X_2. Next, Gaussian noises were added to X_1 and X_2 as $X_1=X_1+\rho_1 E$, $X_2=X_2+\rho_2 E$, where noise parameter ρ_1 in modal 1 varied from 3 to 5 with an increment 0.5, and noise parameter ρ_2 varied from 0.2 to 1 with an increment 0.2. In total, there are 200 simulated cells, the number of attributes in modal 1 and 2 are 5000 and 2000 respectively. The cell type number is 3.

- Simulation dataset 2.

The data set is obtained from Jin et al. (2020), which consists of two simulated modals (paired scRNA-seq and scATAC-seq) where some clusters that were defined from epigenetic profile do not reflect transcriptomic distinctions. The ground truth data matrices were $X_1=W_1H$, $X_2=W_2H$, where $W_1=W_1+\rho E$, $W_2=W_2+\rho E$, E is the gaussian noise with $\rho=0.5$, $x_j(n)=(j-1)(n-coph)$ (Jin et al. 2020).

$$W_1(i,j)=\begin{cases}1, & 1+x_j(200)\le i\le 200+x_j(200);\\ 0, & \text{otherwise};\end{cases} \tag{11.14}$$

$$W_2(i,j)=\begin{cases}1, & 1+x_j(500)\le i\le 500+x_j(500);\\ 0, & \text{otherwise};\end{cases} \tag{11.15}$$

The rank of W_1 was set to be 3 and the rank of W_2 (denoted as K_2) varied from 3 to 7.

$$H(i,j)=\begin{cases}1, & 1+x_j(c)\le i\le x_j(c), j\le K_2-1\\ 1, & \text{or}\ \ 1+x_j(c)\le i\le n, j=K_2;\\ 0, & \text{otherwise};\end{cases} \tag{11.16}$$

Similar to the procedures mentioned above, dropouts on both X_1 and X_2 were generated with $\lambda_1=0.05$, $\lambda_2=0.025$ and added Gaussian noise with $\rho_1=2$, $\rho_2=1$. In addition, if the values in X_2 with dropouts were greater than 0.7, we set the values to be 1, otherwise 0. In total, there are 500 simulated cells with 4 different cell types, the number of attributes in modal 1 and 2 are 5000 and 2000 respectively.

- mESC data.

The dataset was obtained from 77 mouse embryonic stem cells (mESCs), including 13 cells cultured in "2i" media and 64 serum-grown cells, which were profiled by parallel single-cell methylation and transcriptome sequencing technique scM&T-seq (Angermueller 2016).

- pbmc_inhouse data.
  It is a CITE-seq dataset extracted from a healthy donor under IRB approval from the University of Pittsburgh (Wang et al. 2020). We follow the instructions of cell type identification using well defined markers, and removed those cells with uncertain cell types. In the data set, there are 1242 cells in total, containing 5 different cell types.
- pbmc_10X data.
  The multi-modal single cell data (CITE-Seq dataset) was downloaded from 10X Genomics website. A total of 7865 human peripheral blood mononuclear cells (PBMCs) with 14 surface protein markers are included in the dataset in addition to matched scRNA-Seq data. Cells with uncertain cell types were removed. In total, there are 6661 cells involved, containing 7 different cell types: B cells, CD14+ monocytes, CD16+ monocytes,CD4+ T cells, CD8+ T cells, Dendritic cells, and NK cells.

11.4.2 Methods for Comparison

We compare our proposed method scMoHL with the method scAI (Jin et al. 2020), for deconvoluting cellular heterogeneity from parallel transcriptomic and epigenomic profiles. Apart from that, we introduce a number of methods for dealing with multi-modal data for comparison. The methods for comparison are listed as follows

- SCbest: A single-view spectral clustering applied for all the views with the best clustering for output.
- MSE (Xia et al. 2010): A multi-view spectral embedding method. We set the parameter r in the range of $[2, 3, \ldots, 10]$ and report the best result.
- CoregSC (Kumar and Daumé 2011): A multi-view spectral clustering method based on co-training strategy. We set the parameter $\lambda = 0.01$ for clustering.
- AASC (Huang et al. 2012): A multi-view spectral clustering method for optimizing linear combination of affinity matrices.
- RMSC (Xia et al. 2014): A multi-view spectral clustering combined with Markov chain. The parameter λ is set as 0.005 for clustering.
- AMGL (Nie et al. 2016): A auto-weighted multiple graph learning method for multiple views.
- AWP (Nie et al. 2018): A multi-view spectral clustering based on spectral rotation technique.
- scAI (Jin et al. 2020): A regularized matrix-factorization framework for single-cell multi-omics data integration.
- OPMC (Liu et al. 2021): A multi-view matrix factorization clustering.

11.4.3 Computational Results

For performance evaluation, we introduced two popular measures: Adjusted Rand Index (ARI) and Normalized Mutual Information (NMI) for comparing the clustering accuracy. Table 11.1 reports the ARI measures for the compared methods applying in the considered datasets. Table 11.2 reports the NMI measures for the compared methods applying in the considered datasets. In the construction of scMoHL, there are two parameters involved: the scale parameter σ and the parameter k in KNN graph. We set the scale parameter σ as the sample standard deviation of dataset, and the parameter k required by the KNN matrix is set to 10 for small datasets and 100 when sample size is relatively large. Modal-specific laplacian matrices are computed on the preprocessed data-sets through standard normalization and dimension reduction with principal component analysis. As for the multi-modal integration methods, SCbest, MSE, CoregSC, AASC, RMSC, AMGL, k-means clustering methods are applied on the integrated embedding matrix obtained by these methods, hence we report the averaged ARI and NMI values running 20 times for performance comparison. And the averaged ARI and NMI values with standard deviations are reported. AWP can

Table 11.1 Performance comparisons of different methods in terms of ARI

Algorithm/dataset	Simulation data1	Simulation data2	mESC	pbmc_10X	pbmc_inhouse
SCbest	0.2426 ± 0.0233	0.2323 ± 0.0072	0.3764 ± 0.0000	0.7214 ± 0.0411	0.6679 ± 0.0742
MSE	0.2709 ± 0.0050	0.0111 ± 0.0059	0.3764 ± 0.0000	0.7161 ± 0.0133	0.6807 ± 0.0502
CoregSC	0.2529 ± 0.0080	0.1368 ± 0.0280	0.1716 ± 0.0628	0.7162 ± 0.0164	0.5152 ± 0.1351
AASC	0.1755 ± 0.0044	0.0063 ± 0.0089	0.7022 ± 0.0235	0.6805 ± 0.0799	0.6027 ± 0.0290
RMSC	0.0423 ± 0.0094	0.0745 ± 0.0050	0.3468 ± 0.0000	0.5724 ± 0.0001	0.5212 ± 0.0266
AMGL	0.1424 ± 0.0892	-0.0246 ± 0.0123	0.4869 ± 0.4691	0.6332 ± 0.1047	0.7275 ± 0.1452
AWP	0.3338 ± 0.0000	0.1154 ± 0.0000	0.2416 ± 0.0000	0.7230 ± 0.0000	0.5693 ± 0.0000
OPMC	0.0241 ± 0.0463	0.6927 ± 0.3311	0.2269 ± 0.2012	0.6133 ± 0.0648	0.8778 ± 0.1095
scAI-hc	0.9391 ± 0.0000	0.6587 ± 0.0000	0.5480 ± 0.0000	0.5131 ± 0.0000	0.7875 ± 0.0000
scAI-leiden	0.9539 ± 0.0000	0.8042 ± 0.0000	0 ± 0.0000	0.0738 ± 0.0000	0.3317 ± 0.0000
scHoML	0.9854 ± 0.0000	1 ± 0.0000	0.9350 ± 0.0000	0.8737 ± 0.0000	0.9523 ± 0.0000

Table 11.2 Performance comparisons of different methods in terms of NMI

Algorithm/dataset	Simulation data1	Simulation data2	mESC	pbmc_10X	pbmc_inhouse
SCbest	0.2630 ± 0.0149	0.2572 ± 0.0047	0.3894 ± 0.0000	0.8144 ± 0.0070	0.8456 ± 0.0470
MSE	0.3196 ± 0.0098	0.0404 ± 0.0108	0.3894 ± 0.0000	0.8149 ± 0.0004	0.8536 ± 0.0325
CoregSC	0.2796 ± 0.0026	0.1650 ± 0.0295	0.2742 ± 0.0341	0.8125 ± 0.0057	0.6456 ± 0.1145
AASC	0.2456 ± 0.0027	0.0592 ± 0.0120	0.6198 ± 0.0200	0.7374 ± 0.0398	0.6877 ± 0.0195
RMSC	0.1130 ± 0.0295	0.0688 ± 0.0027	0.3719 ± 0.0000	0.6705 ± 0.0000	0.6179 ± 0.0186
AMGL	0.2313 ± 0.0787	0.1140 ± 0.0231	0.5166 ± 0.4328	0.7106 ± 0.0574	0.8615 ± 0.0701
AWP	0.3704 ± 0.0000	0.1703 ± 0.0000	0.3122 ± 0.0000	0.8078 ± 0.0000	0.7225 ± 0.0000
OPMC	0.0329 ± 0.0450	0.7343 ± 0.3040	0.2372 ± 0.1989	0.6939 ± 0.0149	0.8815 ± 0.0298
scAI-hc	0.9112 ± 0.0000	0.7892 ± 0.0000	0.5003 ± 0.0000	0.6232 ± 0.0000	0.7906 ± 0.0000
scAI-leiden	0.9348 ± 0.0000	0.8080 ± 0.0000	0.3233 ± 0.0000	0.5128 ± 0.0000	0.7170 ± 0.0000
scHoML	0.9764 ± 0.0000	1 ± 0.0000	0.8729 ± 0.0000	0.8374 ± 0.0000	0.9470 ± 0.0000

ensure a stable clustering result, hence the standard deviation is 0. In scAI method, a low-dimensional representation matrix H for the multi-omics single cell data was obtained through regularized matrix factorization framework. The heterogeneity of cells is then identified by clustering through the low-dimensional representation matrix H using the Leiden community detection method, with default resolution parameter setting of 1. The resolution parameter has a great effect on the cluster number evaluation for the data set. When we set the default resolution parameter 1 in experiments, most clustering results turned to be single cluster instead, distorting the original heterogeneity in data sets. Hence we use resolution parameter 0.1 in leiden algorithm(scAI-leiden) on the best H chosen (scAI is applied to each dataset 10 times with different seeds) in the comparisons. Besides, we also introduce consensus hierarchical clustering method on the matrix H obtained by scAI(scAI-hc). Regarding the cluster number, if the cluster number is a parameter as input including scAI-hc, we use the true cluster number for comparison. In simulation_data1, the true cluster number is 3, and the estimated cluster number by leiden algorithm ans scHoML are both 3. For simulation_data2 where the true cluster number is 4, the estimated cluster number by scHoML is 4. But for leiden algorithm, the estimated cluster number is 5. mESC data set has 2 different cell states, but in leiden algorithm, the estimated cluster number is equal to the number of cells in the data set, namely, 77. scHoML can accurately estimate the cluster number. For pbmc_inhouse and pbmc_10X data, where the true cluster numbers are 5 and 7, respectively, scAI-leiden estimated the cluster number to be 13 and 77 instead. Overall, scAI-leiden tends to overestimate the heterogeneous groups inside datasets.

11.4.3.1 Overall Performance Comparison

Aside from scMoHL, all the compared algorithms demonstrate specific patterns, with no dominant methods.

scAI demonstrates obvious superiority compared to SCbest, MSE, CoregSC, AASC, RMSC, AMGL, AWP, OPMC for simulated data sets. But the performance of scAI is not satisfactory when applied in mESC and pbmc data sets. SCbest as a single view clustering method performs in a unstable way, where the ARI values obtained for the two simulated datasets and mESC dataset are unsatisfactory, revealing the complex structure of multi-modals in the respected data sets. But it is interesting to see that on pbmc data, SCbest outperforms most of the compared methods including scAI, indicating that in this data set there exists some modal showing a clear relationship among data. MSE as a multi-modal integration method performs similarly as SCbest. In particular for simulation data2 when the single view clustering result showing 0.2323 in ARI value on average, MSE cannot learn a better integration of modals, getting only 0.0111 in averaged ARI value. For AASC, the clustering result on mESC data is the best excluding scHoML, showing 0.7022 in averaged ARI value. The performance of RMSC and AMGL resembled with each other on simulated data sets. When applied on real-world datasets, RMSC and AGML cannot compete with scAI in ARI values on mESC data. RMSC and AGML show better performance than scAI in ARI values and NMI values on pbmc data. For AWP algorithm, the best clustering performance is achieved on pbmc_10X data set, 0.7230 in ARI value. OPMC algorithm shows the best clustering performance in pbmc_inhouse data, while has poor discrimination power in other data sets.

When we compare single view clustering based algorithm (SCbest) with the other multi-modal clustering methods, some conclusions can be made as follows. Firstly, different modal may reveal the data in different perspectives, there are cases when some particular modal shows a clear relationship among data. Secondly, integration methods may not fully integrate the proper information embedded in modals, showing unsatisfactory result compared to single-view based clustering method. Taking CoregSC for example, the results in mESC data, pmbc_inhouse and pbmc_10X data are inferior to that of SCbest. Thirdly, appropriate evaluation of the data relationship is of critical significance for entangling the heterogeneity described by multi-modals. Among all the compared methods, scHoML as a graph based embedding method provides a better description on the relationship between cells, showing that the incorporation of high-order correlation contributes in a positive manner for relationship description.

11.4.3.2 Comparison with scAI: Aggregation and Integration Method for Parallel Single Cell Multi-omics Data

scAI demonstrates explicit superiority compared to other traditional multi-view data clustering methods for simulation data sets. For simulation data sets, scAI ranks the second best, slightly inferior to scHoML. In real-world datasets such as mESC data, scAI with consensus hierarchical clustering method ranks the third in clustering accuracy in terms of ARI and NMI values. It is interesting to see that in pbmc-inhouse data and pbmc-10X data, scAI is not satisfactory. The computational efficiency is also restricted in scAI when the data sets contain large population of cells. When we compare different clustering methods in conjunction with scAI, we have the following findings. scAI with consensus hierarchical clustering (scAI-hc) outperforms scAI with leiden clustering (scAI-leiden) in cellular population heterogeneity analysis in a overall manner. For simulation data sets, scAI-leiden perform in a similar way with scAI-hc. While for real-world datasets, scAI-leiden perform in a unsatisfactory way. One possible explanation may be that the resolution parameter play an important role in the performance of scAI-leiden method, especially in tuning the number of clusters to be detected. In the experiments with resolution parameter 0.1, the tuned number of clusters is more reasonable compared to default resolution parameter 1 for many data sets. Hence we used resolution parameter 0.1 for performance illustration. Secondly, we further checked the influence of resolution parameter on the clustering performance for datasets as shown in Table 3 in supplementary file. We found that default resolution parameter 1 would be appropriate in traditional cases, but may also fail in many new cases. In our experiments with the considered datasets, they all perform unsatisfactory results. Besides, different datasets have different optimal resolution parameters. The estimation and determination of optimal resolution parameter would become an interesting problem.

In the comparison, scHoML shows the best performance for integration in both simulation data sets and real world single cell multi-omics data when the performance is evaluated in ARI and NMI measures. As a nonlinear relationship modeling framework, scHoML used Laplacian matrix to model the relationship in multi-modal single cell data. In particular, the incorporation of high-order neighborhood Laplacian matrix in optimization contribute to a better description of the geometric structure of the complex multi-modal data. Besides, scHoML can robustly represent the noisy, sparse multi-omics data in a unified low-dimensional embedding space. The cluster number determination strategy with sample specific silhouette coefficient for small sample problems as well as variance based statistical measure offers a flexible way for accurately estimating the intrinsic clusters in the data. However, the computational complexity would become an unavoidable issue if the involved number of cells is large, because the time complexity is proportional to the number of cells n, which is $O(n^3)$.

11.4.3.3 Common Embedding Performance Evaluation

All the compared methods attempt to find a common low-dimensional embedding for the single-cell multi-omics data, hence we compared 2D visualization of aggregated low-dimensional embeddings by different methods to evaluate the embedding capabilities of the considered methods. All the figures are attached in supplementary files.

Figures 11.1, 11.2, 11.3, 11.4 and 11.5 show the visualization of aggregated low-dimensional embeddings by different methods using tSNE. Different color represents different true clusters in the data set. Figures 11.1 and 11.2 refer to the tSNE plots for simulation data sets with considered methods. Traditional multi-view clustering methods SCbest, MSE, CoregSC, AASC, RMSC, AMGL, AWP, OPMC failed to decipher the heterogeneity in the cells, where the cell sub-populations were indistinguishable in the recovered low-dimensional space by those methods. However, scAI can obtain a proper low-dimensional embedding matrix H showing appropriate relationship in the cells, where the cells are almost distinguishable. scHoML demonstrates clear superiority in getting common embedding information for the two simulation datasets, and the cell sub-populations were clearly distinguishable in the low-dimensional space when using the aggregated data.

Figure 11.3 shows tSNE plot of different methods in obtaining low-dimensional embeddings for mESC data. AASC and AMGL perform similarly, and the cells tend to show distinguishable properties. scHoML clearly help recover a satisfactory low-dimensional embedding for mESC data generated by parallel single-cell methylation and transcriptome sequencing technique scM&T-seq. Other methods including scAI cannot guarantee a proper embedding for mESC data, where different types of cells tend to mix with each other.

As shown in Fig. 11.4, for pbmc_inhouse data, AMGL, SCbest and MSE perform quite similarly and the tSNE plots for the three methods share similar pattern formations, where most of the cells are distinguishable. scHoML undoubtedly demonstrates superiority compared to the remaining 9 methods in aggregated low-dimensional representation for the 1242 pbmc cells profiled by CITE-seq.

Figure 11.5 corresponds to the aggregated low-dimensional embedding for PBMC_10X data, where the multi-modal single cell data (CITE-Seq dataset) was downloaded from 10X Genomics website containing 6661 human peripheral blood mononuclear cells (PBMCs) cells. When the number of cells increase, the data become more complicated and the cells are more heterogeneous. Methods include OPMC and RMSC, AWP tend to mix the cells. Apart from scHoML, CoregSC shows the best aggregation performance where the same type of cells are more compactly scattered though for some particular type the cells are diversely scattered.

Take a further look at the intrinsic complexity of the multi-omics data, we analyze the tSNE plots for original data in all considered modals. Due to the inherent sparsity and noise in the data, the cells were not well separated in the scRNA-seq data and the scATAC-seq data using t-SNE, for simulation datasets as shown in sub-figures a and b for simulation data1 and c, d for simulation data2 in Fig. 11.6. Also, for mESC data, the cell populations are mixed, as shown in sub-figures e and f. However, the

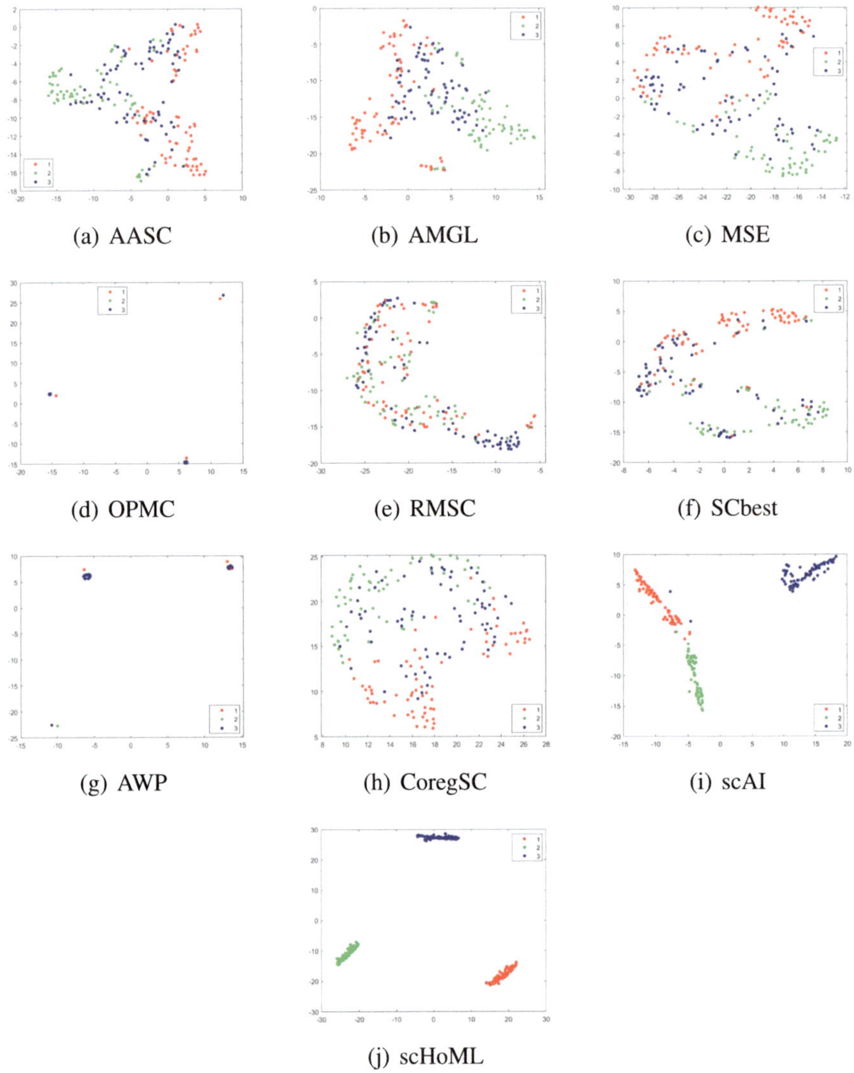

Fig. 11.1 tsne plots of different methods in obtaining low-dimensional embeddings for simulation data1

aggregated low dimensional data generated by scHoML help capture heterogeneity between different types of cells, as shown in subfig j in Figs. 11.1, 11.2 and 11.3. For pbmc_inhouse data, the modal described by ADT features can clearly differentiate cell types, while the modal described by RNA is quite noisy and makes the data analysis complicated. It is interesting to see that for scAI and many of the traditional multi-view data integration methods MSE, AASC, RMSC and OPMC, the aggregated matrix H obtained by those methods failed to give play to the descriptive advantages

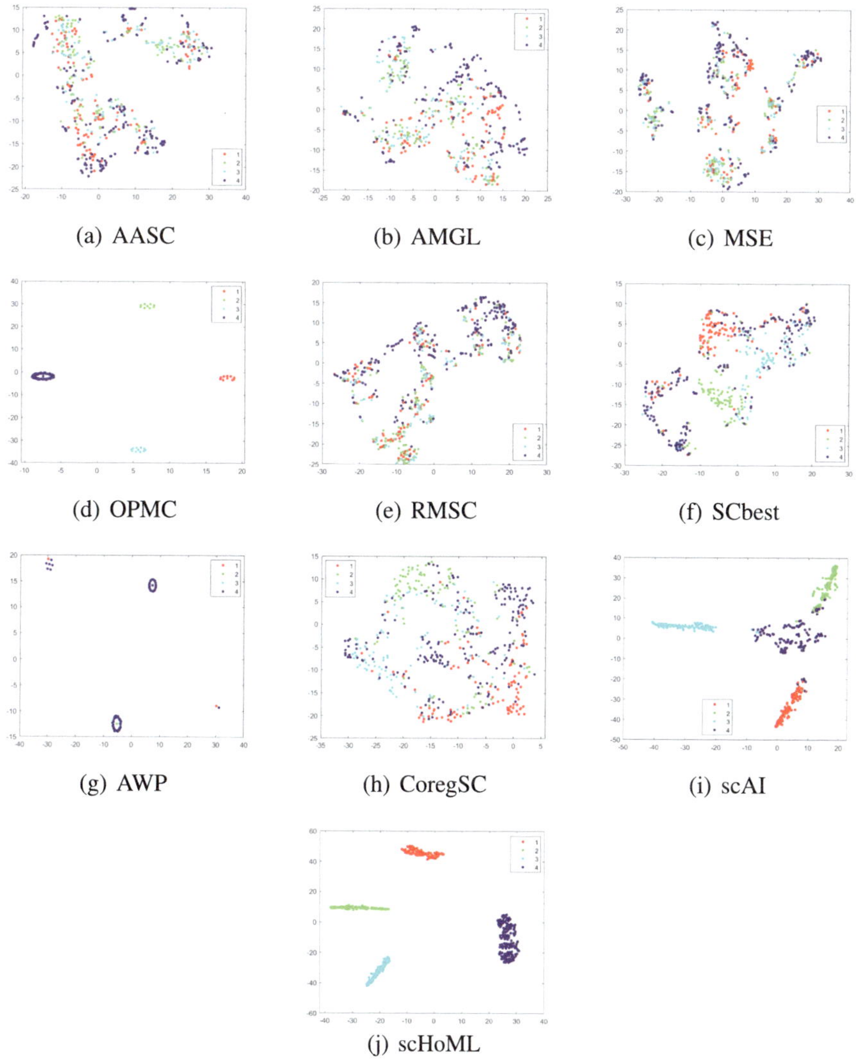

(a) AASC (b) AMGL (c) MSE (d) OPMC (e) RMSC (f) SCbest (g) AWP (h) CoregSC (i) scAI (j) scHoML

Fig. 11.2 tsne plots of different methods in obtaining low-dimensional embeddings for simulation data2

of ADT features, but quite influenced by the noisy RNA data. scHoML tends to obtain the satisfactory common embedding for pbmc_inhouse data. Similar results can be discovered by pbmc_10X data.

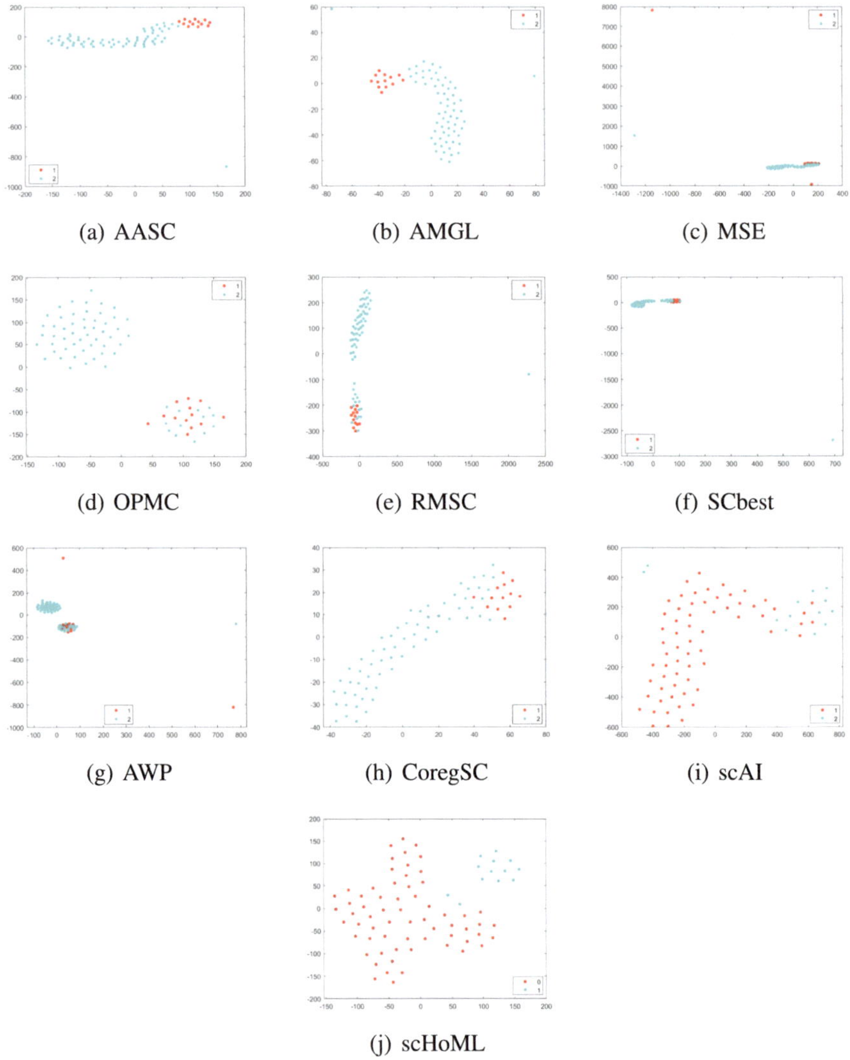

(a) AASC (b) AMGL (c) MSE (d) OPMC (e) RMSC (f) SCbest (g) AWP (h) CoregSC (i) scAI (j) scHoML

Fig. 11.3 tsne plots of different methods in obtaining low-dimensional embeddings for mESC data

11.5 Discussions

From the computational results, we can confirm the robustness and effectiveness of scHoML in dealing with single cell multi-omics data under different signal-to-noise ratio scenarios. In the following, we discuss the feasibility and effectiveness of multi-modal and high-order Laplacian matrix optimization in scHoML. While only considering one mode of single cell data, we have the following observations. Dif-

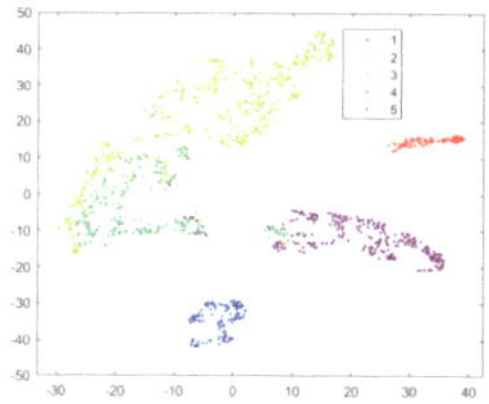

(a) AASC

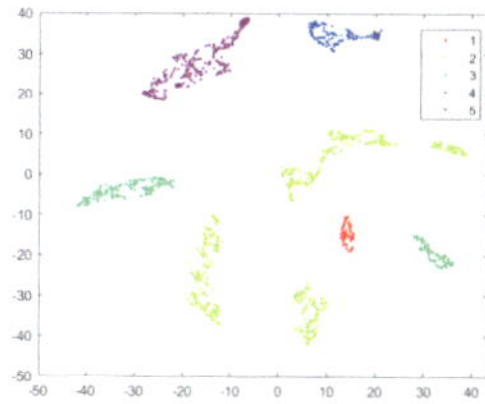

(b) AMGL

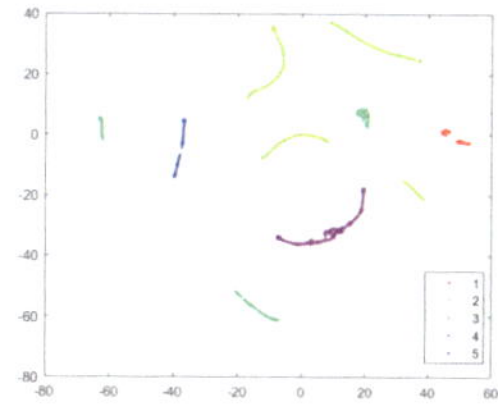

(c) MSE

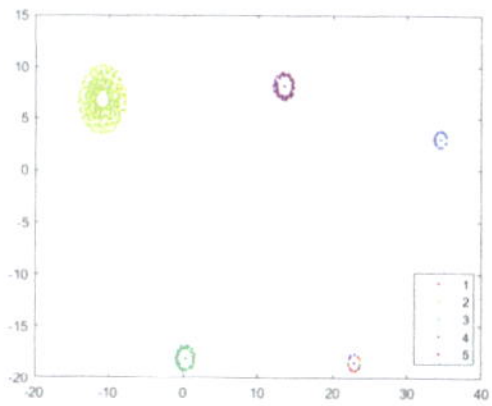

(d) OPMC

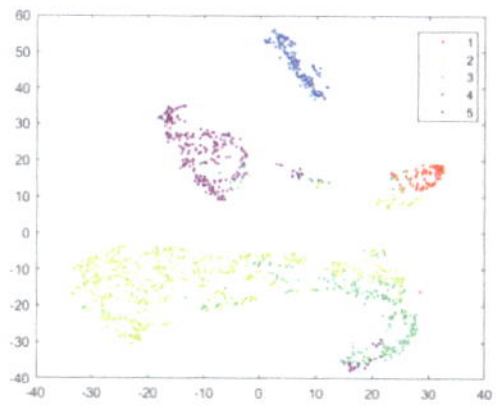

(e) RMSC

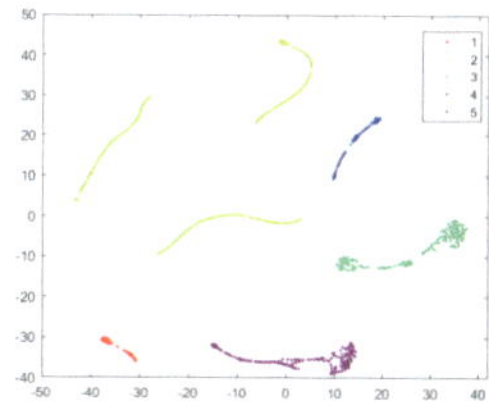

(f) SCbest

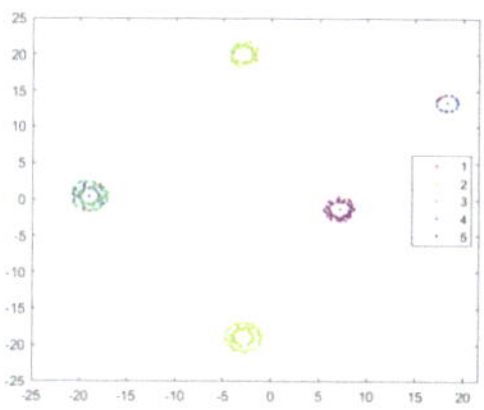

(g) AWP

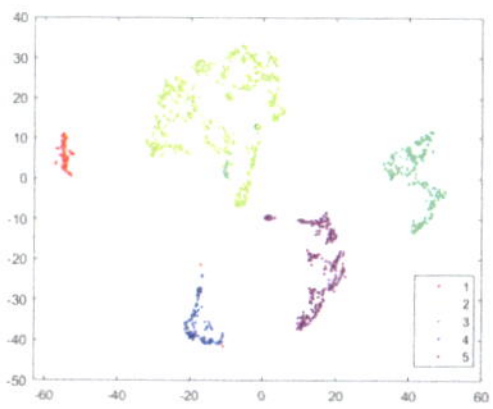

(h) CoregSC

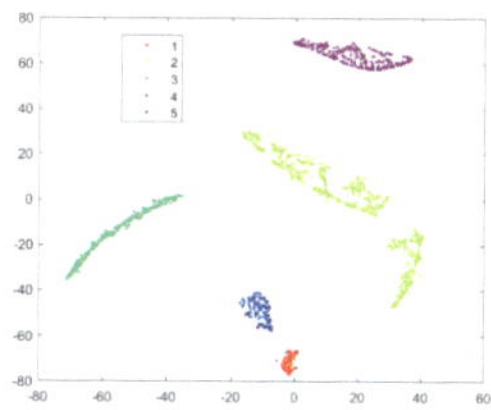

(i) scAI

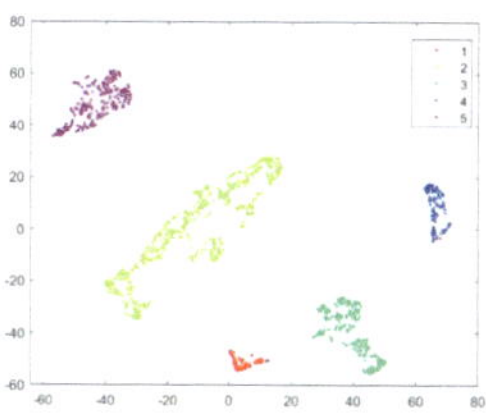

(j) scHoML

Fig. 11.4 tsne plots of different methods in obtaining low-dimensional embeddings for pbmc_inhouse data

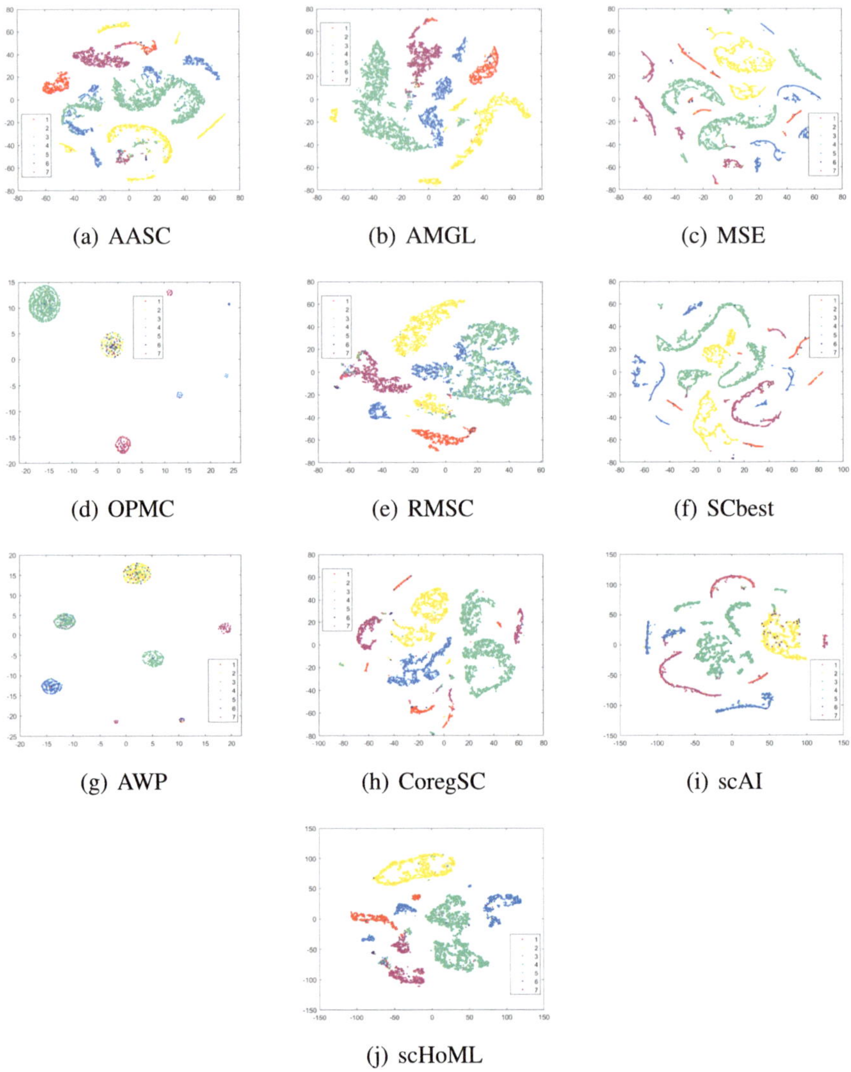

Fig. 11.5 tsne plots of different methods in obtaining low-dimensional embeddings for pbmc_10X data

ferent data sets demonstrate different characteristics. For simulation data1 (subfigs a, b), simulation data2 (subfigs c, d) and mESC data (subfigs e, f) as shown in Fig. 11.6, both modals are noisy. scHoML, however, can overcome the influence of noise effect, robustly integrate the noisy modals to generate a clear common embedding in low dimensions as shown in Figs. 11.1, 11.2 and 11.3j. Slightly inferior to scHoML, scAI can similarly recover the geometric distribution of cells after data integration, shown in Figs. 11.1, 11.2 and 11.3i. The multi-view clustering based algorithms

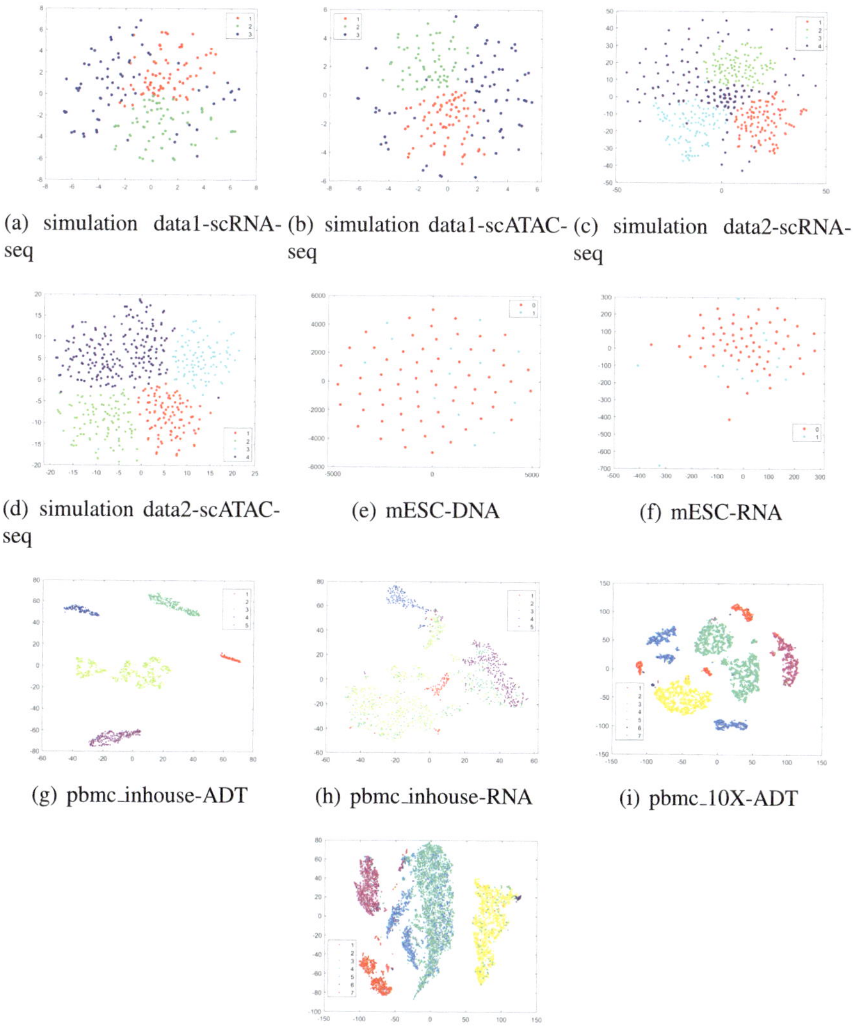

(a) simulation data1-scRNA-seq (b) simulation data1-scATAC-seq (c) simulation data2-scRNA-seq

(d) simulation data2-scATAC-seq (e) mESC-DNA (f) mESC-RNA

(g) pbmc_inhouse-ADT (h) pbmc_inhouse-RNA (i) pbmc_10X-ADT

(j) pbmc_10X-RNA

Fig. 11.6 tsne plots for original multi-omics data

seem to be considerably influenced by the noisy data, and the performance of integration sometimes cannot compete with single-mode clustering method SCbest. For pbmc_inhouse data or pbmc_10X data, the ADT modal is relatively clear for cell type differentiation on tSNE showings in Fig. 11.6g, i. It is shown in Figs. 11.4 and 11.5 that multi-view clustering based algorithms such as AWP, CoregSC can learn the clear relationship revealed by the ADT modal, demonstrating a relatively acceptable performance. However, scAI seems to be influenced by the clustering algorithm, in particular for leiden algorithm. When the resolution parameter differs, the performance fluctuates with large variance. scHoML among all the compared partners shows the stable and robust performance. We conclude that when modals are noisy, scHoML can dig inside the intrinsic geometric relationship and learn a clear common embedding; when multi-modal data contains clear modal information, scHoML has the ability of not being influenced by noisy modals. When only considering the first order laplacian matrix optimization, we can check the performance of MSE whose optimization objective is $\text{argmin}_{H,a} \sum_{p=1}^{V} a_p^r \text{tr}(H^T L_p H)$. From the tSNE plots in Figs. 11.1, 11.2, 11.3, 11.4 and 11.5 as well as Tables 11.1 and 11.2, we came to know that when all the involved modals are noisy, MSE did not have the ability to extract the intrinsic relationship of cells accurately. However, when incorporating high-order Laplacian information, we model the hidden high-order connection information among data in scHoML, and the learned low dimensional data provides a better representation of the original noisy modals.

Besides, we compared scHoML to a robust single cell muti-omics integration method UnionCom (Cao et al. 2020) in terms of embedding capability. In UnionCom, a reference modal within the data set should be given in advance for further processing. We therefore have included all the cases when each modal is regarded as reference modal in the comparison. It can be shown in Figs. 11.7 and 11.8 that the projected low dimensional modals cannot compete with scHoML in tsne showing. When all the modals are noisy, the common low dimensional space learned by UnionCom is also noisy. However, if some modal shows high data quality in the multi-omics data, UnionCom can guarantee a relative clear representation of the multi-omics data.

- **Heterogeneity Analysis**
  We further hope to dissect the heterogeneity analysis results provided by scHoML. It is interesting to see that, for pbmc_10X data, the original data contains 1112 CD8+ Tcells as a single cluster. However, scHoML divides the 1112 cells into 2 major clusters, with one cluster containing 766 cells, the other cluster containing 322 cells. We hence conduct statistical analysis to compare the differences between the 2 sub-clusters. In the ADT based data, we did one-sided two-sample Kolmogorov-Smirnov goodness-of-fit hypothesis test on the two populations generated by scHoML, and select the representative markers which rejects the null hypothesis that $F1(x) = F2(x)$ as the corresponding true (but unknown) population CDFs at the 5% significance level. The representative markers in subcluster 1 (766 cells) include 'TIGIT', 'CD3+', 'CD4+' and 'CD8+', which are reported marker genes for annotating exhausted CD8+ Tcells (Deng et al. 2021). A further analysis on the representative genes for cluster one through one-sided two-sample Kolmogorov-Smirnov goodness-of-fit hypothesis test leads to a filtration of top ranked genes 'CCL5', 'HLA-DRB1', 'GZMH', 'HLA-DPA1' and 'NKG7'. It is well established (Ren and Wang 2021) that for CD8+ T cells, the major pTRTs were exhausted T cells and exhibited high heterogeneity. And in our data set, we successfully identify the subcluster that is consistent with cluster C7 harboring a low frequency of terminal Tex cells and high frequency of 'CD8+ZNF683+CXCR6+'

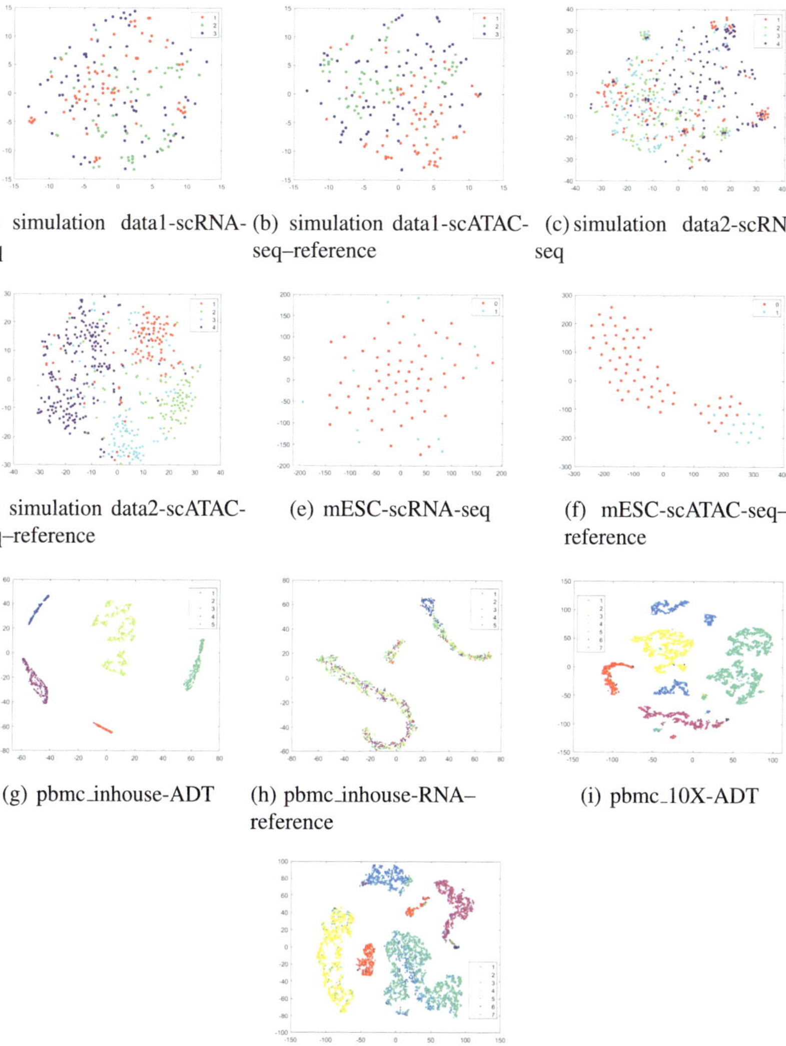

(a) simulation data1-scRNA-seq (b) simulation data1-scATAC-seq–reference (c) simulation data2-scRNA-seq

(d) simulation data2-scATAC-seq–reference (e) mESC-scRNA-seq (f) mESC-scATAC-seq–reference

(g) pbmc_inhouse-ADT (h) pbmc_inhouse-RNA–reference (i) pbmc_10X-ADT

(j) pbmc_10X-RNA–reference

Fig. 11.7 tsne plots for embedding data by UnionCom: Case 1

Trm cells, dominated by naive T cells. It demonstrates the capability of scHoML in identifying the heterogeneity pattern embedded in the noisy single cell multi-omics data.

- **Cellular State Identification**
  We conduct statistical analysis to compare the differences between specific cluster and the remaining clusters by scHoML, to investigate the potential of scHoML in cellular state identification. We performed t-test of the hypothesis that the two

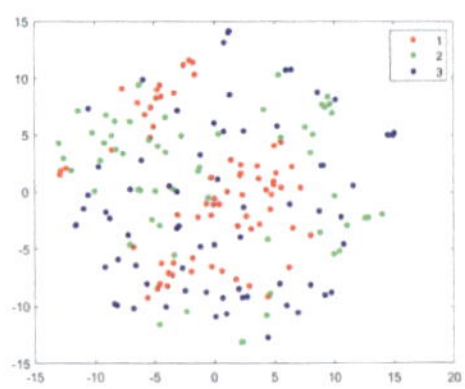

(a) simulation data1-scRNA-seq–reference

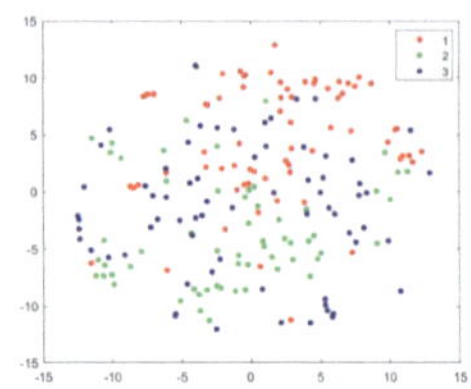

(b) simulation data1-scATAC-seq

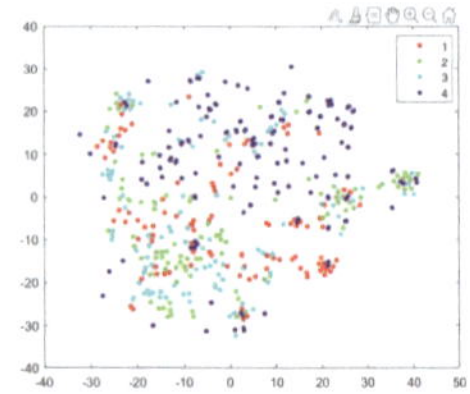

(c) simulation data2-scRNA-seq–reference

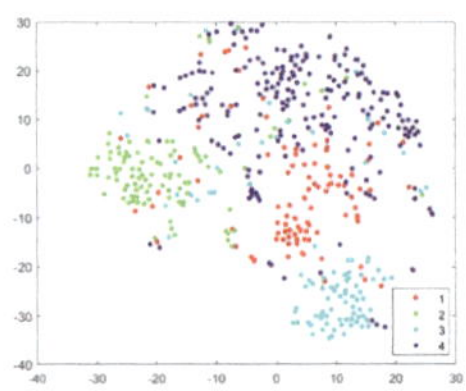

(d) simulation data2-scATAC-seq

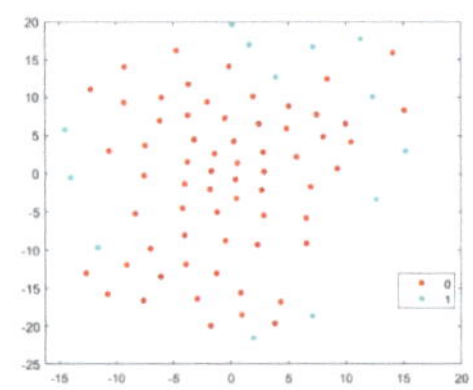

(e) mESC-scRNA-seq–reference

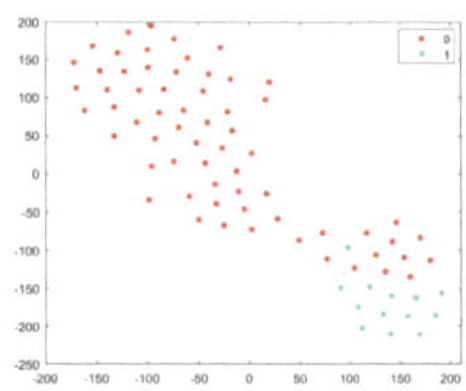

(f) mESC-scATAC-seq

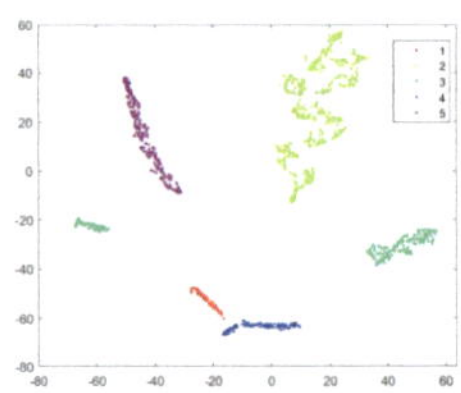

(g) pbmc_inhouse-ADT–reference

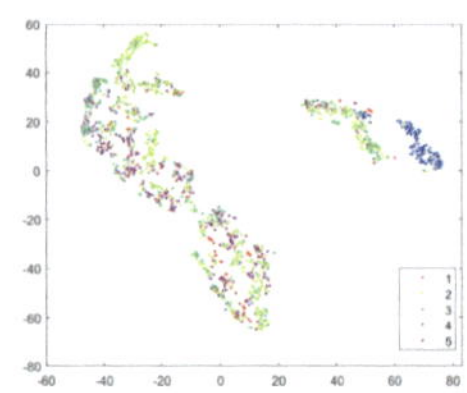

(h) pbmc_inhouse-RNA

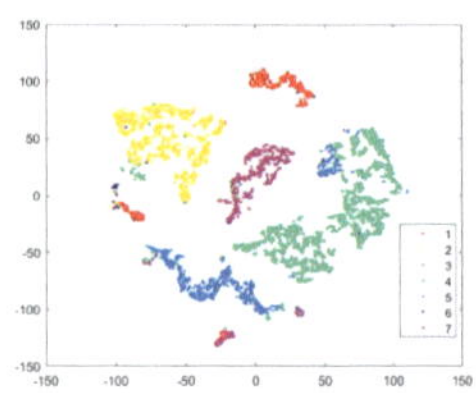

(i) pbmc_10X-ADT–reference

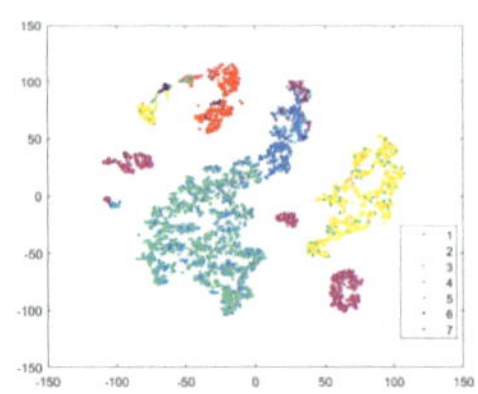

(j) pbmc_10X-RNA

Fig. 11.8 tsne plots for embedding data by UnionCom: Case 2

independent samples generated by the specific cluster and the remaining clusters come from distributions with equal means, and returns the result of the test in H. Here $H = 0$ indicates that the null hypothesis ("means are equal") cannot be rejected at the 5% significance level. Here $H = 1$ indicates that the null hypothesis can be rejected at the 5% level. To be specific, when we consider hypothesis test on cluster 3 and the remaining clusters, in the ADT data with 14 attributes, we filter the differentially expressed attributes for cluster 3 through hypothesis testing. They are 'CD16', 'CD56', 'CD45RA' etc. It is well verified that 'CD16' and 'CD56' are classical markers for NK cells (Justin 2021; Dege et al. 2020). A further analysis on the representative genes for cluster 3 through t-test leads to a filtration of top ranked genes 'FCGR3A', 'GNLY', 'SPON2', 'FGFBP2' and 'TKTL1'. 'FCGR3A', according to UniProtKB/Swiss-Prot, mediates IgG effector functions on natural killer (NK) cells (Lee et al. 2015). The protein product of 'GNLY' is present in cytotoxic granules of cytotoxic T lymphocytes and natural killer cells, revealing the relationship between 'GNLY' and NK cells. These findings indicate the capability of scHoML in extracting key molecules for cellular type/state identification. Besides, we further conducted analysis on the downstream feature selection capability for the compared methods. The comparison methods include OPMC, AWP and scAI, because the clustering results are relatively stable and robust, which are more suitable for stable feature selection. Similarly, we performed t-test on cluster $i, i = 1, 2, \ldots$ and the remaining clusters, in the ADT data with 14 attributes, to annotate the cluster specific markers by the compared methods. In OPMC method, the markers identified using 't-test' for clusters 1–7 are as follows: cluster 1: 'CD8a', 'CD45', 'CD3', 'CD127', 'TIGIT'; cluster 2: 'CD8a', 'CD45', 'TIGIT', 'PD-1', 'CD3'; cluster 3: 'CD19', 'CD45', 'CD56', 'CD16', 'TIGIT'; cluster 4: 'CD3', 'CD4', 'CD127', 'CD45', 'CD25'; cluster 5: 'CD14'; cluster 6:'CD56', 'CD45', 'CD16', 'TIGIT', 'CD19'; cluster 7: 'CD8', 'CD127', 'CD45', 'CD3', 'PD-1'. We can see that in the identified markers, cluster 1 and cluster 2 have many common markers, indicating that OPMC cannot distinguish the cells in a clear manner where some clusters share similar patterns. In AWP method, the markers identified using 't-test' for clusters 1–7 are as follows: cluster 1: 'CD8a', 'CD127', 'CD3', 'TIGIT', 'PD-1'; cluster 2: 'CD4', 'CD45', 'PD-1', 'CD127'; cluster 3: 'CD14'; cluster 4: 'CD19', 'CD45', 'CD56', 'CD16', 'TIGIT'; cluster 5: 'CD19', 'CD45'; cluster 6: 'CD16', 'CD56', 'CD45', 'TIGIT', 'CD15'; cluster 7: 'CD3', 'CD4', 'CD127', 'CD45', 'CD15'. We can see that the identified markers in cluster 5 are a subset of markers, meaning that AWP cannot distinguish the cells in a clear manner as well. In scAI-hc, the markers identified using 't-test' for clusters 1–7 are as follows: cluster 1: ; cluster 2: 'CD4', 'CD3', 'CD45', 'CD14', 'CD25', 'CD127', 'PD-1'; cluster 3: 'CD56', 'CD45'; cluster 4: 'CD56', 'CD45', 'CD19', 'CD16', 'TIGIT', 'CD15'; cluster 5: 'CD45'; cluster 6: 'CD14'; cluster 7: 'CD8a', 'CD127', 'CD3', 'TIGIT', 'PD-1', 'CD45', 'CD15'. We can see that the identified markers in cluster 5 are a subset of markers cluster 3, the identified markers in cluster 3 are a subset of markers, cluster 4, cluster 2 and cluster 7 have a lot of common markers, indicating that scAI-hc cannot help distinguish the cells in a clear manner as well. In scHoML method, the markers identified using 't-test' for clusters 1–7 are as follows: cluster 1: 'CD19', 'CD45'; cluster 2: 'CD8a', 'CD127', 'CD3', 'CD45'; cluster 3: 'CD16', 'CD56', 'CD45', 'TIGIT', 'CD15'; cluster 4: 'CD3', 'CD4', 'CD127', 'CD45', 'CD25'; cluster 5: 'CD14'; cluster 6: 'CD8a', 'CD45', 'TIGIT', 'PD-1', 'CD3'; cluster 7: 'CD19'. Cluster 7 only contain 0.02% number of cells. We can see that the identified markers in each cluster have distinct characteristics, for example, 'CD16', 'CD56', 'TIGIT' in cluster 3 are typical biomarkers for natural killer cells, demonstrating the ability of scHoML in identifying meaningful biomarkers.

11.6 Conclusions

In this study, we propose a multi-modal high-order neighborhood Laplacian matrix optimization framework for integrating the multi-omics single cell data: scMoHL. scHoML can robustly model the complex data structures and represent the noisy, sparse multi-omics data in a unified low-dimensional embedding space. Experiments on simulated data sets as well as real single-cell multi-omics data reveal that scHoML faithfully aligned heterogeneous modalities. The embedded data can further be utilized for heterogeneity analysis as well as cellular state identification, expecting to shed light on intriguing studies for revealing significant mechanisms among cells.

References

Angermueller C, Clark, SJ, Lee HJ et al (2016) Parallel single-cell sequencing links transcriptional and epigenetic heterogeneity. Nat Methods 13(3):229

Bautista J, Cramer N, Miller C et al (2021) Single-cell transcriptional profiling of human thymic stroma uncovers novel cellular heterogeneity in the thymic medulla. Nat Commun 12:1096. https://doi.org/10.1038/s41467-021-21346-6

Buterez D, Bica I, Tariq I, Andr s-Terr H, Li P (2021) CellVGAE: an unsupervised scRNA-seq analysis workflow with graph attention networks. Bioinformatics 38(5):1277–1286. https://doi.org/10.1093/bioinformatics/btab804

Cao ZJ, Gao G (2022) Multi-omics single-cell data integration and regulatory inference with graph-linked embedding. Nat Biotechnol 40:1458–1466

Cao K, Bai X, Hong Y, Wan L (2020) Unsupervised topological alignment for single-cell multi-omics integration. Bioinformatics 36(Suppl1):48–56

Cheng Y, Ma X (2022) scGAC: a graph attentional architecture for clustering single-cell RNA-seq data. Bioinformatics 38(8):2187–2193. https://doi.org/10.1093/bioinformatics/btac099

Chen L, He Q, Zhai Y, Deng M (2020) Single-cell RNA-seq data semi-supervised clustering and annotation via structural regularized domain adaptation. Bioinformatics 37(6):775–784. https://doi.org/10.1093/bioinformatics/btaa908

Dege C, Fegan KH, Creamer JP, Berrien-Elliott MM, Luff SA, Kim D, Wagner JA, Kingsley PD, McGrath KE, Fehniger TA, Palis J, Sturgeon CM (2020) Potently cytotoxic natural killer cells initially emerge from erythro-myeloid progenitors during mammalian development. Dev Cell 53(2):229–239.e7. https://doi.org/10.1016/j.devcel.2020.02.016. https://www.sciencedirect.com/science/article/pii/S153458072030143X

Deng W, Ma Y, Su Z, Liu Y, Liang P, Huang C, Liu X, Shao J, Zhang Y, Zhang K, Chen J, Li R (2021) Single-cell rna-sequencing analyses identify heterogeneity of cd8+ t?cell subpopulations and novel therapy targets in melanoma. Mol Ther Oncol 20:105–118. https://doi.org/10.1016/j.omto.2020.12.003. https://www.sciencedirect.com/science/article/pii/S2372770520301753
Duren Z, Chang F, Naqing F et al (2022) Regulatory analysis of single cell multiome gene expression and chromatin accessibility data with screg. Genome Biol 23:213
Edahiro R, Shirai Y, Takeshima Y et al (2023) Single-cell analyses and host genetics highlight the role of innate immune cells in covid-19 severity. 55:753–767. https://api.semanticscholar.org/CorpusID:258311190
Gavish A, Tyler M, Greenwald AC, Hoefflin R, Simkin D, Tschernichovsky R, Galili Darnell N, Somech E, Barbolin C, Antman T et al (2023) Hallmarks of transcriptional intratumour heterogeneity across a thousand tumours. Nature 1–9
Hao Y, Hao S, Andersen-Nissen S et al (2021) Integrated analysis of multimodal single-cell data. Cell 184(13):3573–3587.e29
Harper J, Huot N, Micci L et al (2021) Il-21 and ifn therapy rescues terminally differentiated nk cells and limits siv reservoir in art-treated macaques. Nat Commun 12:2866
Hashimshony T, Senderovich N, Avital G et al (2017) Cel-seq2: sensitive highly-multiplexed single-cell rna-seq. Genome Biol 17:77
Hashimshony T, Wagner F, Sher N, Yanai I (2012) Cel-seq: single-cell rna-seq by multiplexed linear amplification. Cell Rep 2(3):666–673
Huang HC, Chuang YY, Chen CS (2012) Affinity aggregation for spectral clustering. In: 2012 IEEE conference on computer vision and pattern recognition. IEEE, pp 773–780
Jiang H, Yi M, Zhang S (2021) A kernel non-negative matrix factorization framework for single cell clustering. Appl Math Model 90(1):875–888
Jiang H, Sohn LL, Huang H, Chen L (2018) Single cell clustering based on cell-pair differentiability correlation and variance analysis. Bioinformatics 34(21):3684–3694. https://doi.org/10.1093/bioinformatics/bty390
Jin S, Zhang L, Nie Q (2020) scai: an unsupervised approach for the integrative analysis of parallel single-cell transcriptomic and epigenomic profiles. Genome Biol 21(25)
Kumar A, Daumé H (2011) A co-training approach for multi-view spectral clustering. In: Proceedings of the 28th international conference on machine learning (ICML-11), pp 393–400
Lee J, Zhang T, Hwang I, Kim A, Nitschke L, Kim MJ, Scott JM, Kamimura Y, Lanier LL, Kim S (2015) Epigenetic modification and antibody-dependent expansion of memory-like nk cells in human cytomegalovirus-infected individuals. Immunity 42(3):431–442
Liu J, Liu X, Yang Y, Liu L, Wang S, Liang W, Shi J (2021) One-pass multi-view clustering for large-scale data. In: Proceedings of the IEEE/CVF international conference on computer vision, pp 12,344–12,353
Mei Q, Li G, Su Z (2021) Clustering single-cell RNA-seq data by rank constrained similarity learning. Bioinformatics 37(19):3235–3242. https://doi.org/10.1093/bioinformatics/btab276
Nie F, Li J, Li X et al (2016) Parameter-free auto-weighted multiple graph learning: a framework for multiview clustering and semi-supervised classification. In: IJCAI, pp 1881–1887
Nie F, Tian L, Li X (2018) Multiview clustering via adaptively weighted procrustes. In: Proceedings of the 24th ACM SIGKDD international conference on knowledge discovery & data mining, pp 2022–2030
Peng J, Sun B, Chen C et al (2019) Single-cell rna-seq highlights intra-tumoral heterogeneity and malignant progression in pancreatic ductal adenocarcinoma. Cell Res 29:725–738
Picelli S, Faridani OR, Bjrklund SK, Winberg G, Sagasser S, Sandberg R (2014) Full-length rna-seq from single cells using smart-seq2. Nat Protoc 9(1):171–181
Ramskold D, Luo S, Wang YC et al (2012) Full-length mrna-seq from single-cell levels of rna and individual circulating tumor cells. Nat Biotechnol 30:777–782
Ren L, Wang J, Li Z, Li Q, Yu G (2023) scMCs: a framework for single-cell multi-omics data integration and multiple clusterings. Bioinformatics 39(4):btad133. https://doi.org/10.1093/bioinformatics/btad133

Ren X, Wang L, Wang X et al (2021) Pan-cancer single-cell landscape of tumor-infiltrating t cells. Science 374(6574):abe6474
Sorek M, Oweis W, Nissim-Rafinia M, Maman M, Meshorer E (2021) Pluripotent stem cell derived models of neurological diseases reveal early transcriptional heterogeneity. 22:73
Stoeckius M, Hafemeister C, Stephenson W et al (2017) Simultaneous epitope and transcriptome measurement in single cells. Nat Methods 14:865–868
Stuart T, Butler A, Hoffman P, Hafemeister C, Papalexi E, Mauck WM, Hao Y, Stoeckius M, Smibert P, Satija R (2019) Comprehensive integration of single-cell data. Cell 177(7):1888–1902
Tang F, Barbacioru C, Wang Y, Nordman E, Surani MA (2009) mrna-seq whole-transcriptome analysis of a single cell. Nat Methods 6(5):377–382
Wang X, Sun Z, Zhang Y et al (2020) Brem-sc: a Bayesian random effects mixture model for joint clustering single cell multi-omics data. Nucleic Acids Res 48(11):5814–5824
Welch JD, Hartemink AJ, Prins J (2017) Matcher: manifold alignment reveals correspondence between single cell transcriptome and epigenome dynamics. Genome Biol 18:138
Welch JD, Kozareva V, Ferreira A, Vanderburg C, Macosko EZ (2019) Single-cell multi-omic integration compares and contrasts features of brain cell identity. Cell 177(7):1873-1887.e17
Xia R, Pan Y, Du L, Yin J (2014) Robust multi-view spectral clustering via low-rank and sparse decomposition. In: Proceedings of the AAAI conference on artificial intelligence, vol 28
Xia T, Tao D, Mei T, Zhang Y (2010) Multiview spectral embedding. IEEE Trans Syst Man Cybern Part B (Cybernetics) 40(6):1438–1446
Xiong G, Bekiranov S, Zhang A (2023) ProtoCell4P: an explainable prototype-based neural network for patient classification using single-cell RNA-seq. Bioinformatics btad493. https://doi.org/10.1093/bioinformatics/btad493
Yuan M, Chen L, Deng M (2021) scMRA: a robust deep learning method to annotate scRNA-seq data with multiple reference datasets. Bioinformatics 38(3):738–745. https://doi.org/10.1093/bioinformatics/btab700
Zeng AG, Bansal S, Jin L, Mitchell A, Chen WC, Abbas HA, Chan-Seng-Yue MA, Voisin V, van Galen P, Tierens A, Cheok MH, Preudhomme C, Dombret H, Daver N, Futreal PA, Minden MD, Kennedy JA, Wang JCY, Dick JE (2022) A cellular hierarchy framework for understanding heterogeneity and predicting drug response in acute myeloid leukemia. Nat Med 28:1212–1223. https://api.semanticscholar.org/CorpusID:249095424
Zhana D, Chen X, Mahdi Z, Zeng W, Satpathy AT, Chang HY, Yong W, Hung WW (2018) Integrative analysis of single-cell genomics data by coupled nonnegative matrix factorizations. Proc Natl Acad Sci 115:7723–8
Zhang Q, Jin S, Zou X (2022) scAB detects multiresolution cell states with clinical significance by integrating single-cell genomics and bulk sequencing data. Nucleic Acids Res 50(21):12112–12130
Zhou S, Liu X, Liu J, Guo X, Zhao Y, Zhu E, Zhai Y, Yin J, Gao W (2020) Multi-view spectral clustering with optimal neighborhood Laplacian matrix. In: Proceedings of the AAAI conference on artificial intelligence, vol 34, pp 6965–6972
Zong C, Lu S, Chapman A, Xie X (2012) Genome-wide detection of single-nucleotide and copy-number variations of a single human cell. Science 338:1622–1626
Zou Z, Hua K, Zhang X (2021) HGC: fast hierarchical clustering for large-scale single-cell data. Bioinformatics 37(21):3964–3965. https://doi.org/10.1093/bioinformatics/btab420

Index

H. Jiang and W.-K. Ching, *Kernel Methods for Omics Data Mining*, Intelligent Control and Learning Systems 10, https://doi.org/10.1007/978-981-95-3129-5